Electrocardiography in Ischemic Heart Disease

Electrocardiography in Ischemic Heart Disease

CLINICAL AND IMAGING CORRELATIONS AND PROGNOSTIC IMPLICATIONS

A. Bayés de Luna, MD, FESC, FACC

Director of Cardiac Dep. Hospital Quiron, Barcelona
Professor of Medicine, Universidad Autonoma Barcelona
Director of Institut Catala de Cardiologia
Hospital Santa Creu I Sant Pau
St. Antoni M. Claret 167
ES-08025
Barcelona
Spain

M. Fiol-Sala, MD

Chief of the Intensive Coronary Care Unit
Intensive Coronary Care Unit
Hospital Son Dureta
Palma
Mallorca
Spain

With the collaboration of A. Carrillo[†], D. Goldwasser[*], J. Cino[*], A. Kotzeva[*], M. Riera[†], J. Guindo[*] and R. Baranowski[*]

[*]From the Institut Catala de Cardiologica, Hospital Santa Creu I Sant Pau, Barcelona, Spain
[†]From the Intensive Coronary Care Unit, Hospital Son Dureta, Palma, Mallorca, Spain

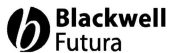

Blackwell
Futura

Blackwell Publishing, Inc., 350 Main Street, Malden, Massachusetts 02148-5020, USA
Blackwell Publishing Ltd, 9600 Garsington Road, Oxford OX4 2DQ, UK
Blackwell Publishing Asia Pty Ltd, 550 Swanston Street, Carlton, Victoria 3053, Australia

First published 2008

1   2008

ISBN: 978-1-4051-7362-9

Library of Congress Cataloging-in-Publication Data

Bayés de Luna, Antonio.
    Electrocardiography in ischemic heart disease : clinical and imaging correlations and prognostic implications / A. Bayés de Luna, M. Fiol-Sala.
        p.   ;   cm.
    Includes bibliographical references and index.
    ISBN 978-1-4051-7362-9
    1. Coronary heart disease–Diagnosis.   2. Electrocardiography. I. Fiol-Sala, M. (Miguel)
II. Title.
    [DNLM: 1. Myocardial Ischemia–diagnosis.   2. Electrocardiography–methods. WG 300 B357s 2007]
    RC685.C6B36 2008
    616.1′2307543–dc22
                                     2007005641

A catalogue record for this title is available from the British Library

Commissioning Editor: Gina Almond
Development Editor: Fiona Pattison
Editorial Assistant: Victoria Pitman
Production Controller: Debbie Wyer

Set in 9.5/12pt Minion by Aptara Inc., New Delhi, India
Printed and bound in Singapore by Fabulous Printers Pte, Ltd

For further information on Blackwell Publishing, visit our website:
www.blackwellcardiology.com

Contents

Foreword by Günter Breihardt

It is a great pleasure and honour for me to present this foreword to this new and exciting book.

Until recently, correlations between the ECG and the structural changes of the heart have relied on experimental studies and on studies done at autopsy, and only to a limited degree on modern imaging techniques. When invasive coronary angiography came into broad use, the general interest shifted away from the simple tool of the ECG that was considered as low technology, leading to a gradual decline in interest in and knowledge of the ECG in ischaemic heart disease. This is in contrast to what has happened over many years in the field of arrhythmias where there has been a continuing learning process with increasingly better interpretation of arrhythmias based on more and more sophisticated invasive electrophysiological studies.

Fortunately, some prominent and expert clinical researchers have kept their interest in the ECG alive. Among them is Antoni Bayés de Luna who, jointly with Miquel Fiol Sala, now can be congratulated for the present book on clinical and imaging correlations and the prognostic implications of the surface ECG in ischaemic heart disease. Both authors rightly state that they are authors and not editors of a multi-author book. Look at the result: This book has a quite homogenous and unified presentation which can only be achieved if there is a common genius behind it.

The aim of this book is to present better correlations between the structure of the heart, its various walls, especially those of the left ventricle, and their relationship with the torso. This will help to eliminate much of the confusion in the interpretation of the ECG and the terms used, which has arisen over several decades and still continues today. The authors not only point to the limitations of still used classifications and correlations but they also present solutions to these problems based on recent anatomic–electrocardiographic correlations. Their presentation is based on the recent pioneering work, initiated by Antoni Bayés de Luna, on the use of magnetic resonance imaging and its correlations with the ECG.

This book deserves the attention of all those who take care of the ever-increasing number of patients with ischaemic heart disease. It is a treasure and a must for everyone who is involved in managing patients with ischaemic heart disease, be it as practitioner, internist, cardiologist or as intensive care physician or interventionalist, as teacher or as student – all will benefit from the vast experience of the authors and from the information from their own studies and the literature that they have assembled.

The reader and eager student of this book will appreciate that the most important messages of each chapter are summarised in a box that emphasises the didactic claim of this work.

This book has the potential to become the 'bible' in this field for generations to come, hopefully worldwide.

Günter Breithardt, MD, FESC, FACC, FHRS
Professor of Medicine (Cardiology)
Head of the Department of Cardiology
and Angiology; *and*
Head of the Department of
Molecular Cardiology of the
Leibniz-Institute for Arteriosclerosis Research,
Westphalian Wilhelms – University of Münster,
Münster, Germany

May 2007
Münster, Germany

Foreword by Elliott M. Antman

Medical decision-making consists of a five-step process including obtaining a medical history from the patient, selecting the appropriate diagnostic tests, interpreting the results of the diagnostic tests, weighing the risks and benefits of additional testing or potential therapeutic interventions, and agreeing on a plan of a therapeutic approach in conjunction with the patients wishes. A diagnostic test that optimizes sensitivity and specificity is particularly attractive clinically, since it is used to amplify the prior probability that a particular diagnostic condition is present. Given the escalating cost of health care, a diagnostic test is especially attractive if it is inexpensive. Diagnostic tests that contain these features and utilize equipment that is universally available are more likely to stand the test of time in clinical medicine. One such diagnostic test – the electrocardiogram – stands out as a shining example of a successful diagnostic test. It is a well accepted component of the diagnostic toolbox of health care professionals around the world.

Einthoven is often credited as the individual who introduced the electrocardiogram to clinical medicine. After applying a string galvanometer to record the hearts electrical signals on the surface of the body, it was in 1895 that he introduced the five deflections P, Q, R, S, and T. Willem Einthoven was honored in 1924 for his invention of the electrocardiograph by receiving the Nobel Prize in Physiology or Medicine. In 1934, Frank Wilson introduced the concept of unipolar leads, and in 1938 the American Heart Association and Cardiac Society of Great Britain defined the standard positions and wiring of the chest leads V1–V6. In 1942, Goldberger introduced the technique for increasing the voltage of Wilsons unipolar leads, thus creating the augmented limb leads aVR, aVL, and aVF. In combination with Einthovens three limb leads, the six precordial leads, and the augmented unipolar leads form the 12-lead electrocardiogram recording pattern as we know it today.

With the passage of time, many new and highly sophisticated imaging and biochemical test have been introduced into clinical medicine. Some might argue that the 12-lead electrocardiogram has lost some its luster but a more penetrating analysis of the situation shows that this is not the case. The new imaging and biochemical tests amplify and extend our ability to interpret the 12-lead electrocardiogram in ways that we did not realize were possible in the past.

One of the most important applications of the surface electrocardiogram is in evaluation of patients with ischemic heart disease. This elegant textbook by Drs. A. Bayes de Luna and M. Fiol-Sala is a refreshing modernistic look at the surface electrocardiogram by two internationally recognized experts in the field. They provide the reader, in a single volume, a richly illustrated resource that integrates clinical findings, contemporary imaging modalities, cutting edge biomarker findings with a 100-year old diagnostic test – the 12-lead surface electrocardiogram. The book is divided into two parts. First, electrocardiographic patterns of ischemia, injury, and infarction are discussed. Polar maps, vectorial illustrations, and simple diagrams illustrating the relationship between myocyte action potentials and the surface electrocardiogram are appealing for both the novice and experienced reader. The second part of the book explores the use of the surface electrocardiogram in a variety of clinical settings of ischemic heart disease, touching on the correlations with coronary anatomy and the prognostic implications that can be gleaned from the ECG.

This textbook by Bayes de Luna and Fiol Sala is a marvelous example of what can be accomplished when clinicians who are comfortable at the patient's bedside also have the visionary insight to incorporate new knowledge from contemporary cardiac imaging procedures into a fresh view of an older, but still extremely useful, diagnostic test. As with the classical 12-lead electrocardiogram itself, readers of this textbook will find themselves returning to it over and over again because of the depth and breadth of its clinical usefulness.

Elliott M. Antman
Senior Investigator, TIMI Study Group
Professor of Medicine, Harvard Medical School; *and*
Director of the Samuel A. Levine Cardiac Unit
at the Brigham & Women's Hospital
Cardiovascular Division
Brigham & Women's Hospital
Boston
USA

May 2007
Boston, USA

Introduction

The electrocardiogram (ECG), which was discovered more than 100 years ago and has just celebrated its first century, appears to be more alive than ever. Until recently its utility was especially important for identifying different ECG morphological abnormalities, including arrhythmias, blocks at all levels, pre-excitation, acute coronary syndromes, as well as Q-wave acute myocardial infarction, for which ECG was the 'gold-standard' diagnostic technique.

An authentic re-evaluation of ECG has been evidenced in the last years as a result of the great importance it acquired in the risk stratification and prognosis of different heart diseases. Every year there is more and more information that demonstrates that ECG provides new and important data, and its applications are growing and will be expanded in the future. It has been recently confirmed that ECG allows us to approach with high reliability the molecular mechanisms that explain some heart diseases, such as chanellopathies. For example, the correlation between ECG changes and the genes involved in long QT syndrome is well known.

Although the usefulness of the surface ECG is important in all types of heart diseases, it stands out particularly in the case of ischaemic heart disease (IHD), for various reasons. The ECG is the key diagnostic tool both in the acute phase of IHD (acute coronary syndromes, ACSs) and in the chronic one (Q-wave infarction). Furthermore, it is crucial for risk stratification in patients with acute ischaemic pain. The ACSs are nowadays divided into two types: with or without ST-segment elevation. This is extremely important in the decision making to use fibrinolytic therapy. In the case of an ACS, especially with ST-segment elevation (STE-ACS), a careful evaluation of ST-segment deviations in different leads allows us to ascertain not only the occluded artery but also the site of occlusion. Therefore, it helps to stratify the risk and, consequently, to take the most appropriate therapeutic decision.

In the chronic phase of Q-wave infarction, the ECG is also very useful, since the identification of different ECG patterns of infarction permits us to have a reliable approximation of the infarcted area.

Lastly, the ECG is of great importance, as the number of patients with IHD is very large, and therefore the repercussion to properly understand the ECG changes may have an extraordinary social and economic impact.

Nevertheless, in spite of all above-mentioned arguments, there are few books that have dealt in a global manner with the value of ECG in IHD. Over 30 years ago Schamroth and Goldberger wrote two important works, dedicated more to the chronic phase of IHD, which have inevitably become outdated in many aspects. More recently, two groups, those of Wellens and Sclarovsky, which have published pioneer studies on the importance of the ECG in the acute phase of IHD, have published two excellent books that brilliantly deal with the ECG's role in the acute phase of this disease. We nevertheless considered that in the overall context of the ECG's importance in IHD there remained a space to fill in this field. That is what we intend to do with this publication.

One of the most important and new aspects of the book is the great number of correlations not only with coronariography but also with echocardiography, isotopic studies and new imaging techniques, especially cardiovascular magnetic resonance (CMR), and also in some cases with coronary multidetector computer tomography (CMDCT). All these correlations have given us a huge amount of important and new information.

We explain the ECG pattern of chronic Q-wave myocardial infarction (MI) based on the correlation with the VCG loops. We consider that the ECG-VCG correlation is the most didactic way to explain ECG (Bayes de Luna 1977, 1999). However, we only comment in this book the ECG criteria for diagnosis of chronic-Q wave MI because there is not agreement supporting that the VCG criteria present better accuracy than ECG criteria (Hurd 1981, Warner 1982) T and the use of VCG is more time-consuming and has not become popular in clinical practice. In order to set up its real importance could be mandatory in the era of imaging techniques to perform a comparative study of ECG and VCG criteria with the standars of cardiovascular magnetic resonance.

When necessary, we also comment on the role of other non-invasive electrocardiographic techniques, especially exercise ECG and Holter monitoring. Just a few remarks are given on other non-invasive electrocardiological techniques. The invasive electrophysiological techniques are usually not useful for risk stratification but are necessary in case of resynchronisation and implantable cardioverter-defibrillator implantation or ablation procedures.

We have two parts in this book. In the first one, following comments on the most important aspects of the heart's anatomy related to IHD on the basis of coronariographic and imaging correlations, we discuss the concept of the ECG patterns of ischaemia, injury and infarction, the electrophysiological mechanisms that explain them and the correlation that exists between the presence of these patterns in different leads and the myocardial area involved. Correlations between ECG curves and vectorcardiographic loops constitute the key to understand the ECG morphologies. For this reason, the two above-mentioned techniques of electrical activity recording are often represented together in this book. Nevertheless, in clinical practice the surface ECG alone allows for making a correct diagnosis in most cases. Of particular interest is the possibility to locate the place of coronary occlusion in patients with STE-ACS, thanks to the application of sequential algorithms, and to identify the typical and atypical ECG patterns of STE-ACS, and to define properly the classification of non (N) STE-ACS. Also important is the new classification of infarction in case of Q-wave MI based on our experience with contrast-enhanced (CE)-CMR correlations. All this represents a new approach to

understand the ECG curves generated during acute and chronic ischaemia.

In the second part we explain a detailed global approach that has to be done in patients with acute precordial pain, emphasising on the importance of ECG changes, first to diagnose the ischaemic origin and later to stratify the risk in different types of ACS. Other electrocardiographic features of ACS, such as coexisting arrhythmias, conduction disturbances, ECG changes following fibrinolytic treatment and mechanical complications and the ECG characteristics of atypical ACSs, are also presented. Furthermore, we comment on the new, current concepts of MI with and without Q wave, the ECG markers of poor prognosis in chronic IHD and the ECG characteristics of other clinical settings with anginal pain outside the acute phase of ACS as chronic stable angina, X syndrome, silent ischaemia, etc. Finally, the capacity of ECG as marker of IHD is also discussed.

The information given in this book may help to perform the best diagnosis in patients with acute thoracic pain and to take decisions, sometimes in an urgent manner, for the best approach of management in patients with acute and chronic IHDs. We would like to emphasise that we are not the editors, but the authors of the book. This is important, because all the information is given in a homogeneous manner, without the presence of contradictory opinions that often appear in 'edited' books. Also, the presence of frequent cross-references within the text makes the content of the book easier to follow. We are aware that we are often repetitive, especially when we comment on the new concepts of ACS with or without STE and the new classification of Q-wave MI based on CMR correlations. However, we consider that this may be helpful especially for the readers who are not too much involved in the topic and also for consultants of some specific topic.

We express our gratitude to E. Antman, pioneer in many aspects of IHD, who has written a generous Foreword to this book, for his support and collaboration. We have written together a monograph related to the role of surface ECG in patients with acute thoracic pain and ST-segment elevation MI, which has been mostly included in this book, and for that he may also be considered co-author of the book. Also my thanks to Günter Breithardt, an expert and pioneer in electrocardiology, because he has also written an outstanding Foreword emphasising the electrocardiographic aspects of the book. We also appreciate very much the advice and friendship of Y. Birnbaum, J. Cinca, P. Clemensen, A. Gorgels, K. Nikus, O. Pahlm, G. Pohost, W. Roberts, S. Sclarovsky, S. Stern, G. Wagner, H. Wellens and W. Zareba, with whom we shared many aspects of the new ideas expressed in this book.

Finally, we would like to thank the help especially of J. Cino, A. Carrillo, A. Kotzeva, M. Riera, J. Guindo, D. Goldwasser and R. Baranowski for their collaboration, and also of T. Bayés-Genís, A. Boix, R. Elosua, P. Farres, J. Guerra, A. Martinez Rubio, J. Gurri, M. Santaló, J. Puig, I. Ramirez, J. Riba, E. Rodriguez, P. Torner, T. Anivarro, M.T. Subirana and X. Viñolas, who collaborated in the selection of iconography and in many other aspects. A special mention of gratitude to the Cardiovascular Imaging Unit of Saint Paul Hospital (G. Pons, F. Carreras, R. Leta and S. Pujadas) for its outstanding contribution with the CMR and CMDCT figures. Many thanks also to Montserrat Saurí, who gave us her valuable secretarial support; to Josep Sarrió for some of the drawings; and to Prous Science and Blackwell Publishing for their invaluable work in all the printing process of the book in its Spanish and English versions.

Antoni Bayés de Luna
Miquel Fiol-Sala

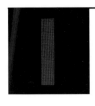

PART I

Electrocardiographic patterns of ischaemia, injury and infarction

CHAPTER 1

Anatomy of the heart: the importance of imaging techniques correlations

The surface electrocardiography (ECG) in both acute and chronic phase of ischaemic heart disease (IHD) may give crucial information about the coronary artery involved and which is the area of myocardium that is at risk or already infarcted. This information jointly with the ECG–clinical correlation is very important for prognosis and risk stratification, as will be demonstrated in this book. Therefore, we will give in the following pages an overview of the anatomy of the heart, especially the heart walls and coronary tree, and emphasise the best techniques currently used for its study.

For centuries, since the pioneering works of Vesalio, Leonardo da Vinci, Lower and Bourgery-Jacob, pathology has been a unique method to study the anatomy of the heart. Since the end of the nineteenth century, the visualisation of the heart in vivo has been possible by **X-ray examination**. The last 40–50 years started the era of invasive imaging techniques with **cardiac catheterisation (angiography and coronary angiography)** and modern non-invasive imaging techniques, first with **echocardiography** and later with **isotopic studies, scanner and cardiovascular magnetic resonance (CMR)**. These techniques open a new avenue to study not only the anatomy of the heart, coronary arteries and great vessels but also the myocardial function and perfusion, and the characterisation of the valves, pericardium, etc.

The coronary angiography (Figure 1.1) is especially important in the acute phase for diagnosing the disease and correlating the place of occlusion with the ST-segment deviations. It is also useful in the chronic phase of the disease. However, in the chronic phase of Q-wave myocardial infarction (MI) the ECG does not usually predict the

state of the coronary tree, because the revascularisation treatment has modified, sometimes very much, the characteristics of the occlusion responsible for the MI. Furthermore, the catheterisation technique may give important information for identifying hypokinetic or akinetic areas. The latter may be considered comparable to infarcted areas (Shen, Tribouilloy and Lesbre, 1991; Takatsu et al., 1988; Takatsu, Osugui and Nagaya, 1986; Warner et al., 1986). Currently, in some cases, the non-invasive **coronary multidetector computer tomography** (CMDCT) may be used (Figure 1.1).

The era of modern non-invasive imaging techniques started with **echocardiography**, which is very easy to perform and has a good cost-effective relation. This technique plays an important role, especially in the acute phase, in the detection of left-ventricular function and mechanical complications of acute MI (Figures 1.2, 8.28 and 8.29). Also, it is very much used in chronic ischaemic-heart-disease patients for the study of left-ventricular function and also detection of hypokinetic and akinetic areas (Bogaty et al., 2002; Matetzky et al., 1999; Mitamura et al., 1981). However, echocardiography tends to overestimate the area that is at risk or necrosed, and thus its reliability is good but not excellent. The techniques of echo stress and especially **isotopic studies (single-photon emission computed tomography, SPECT)** have proved to be very reliable for detecting perfusion defects and necrotic areas (Gallik et al., 1995; Huey et al., 1988; Zafrir et al., 2004) (Figure 1.3). They are very useful in cases where there is dubious precordial pain with positive exercise testing without symptoms (Figure 4.58). It has been demonstrated, however, that in some cases (non-Q-wave infarction) the

(A)

(B)

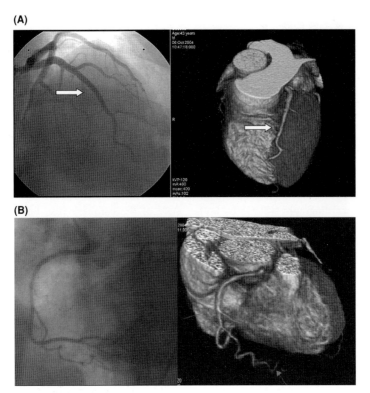

Figure 1.1 (A) Normal case: coronary angiography (left) and three-dimensional volume rendering of CMDCT (right) showing normal LAD and LCX artery. The latter is partially covered by left appendix in CMDCT. The arrow points out LAD. (B) Normal case: coronary arteriography (left) and three-dimensional volume rendering of CMDCT (right) showing normal dominant RCA. (C) 85-year-old man with atypical anginal pain: (a) Maximal intensity projection (MIP) of CMDCT with clear tight mid-LAD stenosis that correlates perfectly with the result of coronary angiography performed before PCI (b). (D) Similar case as (C) but with the stenosis in the first third of RCA ((a–d) CMDCT and (e) coronary arteriography). (E) Similar case as (C) and (D) but with the tight stenosis in the LCX before the bifurcation ((a) and (b) CMDCT and (c) coronary angiography). (F) These images show that CMDCT may also demonstrate the presence of stenosis in distal vessels, in this case posterior descending RCA ((a–b) CMDCT and (c) coronary angiography). (G) These images show that CMDCT (a, b) may delimitate the length of total occlusion and visualise the distal vessels (see arrows in (b), the yellow ones correspond to distal RCA retrograde flow from LAD) that is not possible to visualise with coronary angiography (c). (H) A 42-year-old man sports coach with a stent implanted in LAD by anginal pain 6 months before. The patient complains of atypical pain and present state of anxiety that advises to perform a CMDCT to assure the good result and permeability of the stent. In the MIP of CMDCT (a–c) was well seen the permeability of the stent but also a narrow, long and soft plaque in left main trunk with a limited lumen of the vessel (see (d) rounded circle) that was not well seen in the coronary angiography (e) but was confirmed by IVUS (f). The ECG presents not very deep negative T wave in V1–V3 along all the follow-up. This figure can be seen in colour, Plate 1.

extension of the infarction may be underestimated and that in presence of the left bundle branch block (LBBB) the estimation of some perfusion defects is doubtful.

The most recent imaging techniques are **CMR** (Figure 1.4) and **CMDCT** (Figure 1.1). The latter is used for non-invasive study of coronary tree. CMR, which may also be used for perfusion and func-tion studies of the myocardium, gives us the best 'in vivo' anatomic information about the heart. Thus, this technique, in conjunction with gadolinium in-jection and contrast-enhanced CMR (CE-CMR), is very useful for identifying and locating MI, as well as for determining its transmurality with ex-traordinary reliability, comparable to pathological studies (Bayés de Luna et al., 2006a–c; Cino et al.,

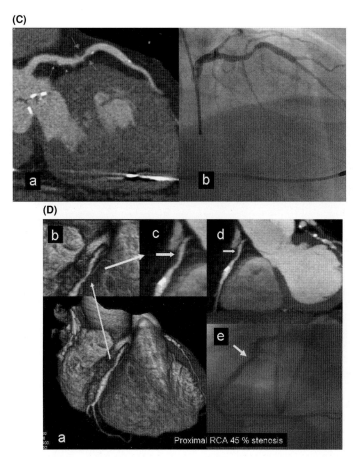

Figure 1.1 (*Continued*)

2006; Moon et al., 2004; Salvanayegam, 2004; Wu et al., 2001). This is why CE-CMR has become the gold-standard technique for studying correlations between ECG findings and infarcted myocardial areas in the chronic phase of IHD (Bayés de Luna et al., 2006a–c; Cino et al., 2006; Engblom et al., 2002, 2003). Also, CE-CMR may distinguish according to location the hyperenhancement areas between ischaemic and non-ischaemic patients (Figure 1.5) and may show in vivo the sequence of the evolving transmural MI (Mahrholdt et al., 2005a, b) (Figure 8.5). The reproducibility of CE-CMR along time, especially after the acute phase, is very good. It also has the advantage of not producing radiation. The current limitation of CMR, which will probably be solved in the next few years, is the study of coronary tree. Currently, this may be performed non-invasively by CMDCT (see above Fig 1.1).

The heart walls and their segmentation: cardiac magnetic resonance (Figures 1.4–1.14)

The heart is located in the central-left part of the thorax (lying on the diaphragm) and is oriented anteriorly, with the apex directed forwards, and from right to left (Figure 1.4).

The left ventricle (LV) is cone shaped. Although its borders are imprecise, classically (Myers et al., 1948a, b; Myers, Howard and Stofer, 1948), it has been divided, except in its inferomost part the apex, into four walls, till very recently named septal, anterior, lateral and inferoposterior. In the 1940s–1950s the inferoposterior wall was named just posterior (Goldberger, 1953) (Figure 1.6A), probably because it was considered opposed to the anterior wall. Later on (Perloff, 1964), only the basal part of this wall, which was thought to bend upwards, was considered really a posterior wall (Figure 1.6B). Therefore,

(E)

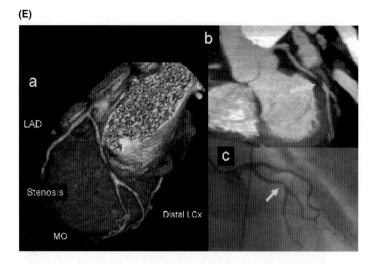

(F)

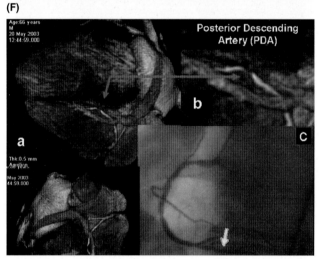

Figure 1.1 (*Continued*)

it was named 'true posterior' and the rest of the wall just 'inferior wall' (Figure 1.6). According to that, for more than 40 years the terms 'true' or 'strict posterior infarction', 'injury' and 'ischaemia' have been applied, when it was considered that the basal part of the inferoposterior wall was affected. The committee of the experts of the International Society of Computerised ECG (McFarlane and Veitch Lawrie, 1989), in accordance with the publications of Selvester and Wagner, has named these walls anterosuperior, anterolateral, posterolateral and inferior, respectively. However, this nomenclature has not been popularised, and the classical names (Figure 1.7A) are still mostly used in the major-

ity of papers (Roberts and Gardin, 1978), ECG books (Figure 1.7B to D), task force (Surawicz et al., 1978) and statements (Hazinsky, Cummis and Field, 2000).

Later on, in the era of imaging techniques, the heart was transected into different planes (Figure 1.7) and different names were given to the heart walls by echocardiographists and experts in nuclear medicine. However, recently, the consensus of the North American Societies for Imaging (Cerqueira, Weissman and Disizian, 2002) divided the LV in 17 segments and **4 walls: septal, anterior, lateral** and **inferior** (Figures 1.8 and 1.9). This consensus states that the classical inferoposterior wall should

(G)

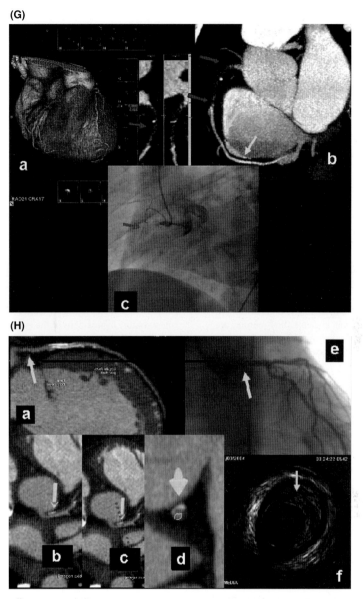

Figure 1.1 (*Continued*)

be called inferior 'for consistency', and segment 4 should be called inferobasal instead of posterior wall. Therefore the word 'posterior' has to be suppressed. Figures 1.8 and 1.9 show the 17 segments into which the four left-ventricular walls are divided (6 basal, 6 medial, 4 inferior and the apex), and the right side of Figure 1.9 shows the heart walls with their corresponding segments on a polar 'bull's-eye' map, as used by specialists in nuclear medicine. Now

we will explain, thanks to correlations with CMR, why we consider that this terminology (Cerqueira, Weissman and Disizian, 2002) is the best and it will be used further in this book. Page 16 shows the evolution of the terminology given to the wall that lies on the diaphragm.

If we consider that the heart is located in the thorax in a strictly posteroanterior position, as is presented by anatomists and by experts in nuclear

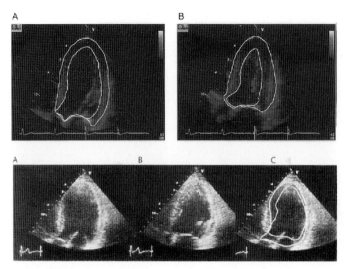

Figure 1.2 Echocardiography: see example of volumes, wall thickening and myocardium mass in a normal case and in a patient with post-MI. Above: (A) End-diastolic and (B) end-systolic apical long-axis views of a normal left ventricle. The endocardial and epicardial contours are traced and the built-in computer software of the ultrasound system allows calculation of volumes, wall thickening and myocardial mass. Below: Segmental wall function analysis: post-infarct lateral wall hypokinesis shown in the four view. The left ventricle is dilated. Superposition of the traced endocardial contours at end diastole (A) and end systole (B) shows the hypokinesis and compensatory hyperkinesis of the interventricular septum. (C) It shows the superimposed end-diastolic and end-systolic contours. (Adapted from Camm AJ, Lüscher TF and Serruys PW, 2006.)

medicine, and in the transverse section of CMR images (Figure 1.10A–C), we may understand that in case of involvement (injury or infarction) of basal part of inferior wall (classically called posterior wall) especially when in lean individuals the majority of inferior wall is placed in a posterior position (Figure 1.13C), an RS (R) and/or ST-segment depression in V1 will be recorded (Figure 1.10D). However, now, thanks to magnetic resonance correlations (Figure 1.11), we have evidence that the sagittal view of the heart is, in respect to the thorax, located with an oblique right-to-left inclination and not in a strictly posteroanterior position, as was usually presented by anatomists, nuclear medicine and the transverse section of CMR (Figure 1.10). This helps us to understand how the RS (R) or predominant ST-segment depression patterns in V1 is the consequence of the infarction of or injury to the lateral, not the inferobasal, segment (classical posterior wall) (Figure 1.12). However, we have to remind

---

The usefulness of invasive and non-invasive imaging techniques and their correlations with ECG in IHD:

• Non-invasive imaging techniques, especially SPECT, are very useful in detecting perfusion defects during exercise test.

• We will present in this book the importance of ECG–coronary angiography correlations to identify the artery occlusion site and the myocardial area at risk.

• The role of coronary angiography, and in special circumstances, of non-invasive detection of coronary tree by CMDCT in chronic-heart-disease patients, will be commented.

• In chronic Q-wave MI we will emphasise the importance of the ECG–CMR correlations to identify and locate the area of infarction.

• ECG is very useful in coronary care unit and is also used routinely in the chronic phase.

• X-ray examination still plays some role especially in the acute phase (heart enlargement and pulmonary oedema) and in the detection of aneurysms and calcifications, visualisation of heart valves, pacemakers, etc.

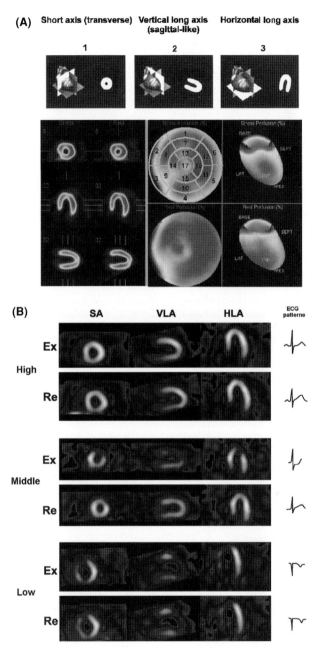

Figure 1.3 Examples of correlation exercise test – isotopic images (SPECT). (A) Above: Observe the three heart planes (see Figure 1.4B) used by nuclear medicine experts (and other imaging techniques) to transect the heart: (1) short-axis (transverse) view (SA), (2) vertical long-axis view (VLA) (oblique sagittal-like) and (3) horizontal long-axis (HLA) view. Below: Normal case of perfusion of left ventricle. On the middle is (B) the bull's-eye image of this case. The segmentation of the heart used in this book is shown (Cerqueira, Weissman and Disizian, 2002). On (A) transections of the three axes are shown. The short-axis transections is at the mid-apical level (see Figure 1.8 for segmentation). (B) Above: In the three planes (SA, VLA and HLA) see (A) normal uptake at rest (Re) and during exercise (Ex) can be observed. Middle: Abnormal uptake only during exercise of segments 7, 13 and 17 (see Figure 1.8) in a patient with angina produced by distal involvement of not long LAD. The basal part of the anterior wall of left ventricle is not involved. Below: Abnormal uptake during rest and exercise in a patient in chronic phase of MI produced by distal occlusion of very long LAD that wraps the apex involving part of inferior wall (segments 7, 13 and 17 and also 15) (see Figure 1.8), without residual ischaemia on exercise. In this case the image of abnormal uptake is persistent during rest. See in all cases the ECG patterns that may be found. This figure can be seen in colour, Plate 2.

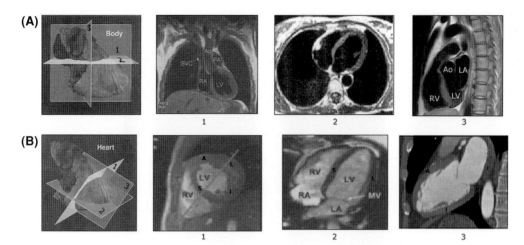

Figure 1.4 Cardiac magnetic resonance imaging (CMR). (A) Transections of the heart following the classical human body planes: (1) frontal plane, (2) horizontal plane and (3) sagittal plane. (B) Transections of the heart following the heart planes that cut the body obliquely. These are the planes used by the cardiac imaging experts: (1) short-axis (transverse) view, in this case at mid-level (see B(1)); (2) horizontal long-axis view; (3) vertical long-axis view (oblique sagittal-like). Check the great difference between the sagittal plane according to human body planes (A(3)) and the heart planes (B(3). (B) It shows the four walls of the heart with the classical names: septal (S), anterior (A), lateral (L) and inferoposterior. Currently, the inferoposterior wall is named for consistency just inferior (I) (see p. 16 and Figure 1.8).

Hyperenhancement patterns

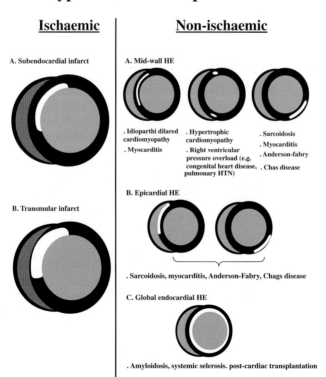

Figure 1.5 Hyperenhancement patterns found in clinical practice. If hyperenhancement is present, the subendocardium should be involved in patients with ischaemic disease. Isolated mid-wall or subepicardial hyperenhancement strongly suggests a 'non-ischaemic' etiology. (Taken from Marhrholdt, 2005.)

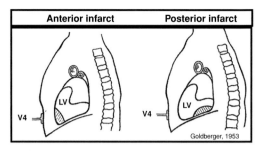

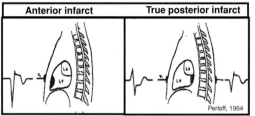

Figure 1.6 Above: The concept of anterior and posterior infarction according to Goldberger (1953). Below: The concept of anterior and true or strict posterior infarction is shown according to Perloff (1964). The other part of the wall that lies on the diaphragm became to be named inferior (see p. 16).

that in the majority of cases except for very lean individuals (see Figure 1.13C), the part of the inferior wall that is really posterior just involves the area of late depolarisation (segment 4, or inferobasal). Therefore, in case of MI of this area, there would not be changes in the first part of QRS, because this MI does not originate a Q wave or an equivalent wave (Durrer et al., 1970).

The CMR technique gives us real information about the in vivo heart's anatomy (Blackwell, Cranney and Pohost, 1993; Pons-Lladó and Carreras, 2005) (Figure 1.4). In this regard, the following are important:

(a) CMR patterns of the frontal, horizontal and sagittal planes of the heart following the human body planes are shown in Figure 1.4A. This allows us to know with precision the heart's location within the thorax. In this figure we can observe these transections, performed at the mid-level of the heart.

(b) Nevertheless, bearing in mind the three-dimensional location of the heart within the thorax, in order to correlate the left ventricular walls amongst themselves and, above all, to locate the different segments into which they can be divided, it is best to perform transections following the

heart planes that are perpendicular to each other (see Figure 1.4B), as has been already done in nuclear medicine (Figure 1.3; see Plate 2). These planes transect the heart following the heart planes (Figure 1.4B) and are the following: horizontal long-axis view, short-axis view (transverse) and vertical long-axis view (oblique sagittal-like). In reality the oblique sagittal-like view (Figure 1.11B) presents, as we have said, an oblique right to left and not a strict posteroanterior direction (compare Figure 1.4A(3) with Figures 1.4B(3) and 1.11B). Therefore in the presence of infarction of the inferobasal part of inferior wall (classically called posterior wall) and especially when the infarction involves the mid-inferior wall if it is located posteriorly, as happens in very lean individuals (Figure 1.13C), the vector of infarction generated in this area is directed forwards and from right to left and is recorded as RS morphology in V2–V3, but not in V1 where it presents a normal rS morphology (Figure 1.12B). On the contrary, the vector of infarction, in the case of infarction involving the lateral wall, may generate an RS pattern in V1 (Bayés de Luna, Batchvarov and Malik, 2006; Bayés de Luna, Fiol and Antman, 2006; Cino et al., 2006) (Figure 1.12C) (see legend Figure 1.12).

(c) The longitudinal vertical plane (Figures 1.3(2), 1.8C and 1.11B; see Plate 2) is not fully sagittal with respect to the anteroposterior position of the thorax, but rather oblique sagittal, as it is directed from right to left. (The sagittal-like axis follows the CD line in Figure 1.11A.) Compare Figures 1.4B(3) and 1.11B with the true sagittal view – Figure 1.4A(3). The view of this plane, as seen from the left side (oblique sagittal), allows us to correctly visualise the anterior and the inferior heart walls (Figure 1.11B). We can clearly see that the inferior wall has a portion that lies on the diaphragm until, at a certain point, sometimes it changes its direction and becomes posterior (classic posterior wall), now called inferobasal segment. This posterior part is more or less important, depending on, among other factors, the body-build. We have found (Figure 1.13) that in most cases the inferior wall remains flat (C shape) (Figure 1.13B). However, sometimes a clear basal part bending upwards (G shape) (Figure 1.13A) is seen. Only rarely, usually in very lean individuals, does the great part of the inferior wall present a clear posterior position (U shape) (Figure 1.13C).

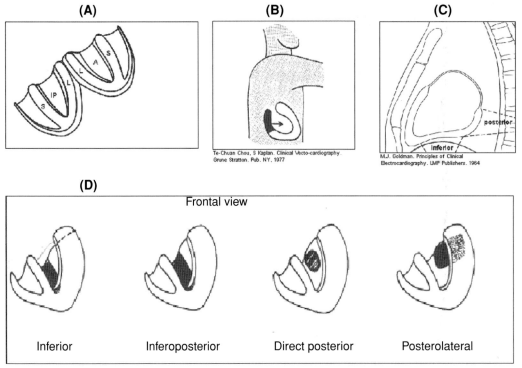

Figure 1.7 (A) The left ventricle may be divided into four walls that till very recently were usually named anterior (A), inferoposterior (IP) or diaphragmatic, septal (S) and lateral (L). However, according to the arguments given in this book, we consider that the 'inferoposterior' wall has to be named just 'inferior' (see p. 16). (B–D) Different drawings of the inferoposterior wall (inferior + posterior walls) according to different ECG textbooks (see inside the figure). In all of them the posterior wall corresponds to the basal part of the wall lying on the diaphragm that was thought to bend upwards. It was considered that the heart was located strictly in a posteroanterior position in the thorax (Figures 1.10D and 1.12A). The cardiovascular magnetic resonance (CMR) gives us the information that the inferoposterior wall lies flat, even in its basal part, in around two-third of cases (Figure 1.13) and make evident that the heart is always placed in an oblique position (Figure 1.12B,C).

Therefore, often, the posterior wall does not exist and for this reason, the name 'inferior wall' seems clearly better than the name 'inferoposterior'. On the other hand, the anterior wall is, in fact, superoanterior, as is clearly appreciated in Figure 1.11B. However, in order to harmonise the terminology with imaging experts and to avoid more confusion, we consider that the names 'anterior wall' and 'inferior wall' are the most adequate for its simplification and also, because when an infarct exists in the anterior wall, the ECG repercussion is in the horizontal plane (HP; V1–V6) and when it is in the inferior wall – even in the inferobasal segment – it is in the frontal plane (FP).

(d) The longitudinal HP (Figures 1.3(3) and 1.8B; see Plate 2) is directed from backwards to forwards from rightwards to leftwards, and slightly cephalocaudally. In Figure 1.8A (arrows), one can appreciate how, following the line AB, the heart can be opened like a book (Figure 1.8B).

(e) The transverse plane (Figures 1.4B(1), 1.3A(1) and 1.8A), with respect to the thorax, is directed predominantly cephalocaudally and from right to left, and it crosses the heart, depending on the transection performed, at the basal level, mid-level or apical level (Figure 1.8A). Thanks to these transverse transections performed at different levels, we are able to view the right ventricle (RV) and the left-ventricular

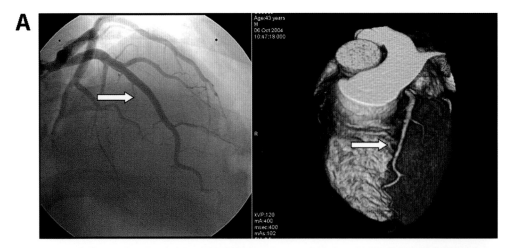

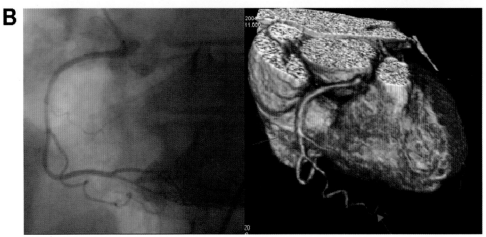

Plate 1 (A) Normal case: coronary angiography (left) and three-dimensional volume rendering of CMDCT (right) showing normal LAD and LCX artery. The latter is partially covered by left appendix in CMDCT. The arrow points out LAD.
(B) Normal case: coronary arteriography (left) and three-dimensional volume rendering of CMDCT (right) showing normal dominant RCA. (C) 85-year-old man with atypical anginal pain: (a) Maximal intensity projection (MIP) of CMDCT with clear tight mid-LAD stenosis that correlates perfectly with the result of coronary angiography performed before PCI (b). (D) Similar case as (C) but with the stenosis in the first third of RCA ((a–d) CMDCT and (e) coronary arteriography). (E) Similar case as (C) and (D) but with the tight stenosis in the LCX before the bifurcation ((a) and (b) CMDCT and (c) coronary angiography). (F) These images show that CMDCT may also demonstrate the presence of stenosis in distal vessels, in this case posterior descending RCA ((a–b) CMDCT and (c)) coronary angiography). (G) These images show that CMDCT (a, b) may delimitate the length of total occlusion and visualise the distal vessels (see arrows in (b), the yellow ones correspond to distal RCA retrograde flow from LAD) that is not possible to visualise with coronary angiography (c). (H) A 42-year-old man sports coach with a stent implanted in LAD by anginal pain 6 months before. The patient complains of atypical pain and present state of anxiety that advises to perform a CMDCT to assure the good result and permeability of the stent. In the MIP of CMDCT (a–c) was well seen the permeability of the stent but also a narrow, long and soft plaque in left main trunk with a limited lumen of the vessel (see (d) rounded circle) that was not well seen in the coronary angiography (e) but was confirmed by IVUS (f). The ECG presents not very deep negative T wave in V1–V3 along all the follow-up.

C

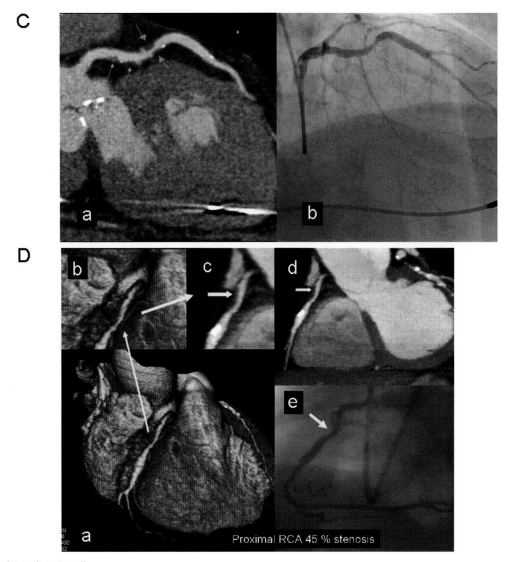

D

Proximal RCA 45 % stenosis

Plate 1 (*Continued*)

E

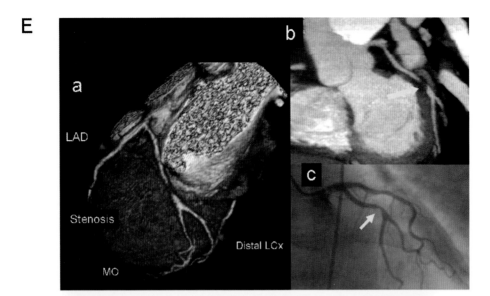

F

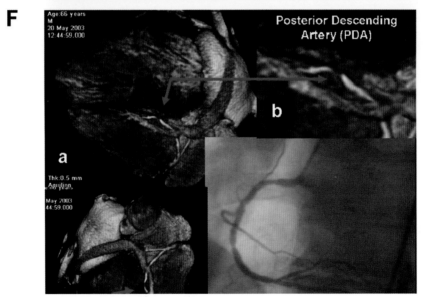

Plate 1 (*Continued*)

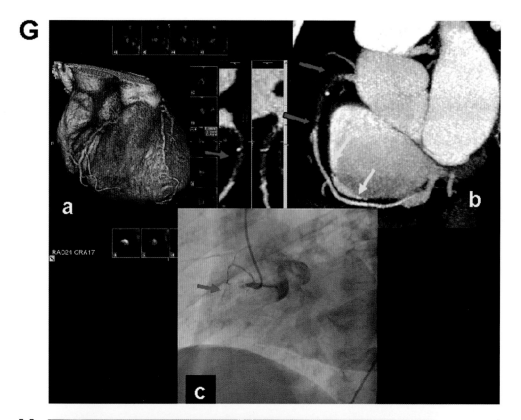

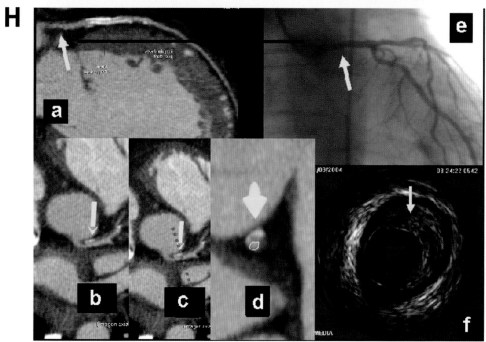

Plate 1 (*Continued*)

(A)

Short axis (transverse) | **Vertical long axis (sagittal-like)** | **Horizontal long axis**

1   2   3

A   B   C

(B)

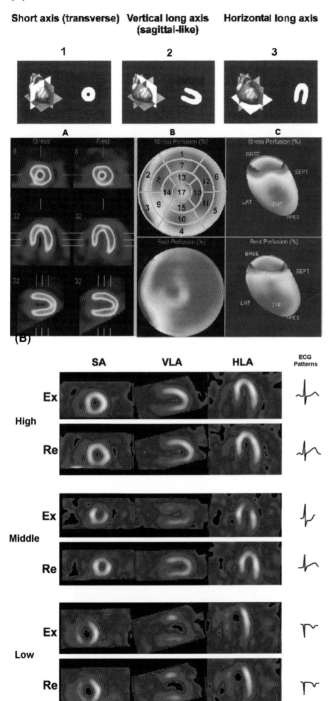

Plate 2 Examples of correlation exercise test – isotopic images (SPECT). (A) Above: Observe the three heart planes (see Figure 1.4B) used by nuclear medicine experts (and other imaging techniques) to transect the heart: (1) short-axis (transverse) view (SA), (2) vertical long-axis view (VLA) (oblique sagittal-like) and (3) horizontal long-axis (HLA) view. Below: Normal case of perfusion of left ventricle. On the middle is (B) the bull's-eye image of this case. The segmentation of the heart used in this book is shown (Cerqueira, Weissman and Disizian, 2002). On (A) transections of the three axes are shown. The short-axis transections is at the mid-apical level (see Figure 1.8 for segmentation). (B) Above: In the three planes (SA, VLA and HLA) see (A) normal uptake at rest (Re) and during exercise (Ex) can be observed. Middle: Abnormal uptake only during exercise of segments 7, 13 and 17 (see Figure 1.8) in a patient with angina produced by distal involvement of not long LAD. The basal part of the anterior wall of left ventricle is not involved. Below: Abnormal uptake during rest and exercise in a patient in chronic phase of MI produced by distal occlusion of very long LAD that wraps the apex involving part of inferior wall (segments 7, 13 and 17 and also 15) (see Figure 1.8), without residual ischaemia on exercise. In this case the image of abnormal uptake is persistent during rest. See in all cases the ECG patterns that may be found.

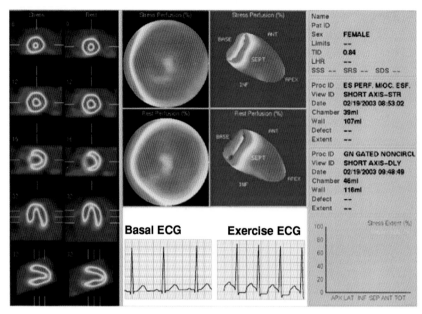

Plate 3 Patient with atypical precordial pain and a clearly positive exercise test (marked ST-segment depression) without pain during the test. The SPECT test was normal (see homogeneous uptake in red), as well as coronary angiography. It is a clear example of a false-positive exercise test.

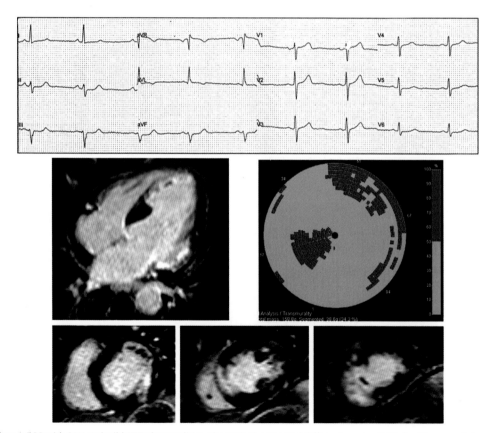

Plate 4 ECG with SAH and mild ST/T abnormalities. The patient presented different myocardial infarctions – septal, anterior and lateral detected by CE-CMR that masked each other.

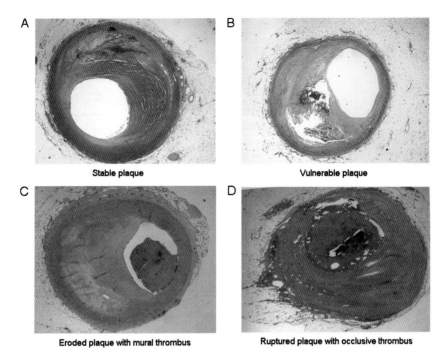

A   Stable plaque

B   Vulnerable plaque

C   Eroded plaque with mural thrombus

D   Ruptured plaque with occlusive thrombus

Plate 5 Different examples of (A) stable plaque, (B) vulnerable plaque, (C) eroded plaque with small thrombus and (D) ruptured plaque with occlusive thrombus.

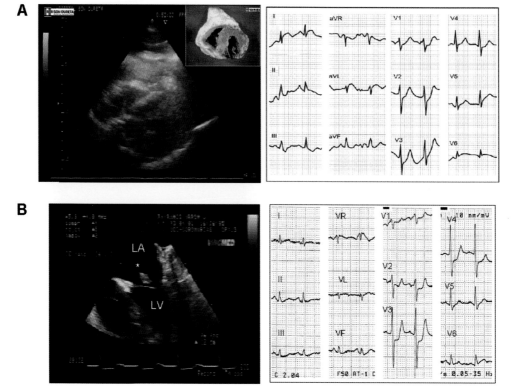

Plate 6 (A) Rupture of inferior wall in a patient after 7 days of inferior MI due to LCX occlusion. See the echocardiography with great haematic pericardial effusion and the pathological aspect of the rupture. In spite of that, the ECG shows relatively small ECG changes (mild ST-segment elevation in I and VL and mirror image of ST-segment depression in V1–V3 that remains after a week of MI). (B) Rupture of posteromedial papillary muscle (see asterisk in the echocardiography) in a patient with inferolateral MI due to LCX occlusion. The ECG shows ST-segment depression in V1–V4 as a mirror image of inferolateral injury without ST-segment elevation in inferior leads, just mild ST-segment elevation in lateral leads (I, VL and V6).

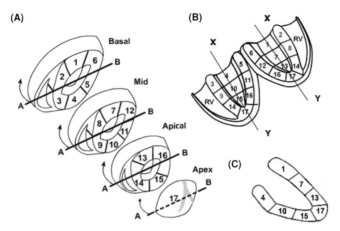

Figure 1.8 (A) Segments into which the heart is divided, according to the transverse (short-axis view) transections performed at the basal, mid and apical levels. The basal and medial transections delineate six segments each, while the apical transection shows four segments. Together with the apex, they constitute the 17 segments in which the heart can be divided according to the classification performed by the American imaging societies (Cerqueira, Weissman and Disizian, 2002). (B) View of the 17 segments with the heart open in a horizontal long-axis view and (C) vertical long-axis (sagittal-like) view seen from the right side. Figure 1.14 shows the perfusion of these segments by the corresponding coronary arteries.

Figure 1.9 Images of the segments into which the left ventricle (LV) is divided according to the transverse transections (short-axis view) performed at the basal, mid and apical levels, considering that the heart is located in the thorax just in a posteroanterior and right-to-left position. Segment 4, inferobasal, was classically named posterior wall. The basal and medial transections delineate six segments each, while the apical transection shows four segments. Together with the apex, the left ventricle can be divided into 17 segments. Note, in the mid-transection, the situation of the papillary muscles is shown. To the right, all 17 segments in the form of a polar map (bull's-eye), just as it is represented in nuclear medicine reports.

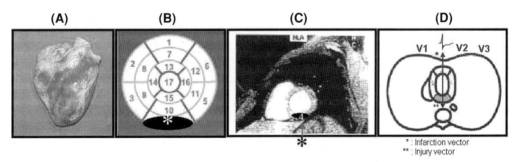

Figure 1.10 (A) The heart, shown out of the thorax by anatomists and pathologists; (B) bull's-eye image as it is shown by nuclear medicine and (C) transverse transection as it is shown by CMR. In both cases the position of the heart is presented as if the heart was located in the thorax in a strictly posteroanterior position. (D) The injury and infarction vectors (Inj. V and Inf. V) with the same direction but different sense may be seen. Compare the differences in the transections of the heart presented in Figure 1.4(above) taking the body as a centre and 1.4(below) taking the heart as a center.

(A)   **(B)**

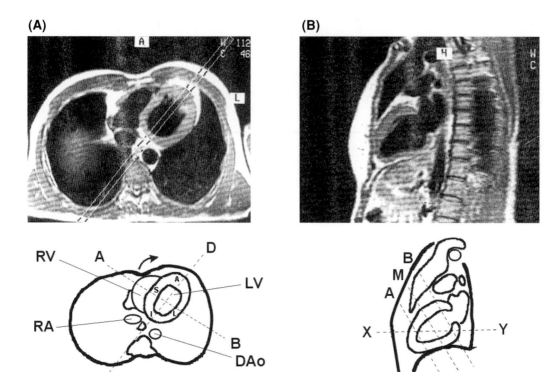

Figure 1.11 Magnetic resonance imaging. (A) Thoracic horizontal axial plane at the level of the '*xy*' line of the drawing on the right side of the figure. The four walls can be adequately observed: anterior (A), septal (S), lateral (L) and inferior (I), represented by the inferobasal portion of the wall (segment 4 of Cerqueira statement) that bends upwards in this case (B). The infarction vector generated principally in segments 4 and 10; in case of very lean individuals (Figure 1.13C) it faces lead V3 and not V1 (line CD). On the contrary, the vector of infarction that arises from segments 5 and 11 (lateral wall) faces V1 and therefore explains RS morphology in this lead (line BA). (B) According to the transection, following the vertical longitudinal axis of the heart (line CD in (A)), we obtain a sagittal oblique view of the heart from the left side. These four walls, anterior, inferior (inferobasal), septal and lateral, are clearly seen in the horizontal axial plane (A), and two walls, anterior and inferior including the inferobasal segment, in sagittal-like plane (B).

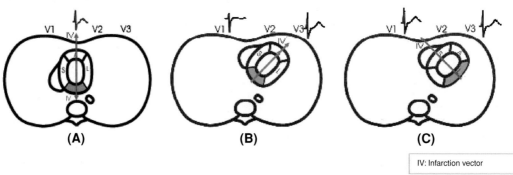

IV: Infarction vector

Figure 1.12 (A) The posterior (inferobasal) wall as it was wrongly considered to be placed. With this location an infarction vector of inferior infarction (segments 4 and 10 in case of very lean individuals) faces V1–V2 and explains the RS pattern in these leads. (B, C) The real anatomic position of inferior wall (inferobasal) and lateral wall infarctions. The infarction vector of inferobasal and mid-segment in lean individuals faces V3–V4 and not V1, and may contribute to the normal RS pattern seen in these leads. On the contrary, the vector of infarction of the lateral wall faces V1 and may explain RS pattern in this lead (see p. 156).

(A)   **(B)**   **(C)**

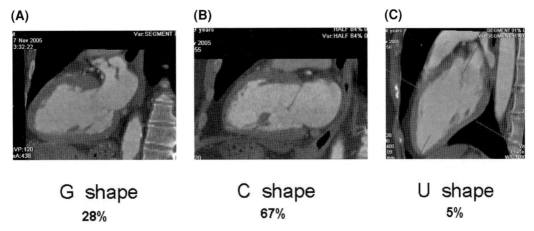

G shape   C shape   U shape
28%   67%   5%

Figure 1.13 Sagittal-oblique view in case of normal-body-build subject (A) (G shape), in a man with horizontal heart (B) (C shape) and in a very lean subject (C) (U shape). We have found that the inferior wall does not bend upward in C shape (two-third of the cases), and only in very lean individuals with U shape, the largest part of the wall is posterior (5% of the cases) (C).

septal, anterior, lateral and inferior walls (Figures 1.3(1) and 1.8A; see Plate 2). Thus, the LV is divided into the basal area, the mid-area, the apical (inferior) area and the strict apex area (Figures 1.8A and 1.9).

In order to clarify the terminology of the heart walls, a committee appointed by ISHNE (International Society Holter Non-invasive Electrocardiography) has made the following recommendations (Bayés de Luna et al., 2006c):

1. Historically, the terms 'true' or 'strictly posterior' MI have been applied when the basal part of the LV wall that lies on the diaphragm was involved. However, although in echocardiography the term posterior is still used in reference to other segments of LV, it is the consensus of this report **to abandon the term 'posterior' and to recommend that the term 'inferior' be applied to the entire LV wall that lies on the diaphragm.**

2. Therefore, the **four walls of the heart are named anterior,septal,inferior** and **lateral.** This decision regarding change in terminology achieves agreement with the consensus of experts in cardiac imaging appointed by American Heart Association (AHA) (Cerqueira, Weissman and Disizian, 2002) and thereby provides great advantages for clinical practice. However, a global agreement, especially with an echocardiographic statement, is necessary.

The coronary tree: coronary angiography and coronary multidetector computed tomography

In the past, only pathologists have studied coronary arteries. In clinical practice, coronary arteriography, first performed by Sones in 1959, has been the 'gold standard' for identifying the presence or absence of coronary stenosis due to IHD, and it provides the most reliable anatomic information for determining the most adequate treatment. Furthermore, it is crucial not only for diagnosis but also for performing percutaneous coronary intervention (PCI). Very recently, new imaging techniques, especially CMDCT, are being used more and more with a great reproducibility compared with coronary angiography (O'Rourke et al., 2000; Pons-Lladó and Leta-Petracca, 2006) (Figure 1.1). CMDCT is very useful for demonstrating bypass permeability and for screening patients with risk factors. Recently, it has even suggested its utility in the triage of patients at emergency departments with dubious precordial (Hoffmann, 2006). In chronic-heart-disease patients, there are some limitations due to frequent presence of calcium in the vessel walls that may interfere with the study of the lumen of the vessel. However the calcium score alone without the visualisation of coronary arteries is important in patients with intermediate risk, in some series even

In the light of current knowledge, we would like to summarise the following:

1. Classically it was considered that the four walls of the heart are named septal, anterior, lateral and inferoposterior. The posterior wall represents the part of inferoposterior wall that bends upwards.

2. Since mid-1960s it was defended that infarction of the posterior wall presents a vector of infarction that faces V1–V2 and therefore explains RS (R) morphology in these leads (Perloff, 1964).

3. However, (a) **infarction of the inferobasal segment (posterior wall) does not usually generate a Q wave** because it depolarises after 40 milliseconds (Durrer et al., 1970) (Figure 9.5). (b) **Furthermore,** the CMR correlations have demonstrated that the **posterior wall often does not exist,** because usually the basal part of the inferoposterior wall does not bend upwards (Figure 1.13). (c) **In cases that the inferoposterior wall bends upwards,** even if the most part of inferior wall is posterior, as may be rarely seen in very lean individuals, **as the heart is located in an oblique right-to-left position, the vector of infarction*** is directed forwards, but to the left, and faces V3 and not V1, and therefore it **originates RS morphology in V3–V4 but not in V1. In reality the vector of infarction that explains the RS morphology in V1 is generated in the lateral wall** (Figures 1.11 and 1.12).

4. Currently, **the four walls of the heart have to be named septal, anterior, lateral** and **inferior.**

---

*The injury vector has approximately the same direction as that of the vector of ischaemia and infarction but opposite sense (see p. 35, 60 and 131 and Figures 3.6, 4.8 and 5.3). Therefore, most probably, in case of injury of the lateral wall, an ST-segment depression will be especially recorded in V1–V2, and in case of injury of the inferobasal wall, the ST-segment depression will be recorded especially in V2–V3. However, further perfusion studies, with imaging techniques in the acute phase have to be done to validate this hypothesis.

Most common names given along the time to the wall that lies on the diaphragm

1940s to 1950s (Goldberger, 1953)	Posterior wall
1960s to 2000s (since Perloff, 1964)	Inferoposterior (basal part = true posterior)
2000s (since Cerqueira, Weissman and Disizian, 2002, and Bayés de Luna, 2006)	Inferior (basal part = inferobasal)

Therefore we consider that the four walls of the heart have to be named anterior, septal, lateral and inferior.

---

better than exercise testing, to predict the risk of IHD. CMDCT has some advantages in case of complete occlusion (Figure 1.1G) and in detecting soft plaques. It is also useful for the exact quantification of the lumen of occluded vessel that is comparable with intravascular ultrasound (see Figure 1.1H). However, it is necessary to realise the need to avoid repetitive explorations form an economical point of view and also to avoid possible side-effects due to radiation. A clear advantage of invasive coronary angiography is that it is possible, and this is very important especially in the acute phase, to perform immediately a PCI.

The perfusion of the heart walls and specific conduction system

The myocardium and specific conduction system (SCS) are perfused by the right coronary artery (RCA), the left anterior descending coronary artery (LAD) and the circumflex coronary artery (LCX). Figure 1.1 shows the great correlation of coronary angiography and CMDCT in normal coronary tree and some pathologic cases.

Figures 1.14B–D show the perfusion that the different walls with their corresponding segments receive from the three coronary arteries. The areas with common perfusion are coloured in grey in

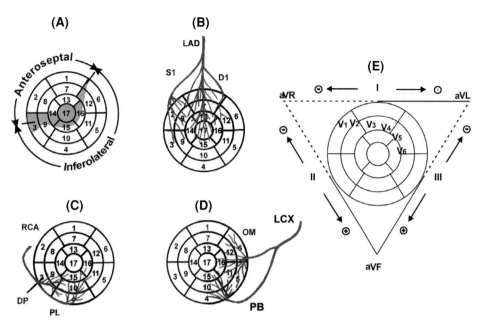

Figure 1.14 According to the anatomical variants of coronary circulation, there are areas of shared variable perfusion (A). The perfusion of these segments by the corresponding coronary arteries (B–D) can be seen in the 'bull's-eye' images. For example, the apex (segment 17) is usually perfused by the LAD but sometimes by the RCA or even the LCX. Segments 3 and 9 are shared by LAD and RCA, and also small part of mid-low lateral wall is shared by LAD and LCX. Segments 4, 10 and 15 depend on the RCA or the LCX, depending on which of them is dominant (the RCA in >80% of the cases). Segment 15 often receives blood from LAD. (E) Correspondence of ECG leads with the bull's-eye image. Abbreviations: LAD, left anterior descending coronary artery; S1, first septal branch; D1, first diagonal branch; RCA, right coronary artery; PD, posterior descending coronary artery; PL, posterolateral branch; LCX, left circumflex coronary artery; OM, obtuse marginal branch; PB, posterobasal branch.

Figure 1.14A. Figure 1.14E shows the correlation of ECG leads with the bull's-eye image (Bayés, Fiol and Antman, 2006). **The myocardial areas perfused by three coronary arteries are as follows** (Candell-Riera et al., 2005; Gallik et al., 1995):

• **Left anterior descending coronary artery (LAD) (Figure 1.14B)**. It perfuses the anterior wall, especially via the diagonal branches (segments 1, 7 and 13), the anterior part of the septum, a portion of inferior part of the septum and usually the small part of the anterior wall, via the septal branches (segments 2, 8 and part of 14, 3 and 9). Segment 14 is perfused by LAD, sometimes shared with the RCA, and also parts of segments 3 and 9 are shared with the RCA. Segments 12 and 16 are sometimes perfused by the second and third diagonals and sometimes by the second obtuse branch of LCX. Frequently, the LAD perfuses the apex and part of the inferior wall, as the LAD wraps around the apex in over 80% of cases (segment 17 and part of segment 15).

• **Right coronary artery (RCA) (Figure 1.14C)**. This artery perfuses, in addition to the RV, the inferior portion of the septum (part of segments 3 and 9). Usually, the higher part of the septum receives double perfusion (LAD + RCA conal branch). Segment 14 corresponds more to the LAD, but it is sometimes shared by both arteries (see before). The RCA perfuses a large part of the inferior wall (segment 10 and parts of 4 and 15). Segments 4 and 10 can be perfused by the LCX if this artery is of the dominant type (observed in 10–20% of all cases), and at least part of segment 15 is perfused by LAD if this artery is long. Parts of the lateral wall (segments 5, 11 and 16) may, on certain occasions, pertain to RCA perfusion if it is very dominant. Sometimes segment 4 receives double perfusion (RCA + LCX). Lastly, the RCA perfuses segment 17 if the LAD is very short.

• **Circumflex coronary artery (LCX) (Figure 1.14D)**. The LCX perfuses most of the lateral wall – the anterior basal part (segment 6) and the mid and low parts of lateral wall shared with the LAD (segments 12 and 16) and the inferior part of the lateral wall (segments 5 and 11) sometimes shared with RCA. It also perfuses, especially if it is the dominant artery, a large part of the inferior wall, especially segment 4, on rare occasions segment 10, and part of segment 15 and the apex (segment 17).

The double perfusion of some parts of the heart explains that this area may be at least partially preserved in case of occlusion of one artery and that in case of necrosis the involvement is not complete (no transmural necrosis).

Both acute coronary syndromes (ACSs) and infarcts in chronic phase affect, as a result of the occlusion of the corresponding coronary artery, one part of the two zones into which the heart can be divided (Figure 1.14A): (1) the **inferolateral** zone, which encompasses all the inferior wall, a portion of the inferior part of the septum and most of the lateral wall (**occlusion of the RCA or the LCX**); (2) the **anteroseptal** zone, which comprises the anterior wall, the anterior part of the septum and often a great part of inferior septum and part of the mid-lower anterior portion of lateral wall (**occlusion of the LAD**). In general, the LAD, if it is large, as is seen in over 80% of cases, tends to perfuse not only the apex but also part of the inferior wall (Figures 1.1 and 1.14).

The occlusion of a coronary artery may affect only one wall (anterior, septal, lateral or inferior) or, more often, more than one wall. ACSs and infarcts in their chronic phase, which affect only one wall, are uncommon. Even the occlusion of the distal part of the coronary arteries usually involves several walls. For example, the distal LAD affects the apical part of anterior wall but also the apical part, even though small, of the septal, lateral and inferior wall (Bogaty et al., 2002), and the distal LCX generally affects part of the inferior and lateral walls. In addition, an occlusion of the diagonal artery, although fundamentally affecting the anterior wall, often also involves the middle anterior part of the lateral wall and even the occlusion of the first septal branch artery, or a subocclusion of the LAD encompassing the septal branches involves part of the septum and often a small part of the anterior wall. Probably, the occlusion of oblique marginal (OM) (part of the lateral wall) or distal branches of a non-dominant RCA and LCX (part of the inferior wall) involves only a part of a single wall.

In fact, **whether ACSs or established infarctions involve one or more walls has a relative importance. What is most important is their extension, related mainly to the site of the occlusion and to the characteristics of the coronary artery (dominance, etc.).** Naturally, on the basis of all that was previously discussed, large infarcts involve a myocardial mass that usually corresponds to several walls, but the involvement of several walls is not always equivalent to a large infarct, as we have already commented. For instance, the apex, although a part of various walls, is equivalent to only a few segments. Therefore **knowing what segments are affected allows us to better approximate the true extension of the ventricular involvement** (Cerqueira, Weissman and Disizian, 2002). Lastly, although in many cases multivessel coronary disease exists, this does not signify that a patient has suffered more than one infarct.

Consequently, in order to better assess the prognosis and the extent of the ACSs, and infarcts in the chronic phase, it is very important in the acute phase to establish the correlation between the ST-segment deviations/T changes and the site of occlusion and the area at risk (p. 66), and in the chronic phase between leads with Q wave and number and location of left-ventricular segments infarcted (p. 139) (Figures 1.8 and 1.9).

The perfusion of SCS structures is as follows:
(a) The sinus node and the sinoatrial zone by the RCA or the LCX (approximately 50% in each case)
(b) The AV node perfused by the RCA in 90% of cases and by the LCX in 10% of cases
(c) The right bundle branch and the anterior subdivision of the left bundle branch by the LAD
(d) The inferoposterior division of the left bundle branch by septal branches from the LAD and the RCA, or sometimes the LCX
(e) The left bundle branch trunk receiving double perfusion (RCA + LAD)

This information will be useful in understanding when and why bradyarrhythmias and/or intraventricular conduction abnormalities may occur during an evolving ACS (see 'Arrhythmias and intraventricular conduction blocks' in ACS p. 250).

CHAPTER 2

Electrocardiographic changes secondary to myocardial ischaemia

The importance of ECG to detect myocardial ischaemia: correlation with imaging techniques

Myocardial ischaemia is the name given to the decrease in the perfusion of a certain area of the myocardium. Therefore whenever the oxygen supply is not sufficient for demands, a state of myocardial ischaemia occurs. This may be caused by (1) acute diminution of a coronary blood flow (ACSs and MI), which is usually secondary to the complete or partial occlusion of a coronary artery due to atherothrombosis,* and (2) when there is an increase of a myocardial oxygen demands. The latter happens with exercise in cases in which impaired myocardial perfusion already exists, especially in the subendocardium when the coronary arteries have a diminished ability to increase a coronary blood flow (exercise angina). We have to remind that the subendocardium is more vulnerable to myocardial ischaemia because its vasodilatory capacity is less, and this vulnerability increases during exercise (tachycardia) (see p. 57).

Generally, the clinical presentation of myocardial ischaemia is the characteristic pain known as angina pectoris or some equivalents (e.g. dyspnoea), although sometimes ischaemia may be silent (see 'Silent ischaemia', p. 302). If the anginal pain is new or if it has increased with respect to previous discomfort (*crescendo angina*), this constitutes the clinical condition called **acute coronary syndrome** (ACS), which may evolve into **myocardial infarction** (MI) (see Section 'Acute coronary syndrome', p. 209). If the angina pain appears with exercise

in a stable form, this constitutes the **typical exercise angina** (see Section 'Classic exercise angina', p. 297).

In case of ACS with ST-segment elevation (STE-ACS), the ECG patterns of ischaemia (subendocardial), injury (transmural) and usually necrosis appear in a sequential way (see Figures 3.7 and 8.5). In the case of exercise angina, the ECG pattern of subendocardial injury is the most frequently found (see Figures 3.9A and 4.57).

Prior to the presentation of clinical symptoms, myocardial ischaemia generates, in a sequential fashion, a successive cascade of changes in relaxation, contractility, haemodynamics and, lastly, electrical changes (Jennings, 1969), known as the ischaemic cascade (Nesto and Kowaldruk, 1987) (Figure 11.3). In clinical practice, in patients without evident chronic ischaemia after complete occlusion of coronary artery as occur in some ACSs, sequentially appear QTc prolongation accompanied by changes in T wave (symmetric and usually taller) and if occlusion persists ST-segment elevation (STE-ACS) evolving to Q-wave MI is recorded. These ECG changes, together with a good history taking and enzymatic (troponin) levels, are crucial to diagnose the ischaemic origin of acute precordial pain. When the complete occlusion is transient (coronary spasm and percutaneous coronary intervention (PCI), all these changes do not occur (p. 270, 271). **In chronic patients with subendocardial ischaemia** due to incomplete coronary occlusion, the ECG may remain normal at rest. In these cases the exercise testing is the first technique used to detect ST/changes, usually ST-segment depression that is generated by the increase in subendocardial ischaemia (injury) that appears during exercise in case of incomplete occlusion. These ECG changes are suggestive of perfusion defects and demonstrate the presence

---

* There do exist infrequent cases of ischaemia without occlusion of the coronary arteries (see 'Atypical coronary syndromes', p. 265 and Table 6.1).

of 'active' ischaemia especially in presence of **symptoms. However, in dubious cases, different imaging techniques, currently the most widely used are isotopic studies (SPECT)** (Figure 1.3), may confirm the evidence of perfusion defects and also give good information about the infarction areas. However, as we have said (p. 6), **CMR is the 'gold standard' for chronic MI identification, location and definition of its transmurality. The electrical changes induced directly by 'active' or 'true' ischaemia or appearing as a consequence of ischaemia but without presence of 'active' ischaemia at this moment, originate the so-called electrocardiographic patterns of ischaemia, injury and necrosis** (Figure 1.14) (see below), which correspond to different types and grades of clinical ischaemia.

The concept of the electrocardiographic patterns of ischaemia, injury and necrosis (Sodi

Pallares, 1956, 1968; Cabrera, 1966)
In the past the experimental occlusion of the coronary arteries in animals was performed with the animals under anaesthesia, with the thorax open and with the electrodes on the pericardial sac (Bayley, 1944a, b). Under these conditions, the ECG changes induced by the occlusion appear in three sequential stages that were considered to be of increased ischaemia (Sodi Pallares and Calder, 1956). First, a **negative T wave** appears, which corresponds to an **ECG pattern of ischaemia**. Later on appears the **ST-segment elevation** that corresponds to **ECG patterns of injury**. Finally, when the ischaemia has produced tissue necrosis, a **Q wave appears**, which corresponds to **ECG pattern of necrosis** (see below in 'Electrophysiological mechanism of the ECG pattern of ischaemia' p. 32 and Figure 3.4). Since then the ECG pattern of ischaemia is linked to T-wave changes, the ECG pattern of injury to ST-segment deviations and the ECG pattern of necrosis to the appearance of Q wave. The areas of injured and ischaemic tissue remain surrounding the necrotic tissue, sometimes during the experimental MI. However in the coronary occlusion in human beings and animals with close thorax, the sequential changes are different (Lengyel et al., 1957): first appears a peaked and taller T wave followed by ST-segment elevation and then a Q wave with negative

T wave (see 'Electrophysiological mechanism of the ECG pattern of ischaemia' p. 32 and Figures 3.4 and 3.7).

We will now briefly define the classical ECG patterns of ischaemia, injury and necrosis, and later on (sections 'Electrophysiological mechanism of the ECG pattern of ischaemia' to 'ECG pattern of necrosis') we will explain these in detail.

The electrocardiograhpic pattern of ischaemia (see p. 30 and Figures 2.1(2) and 3.5) is characterised by changes of T wave generated by prolongation of repolarisation in the affected area. If the ischaemia is predominantes subendocardial, as happens immediately after occlusion of a coronary artery in a heart without previous evident ischaemia, the delay in repolarisation in the subendocardium explains that the T wave is more symmetric (and usually taller) than normal accompanied by prolongation of QTc (**subendocardial ischaemic pattern**) (see Figure 3.5). If experimentally the subepicardium is cooling down – equivalent of ischaemia – or if it exists in animals or clinical practice as a consequence of coronary occlusion, a delay of repolarisation without evident changes of the morphology of TAP, that involves predominantly the subepicardium or even is transmural the ECG expression of this situation is a negative T wave (**subepicardial ischaemic pattern**) (Figure 2.1(2)). This delay of repolarisation is in general more related to previous ischaemia (post-ischaemic changes) than to 'active ischaemia' (see Figures 3.5 and 3.6, section 'Clinical point of view' p. 35 and Table 2.1).

The electrocardiographic pattern of injury (see p. 55, Figures 2.1(3) and 4.5) is characterised by deviations of the ST segment. These changes are recorded in case of evident 'active' ischaemia and are generated because as a consequence of this ischaemia a low-quality TAP of the affected area is generated (Figure 4.5). If the evident 'active' ischaemia predominates in the subendocardium gives rise to ST-segment depression (**subendocardial injury pattern**). If the ischaemia predominates in the subepicardium, in fact clinically is transmural, it generates an ST-segment elevation (**subepicardial injury pattern**) (see 'ECG pattern of injury', p. 55 and Figures 4.5 and 4.8). The ST-segment deviations are often seen in acute IHD as a clear expression of 'active' ischaemia; nevertheless, these may also be observed in the chronic phase, especially as an ST-

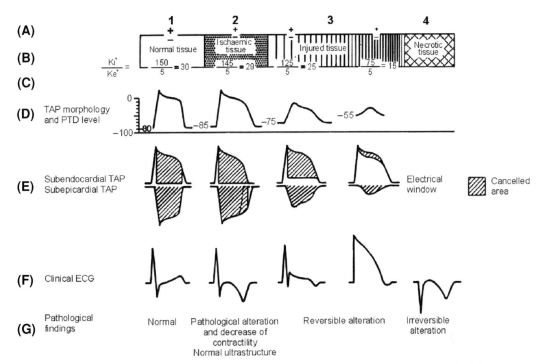

Figure 2.1 Different types of tissues (normal, ischaemic, injured and necrotic – from 1 to 4) (A) and (B). In each of them the corresponding electrical charges are shown – they decrease in a steady fashion. Levels of Ki^+/Ke^+ (C), TAP morphologies and the level of DTP (D), the subendocardial and subepicardial TAP (E), the corresponding patterns that are recorded in the ECG (F), considering that it is a subepicardial involvement (clinically transmural) and the pathological findings that are found (G). Note that necrotic tissue is non-excitable (does not generate a TAP) due to the marked diastolic depolarisation that it shows.

segment depression, and in this case they especially represent 'active' ischaemia if the ST-segment depression presents dynamic changes along the day (Holter technology) or with exercise especially in presence of symptoms (angina).

The electrocardiographic pattern or necrosis (see p. 129, Figures 2.1(4) and 5.3) is characterised by the occurrence of abnormal (pathological) Q wave (see explanation in 'Electrophysiological mechanisms of Q wave of necrosis' p. 130 and Figure 5.3). Today we know that in many cases of MI, this pattern is not present (non-Q-wave infarction). Tissue necrosis is the highest degree of clinical ischaemia.

The electrocardiographic patterns of ischaemia, injury and necrosis are of greatest importance in the diagnosis and prognosis of IHD. They are recorded in different leads as **direct patterns**, according to the affected zone. On the other hand, they may also be recorded in opposite leads as '**mirror patterns**'

(a positive T wave instead of a negative T wave, ST-segment depression instead of ST-segment elevation and a tall R wave instead of a Q wave). From the clinical point of view, these mirror patterns should not be considered only as a passive expression of something happening at a distance but, rather, as the indirect but evident sign that there exists an area of clinical ischaemia in some part of the heart distant from the exploring electrode that generates this pattern. Understanding the significance of the presence of direct or mirror patterns is of great value from the electrocardiographic diagnostic viewpoint (see p. 62 and Figures 4.10–4.12).

When we affirm in daily clinical practice that a patient's ECG shows an electrocardiographic pattern of ischaemia, injury or infarction, it does not mean that we can establish a diagnosis of IHD. **The same patterns can be found in other clinical situations** as well. In fact, the recording of sequential changes of a certain electrocardiographic pattern

Table 2.1 Acute and chronic ischemic heart disease: relationship between degree of ventricular wall involvement and electrocardiographic pattern of ischaemia, injury and necrosis.

A STE-ACS

First predominant subendocardial compromise occurs and then, transmural and homogeneous compromise: ACS with ST-segment elevation evolving to Q-wave infarction or coronary spasm (Prinzmetal angina):

1 Typical patterns

Evolving Q-wave MI:

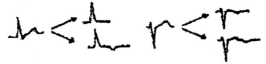

Coronary spasm

2 **Atypical patterns** (see Figure 8.3 and Table 4.1)

B STE-ACS

Compromise is sometimes extensive and even transmural, but not homogeneous.

1 With evident and predominant subendocardial involvement and usually increase of LV telediastolic pressure: **ST-segment depression. 'Active ischaemia'.** ST-segment depression appears or increases during pain, usually in leads with predominant R wave.

2 **Without predominant subendocardial involvement:** flat or negative T wave. Although is not fully known the origin of this pattern, probably in the majority of cases represent a post-ischaemic change.

C Chronic ischaemic heart disease

Pathological Q wave may or may not be present.

Also ST-segment deviations and flat/negative T wave may be present.

The presence of 'active ischaemia' is evident only if ST/T changes occurs during pain or exercise (figure 4.64).

ACS = acute coronary syndrome

and/or its correlation with the clinical setting helps to ensure the diagnosis of IHD. Even though sometimes the patterns themselves allow one to highly suspect, or even ensure, the diagnosis, on certain occasions they can give rise to many doubts, especially in the absence of clinical symptoms. Furthermore, we should remember that myocardial ischaemia is sometimes silent from a clinical point of view (Cohn, 1980, 2001; Cohn, Fox and Daly, 2003; Stern and Tzivoni, 1974) (p. 302), and that on exceptional occasions, neither clinical nor electrocardiographic manifestations exist (supersilent ischaemia) (Stern, 1998).

Location of ECG patterns due to clinical ischaemia: classical classification

Since the pathological studies of Myers et al. (1948a, b), followed by others such as Rodriguez, Anselmi

–ECG pattern of Ischaemia = prolongation of repolarisation (Figures 2.1(2) and 3.5)
–ECG pattern of injury = TAP of 'low quality' (Figures 2.1(3) and 4.5)
–ECG pattern of necrosis = lack of formation of TAP (Figures 2.1(4) and 5.3)

and Sodi Pallares (1953), Dunn, Edwards and Pruitt (1956), Horan, Flowers and Johnson (1971) and Savage et al. (1977), the following relationship between anatomical location of infarcted areas and the leads recording infarction Q waves has been accepted: **Q waves in V1–V2 leads corresponded to the septal wall; in V3–V4 to the anterior wall; in I, VL and/or V5–V6 to the lateral wall (upper and/or lower, respectively); in II, III and VF to the inferior wall (the inferomost part of inferoposterior wall) and V1–V3 (mirror pattern) to the more basal part of the inferoposterior wall (classically called posterior wall and now inferobasal segment)** (see p. 16). This is, sometimes with small changes, the accepted classification for the majority of books, task forces, clinical trials and statements, such as the Task Force of AHA (Surawicz et al., 1978), the most popular ECG books (Bayés de Luna, 1978, 1999; Surawicz, 1996; Wagner, 2001), textbooks of cardiology (Braunwald, Zipes and Lippy, 1998) and the Handbook of Emergency Medicine by the AHA (Hazinsky, Cummis and Field, 2000).

In acute phase, usually the ECG shows at the same time patterns of injury, ischaemia and even necrosis, and in chronic phase there are frequently Q waves and abnormal T waves. These different ECG patterns are not present exactly in the same leads, because although the areas of infarction, injury and ischaemia often coincide, they are not usually identical and especially the injury pattern (ST-segment deviations) in acute phase is present in more leads than is the necrosis pattern (Q wave or equivalent) in chronic phase.

Therefore, in clinical practice, the same correlation 'Q waves of necrosis in ECG leads and necrotic areas' is used to locate injured areas (ST changes) or ischaemic ones (T-wave changes), although, very often in the acute phase, the ECG patterns of ischaemia and injury are usually visible in more leads than the ECG pattern of necrosis. However, in the chronic phase, the ECG pattern of injury usually

disappears and the ECG pattern of ischaemia usually decreases more than ECG pattern of necrosis (Bayés de Luna, 1999) (Figure 8.5).

There exist evidences, some of them known already for many years (Coksey, Massie and Walsh, 1960), which show various limitations to the above-mentioned Q-wave-MI necrotic areas correlation. Later, different papers published on correlations between ECG findings, and various imaging techniques have been key for recognising the limitations of this classical classification. We will now comment on these limitations and propose a new classification based on the standard of CMR correlation (Bayés de Luna, et al., 2006a).

Limitations of classical classification

We will now comment on the most important limitations in the light of current knowledge:

(a) **Limitations due to performing the correlation with pathologic findings**: Pathological correlations only include patients that have died due to infarction, usually the most extensive, and furthermore, the heart is studied outside the thorax in a completely different situation of normal assessment of the heart in humans (Anderson, Razavi and Taylor, 2004; Myers, et al. 1948a,b,c); Sullivan, Klodever and Edwards, 1978).

(b) **Limitations due to technical problems in the recording of the ECG**: Surface ECG leads are indirect leads that are not comparable to direct epicardial leads placed directly over the affected area. Furthermore, precordial leads are frequently located on sites somewhat different from where they should be placed, in their positioning from both right to left and top to down (Herman et al., 1991; Kerwin, McLean and Tegelaar, 1960). Furthermore, frequently, they are not located at the same place while sequential ECG recordings are performed (Surawicz, 1996; Wenger and Kligfield, 1996). On the other hand, even if the leads are properly located, the correlation between recorded ECG changes and the corresponding affected area depends on

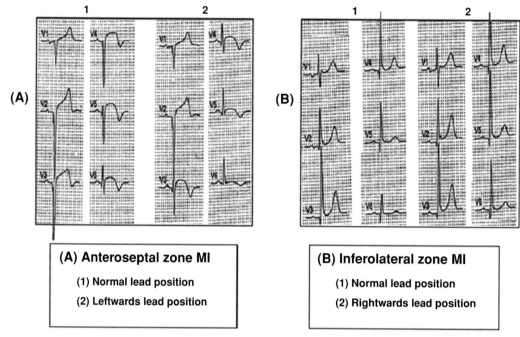

(A) Anteroseptal zone MI

(1) Normal lead position

(2) Leftwards lead position

(B) Inferolateral zone MI

(1) Normal lead position

(2) Rightwards lead position

Figure 2.2 (A) A patient with myocardial infarction of anteroseptal zone in a subacute phase: (1) normal recording that displays extension of Q waves up to V6 (qrs). Small changes in the placement of precordial V3–V6 leads have significantly modified the morphology of QRS, now being qR in a lead V6. Therefore, according to the classical concept we would say that ECG (1) presents low lateral extension, while ECG (2) does not. (B) A patient with an infarction of inferolateral zone (R ≥ S in V1) and QR in V6 (1). After having moved precordial leads a little bit to the right (2) the QR pattern in V6 disappears.

body-build, not being the same in a very lean individual (vertical heart) and a very obese one (horizontal heart). In the former case the heart is usually dextrorotated; therefore, Rs or qRs morphologies are recorded up to V6 lead, while in the latter case it is levorotated such that qR morphology may be observed from V3–V4 leads.

As a consequence, we think that it may often lead to errors to decide that an ACS with ST-segment elevation (STE-ACS) or a chronic MI affect one area or another basing the decision only on the presence of an ST-segment elevation or a Q wave in a determined lead, e.g. ECG changes in V4 and not in V5 lead. One should bear in mind that just a slight change in the placement of precordial leads may significantly modify ECG patterns and therefore the location of presumed affected areas (Figure 2.2).

(c) Limitations due to bad correlation with the electrophysiological data: It is well known since the pioneering study of Durrer et al. (1970) that the basal part of LV depolarises after 40–50 milliseconds and that Q wave does not appear in areas of late depolarisation. In spite of this, it has been accepted till now (2006) that the infarction of inferobasal segment of the inferior wall (old posterior wall) generates R wave (equivalent of Q) in V1 (Perloff, 1964). Therefore, in strict sense, it is not possible that the pathological R wave in V1 (Q-wave equivalent) may be due to infarction of the posterior wall (currently inferobasal segment of the inferior wall).

(d) Limitations related to different types of IHD: The traditional classification was introduced to locate Q-wave infarctions, although in clinical practice it has also been used to identify the injured area at risk for infarction in cases of STE-ACS (ST-segment elevation), as well as the ischaemic area (negative T wave) in an acute or chronic phase of IHD. Nevertheless, there exist many types of IHD in which this classification is less useful, e.g. ACS without ST-segment elevation (NSTE-ACS) or non-Q-wave infarctions that, in addition, are now observed more frequently. However, even in cases of NSTE-ACS some ECG patterns exist, which may help us to identify quite well the location and size of the myocardial area at risk (see STE-ACS: from ECG to the occluded artery') (p. 98).

(e) Limitations due to anatomical variants of coronary arteries: The fact that LAD is long in over 80% of all cases and wraps around the apex to perfuse the inferior wall explains why a distal LAD occlusion (distal to D1 and S1 branches) involves, very often, a relatively important part of the left-ventricular apex. Depending on where the LAD occlusion site is after D1 and S1, myocardial involvement may be limited to no more than the apex and the small inferior parts of four walls (apical area) or may extend to a larger area of the middle segments of the anterior and septal walls and middle segment of lateral wall.

The RCA artery is dominant in 80–90% of all cases and the LCX in the rest. Different QRS morphologies may be observed with similar location of the obstruction according to the degree of artery dominance and the length of their principal branches. Furthermore, the LCX and OM occlusion often result in slight or even no changes in the ECG, as these arteries perfuse areas with late depolarisation.

(f) Limitations due to the structure of the LV: The LV is cone shaped, and, as a consequence, the four heart walls present well-defined borders at the base of the heart. However, these borders become less clear as the walls approach the apex, such that it is difficult to be sure if the infarction limited to apical area involves one or other walls. Furthermore, CMR shows that the inferobasal segment of inferior wall often does not bend upwards (Figure 1.13); thus, very frequently all the inferior walls present the same horizontal or near-horizontal inclination.

(g) Limitations due to coexisting heart diseases: The presence of left-ventricular hypertrophy (LVH) and previous infarctions may affect both the magnitude and the direction of the electrical forces of the heart and, consequently, also their relationship with the precordial leads.

(h) Limitations due to the cancellation of vectorial forces: As will be evidenced throughout this book, infarct vectors of injury and also infarction affecting different areas of the heart may be cancelled. This creates the false impression that the area of infarction or injury is smaller and less important, which it in fact is (see p. 136) (Figure 5.7),

or even infarcted zones may be completely hidden (Figure 5.40). In fact, it is possible that a new infarction mask even completely the Q wave of a previous MI (Figure 5.38) (see p. 170).

(i) Limitations related to anteroseptal zone involvement (precordial leads): Acute and severe ischaemia of the basal part of septal wall (LAD occlusion proximal to the S1 branch) generates ST-segment deviations (ST-segment elevation in V1–V2 and VR and ST-segment depression in V6 and the inferior wall leads) (see p. 72) (Figure 4.12). Nevertheless, it is known (Sodi Pallares et al., 1960) that the infarction of this area is silent because the first vector of ventricular activation (which generates an r wave in V1 and V2) is formed in the mid-to-lower part of the septum, and on the contrary, the basal part depolarises later (after 40 ms). In consequence, although the ST-segment elevation in V1 reflects the high septal involvement, the presence of QS morphology in V1–V4 does not mean that the high septal and high anterior walls are necrosed (Shalev et al., 1995). Therefore in the presence of QS in V1–V4, the infarction may be limited to the lower part of these walls (apical-anterior infarction) (see p. 143).

These findings have been recently confirmed by imaging techniques. It was demonstrated that in case of chronic infarction with QS in V1–V4, usually due to LAD occlusion distal to S1 and D1, in general, the high part of septum shows preserved contractility on echocardiography (Bogaty et al., 2002). This was also confirmed by magnetic resonance imaging with gadolinium (Selvanayagam, 2004), which clearly showed that in these cases the infarction was limited to inferior areas of LV (apical part). On the other hand, in cases of LAD occlusion proximal to D1 and S1, the myocardial involvement is more extensive, including middle and basal areas of the LV's anterior and septal walls. In this case the Q wave (and the ST-segment elevation/negative T wave) is recorded not only up to the V4–V6 lead but generally also in VL and sometimes I (Bayés de Luna et al, 2006a).

(j) Limitations related to lateral wall involvement (so-called lateral leads I–VL and V5–V6): In case of ACS due to selective occlusion of D1, the ST-segment elevation is especially evident in I and VL and often in some precordial leads, and in case of proximal LAD occlusion, before the first diagonal

Although when we speak of leads I, VL and V5–V6 we may continue considering these as 'lateral leads', we should bear in mind that the classical concept relating these leads, respectively, to low lateral involvement (V5–V6) or high lateral involvement (I and VL) should be modified. Lead V5, and particularly V6, more predomi-nantly faces the apical part of the inferior wall than the low lateral wall (Warner et al., 1986), and lead VL faces, in particular, the middle part of the anterior and lateral wall more than the high part of lateral wall. To a lesser degree the same happens with lead I.

branch, but distal to first septal branch, the ST-segment elevation is present in the majority of the precordial leads and is also accompanied by an ST-segment elevation in I and VL. Even in cases in which there is a very long LAD affecting part of inferior wall, an ST-segment elevation in leads I and VL continues to be seen, with a coexisting mirror pattern in the form of an ST-segment depression in the inferior wall (see Figure 4.20). In case of the occlusion proximal to D1 of a long LAD, leading to extensive anterior infarction with inferoapical involvement, the Q wave of infarction is usually recorded not only in the precordial leads but also in I and VL (see 'ECG patterns of the anteroseptal and inferolateral zone') (p. 134). However, on some occasions if the LAD is very long, the vector of infarction of the mid-anterior wall may be counteracted by the vector of infarction of the inferior wall. Thus, despite there being an extensive infarction, in some cases no Q wave in I and VL, nor in II, III and VF, is recorded (Figure 5.7B).

Furthermore, it has been demonstrated, thanks to the correlations between leads recording Q waves and the areas of infarction detected by CE-CMR (Selvanayagam, 2004), the asynergic areas confirmed by echocardiography or angiography (Takatsu, Osugui and Nagaya, 1986; Warner et al., 1986), or non-perfused areas observed by scintig-raphy (Huey et al., 1988), that in case of proximal LAD incomplete occlusion involving diagonal but not septal branches or selective occlusion of D1, a Q wave of necrosis in VL, usually QS pattern, and sometimes in lead I, may appear. These Q-wave patterns are due to infarction of the middle-low anterior wall with certain participation of the middle anteromost part of the lateral wall, but not of the high lateral wall infarction (anterior and posterior part). This is explained because the involved area is perfused by the D1 branch, while the high part of the lateral wall is perfused by the LCX or intermediate artery (see Figure 1.14). Therefore, **the term high lateral infarction applied to QS morphology in VL (and sometimes in lead I) is confusing, as the above-mentioned morphology does not appear in case of infarction of the highest lateral wall. Furthermore, when the infarction affects fundamentally, all the lateral wall (LCX occlusion) QS morphology is not usually recorded in VL, although 'qr' or low-voltage 'r' wave may be seen** (p. 154 and Figure 5.9).

Indeed, it has been also demonstrated that the V5–V6 leads reflect more inferoapical than lateral involvement (Warner et al., 1986) and that the initial 'r' wave ≥1 mm in the lead VR lead is observed in apical lateral infarction (Okamoto et al., 1967).

Furthermore, the rotations of the heart may influence the recording of QS morphology in the lead VL. In patients presenting with more vertical hearts, the lead VL may face the intracavitary potential of the LV. Consequently, in very lean subjects with asthenic body-build, thin and often relatively deep QS morphology may be recorded in VL, usually with negative P and flat or negative T wave. This never happens in case of obese individuals. However, the QS pattern due to mid-anterior MI is usually of low voltage and presents some slurrings.

(k) **Limitations with respect to the inferior wall involvement (so-called inferior leads):** The presence of ST/T changes or of a Q wave in leads II, III, and VF indicates not only the involvement of the inferior wall but also the inferior part of septal wall. On the other hand, it has been traditionally considered that the inferobasal involvement (segment 4), classically known as posterior wall, could be recognised on the basis of morphologies observed in the right precordial leads (V1–V2). Classically, it was considered that the presence of R (RS) in V1–V2 indicated the extension of infarction to the segment 4 (posterior), and therefore the term posterior infarction was used (Perloff, 1964; Tranchesi et al., 1961; Tulloch, 1951). Recently, we have demonstrated, thanks to the correlations with magnetic resonance imaging (Bayés de Luna, et al. 2006a; Cino et al., 2006), that an infarction involving segment 4 generates rS, not RS, in V1, whereas RS morphology in V1 is due to infarctions affecting the lateral wall (segments 5 and 11) (p. 155 and Figures 1.12 and 5.23–5.26).

Furthermore, there is an inferior infarction in cases of occlusion of a large LAD artery that wraps the apex. Usually, the Q waves are only observed in leads II, III and VF when the involvement of inferior wall is equal to or greater than anterior wall (Figure 5.16). In addition, a Q wave or an ST-segment elevation in V5–V6 indicates more inferoapical than anterolateral involvement (Warner et al., 1986).

(1) **Limitations due to the lack of value given to ECG changes in lead VR and other additional leads**: In order to establish a diagnosis and the localisation of the affected area, in both the ACS and the chronic infarction, traditional classification considers the changes detected in surface ECG leads, except for VR. We, nevertheless, would like to emphasise the usefulness of VR and other additional leads.

–**The VR lead** is usually not taken into account by the cardiologist when interpreting an ECG. Nonetheless, ST-segment elevation in VR is very important in the presence of an STE-ACS in the precordial leads because it suggests that LAD occlusion is proximal to S1 (Figures 4.18 and 4.19).

The same pattern (ST↑ in VR) in case of an NSTE-ACS with ST-segment depression in many leads suggests the incomplete occlusion of the left main trunk (LMT) (Yamaji et al., 2001) or its equivalent (very proximal LAD occlusion + LCX) in patients with previous subendocardial ischaemia (Figures 4.59–4.61).

The presence of the initial 'r' wave higher than normal in VR (> 1.5 mm) suggests infarction of apical lateral wall (Okamoto et al., 1967), as we have already mentioned.

Lastly, the VR lead may also be useful in detecting multivessel disease during the exercise stress test (Michaelides et al., 2003).

–**The extreme right precordial leads** (V3R–V5R) are useful for diagnosing an RV infarction and may allow for distinguishing which is the culprit artery (RCA or LCX) in case of inferior MI (Gorgels and Engelen, 2001; Wellens, 1999). Nevertheless, diagnosis based on these leads has some limitations, as the ECG changes observed in the right leads are usually very transient. Furthermore, these leads are frequently not recorded at many centres (Figure 4.31).

–**The posterior leads** may help us to diagnose lateral infarction (Casas, Marriott and Glancy, 1997). However, these leads present the same limitations as seen in right precordial leads; e.g. they are frequently omitted while recording an ECG. Recent studies (Schmitt et al., 2001; Zalenski et al., 1997) have shown that the use of additional extreme right precordial and posterior leads only slightly increases the diagnostic sensitivity obtained with classical leads for diagnosing an acute MI.

–**The 24-lead ECG's** value obtained by adding the 12 opposed parts of the leads has also been postulated (Wagner, Pahlm and Selvester, 2006) to increase the diagnostic value of ECG, using also the reversal leads. However, although with this method an increase of sensitivity is observed, this is accompanied by a decrease of specificity.

–**External body-mapping surface** technique has been used with promising results (Menown, McKenzie and Adgey, 2000) especially to better diagnose MI of laterobasal areas. However, in practice this method has not been popularised.

The need for a new classification in the acute and chronic phases

Due to these limitations it seems worthwhile, with the aim of increasing ECG accuracy, to carry out **new correlations between Q waves and infarcted areas in the chronic phase** of MI and **between ST-segment elevations and depressions in the acute phase and the myocardial area at risk**.

What is important **in the chronic phase of MI** is to recognise with high accuracy, **based on the ECG–CMR correlations, the location of the infarction and the approximate size of the infarcted area**, as these are of significant prognostic value. Nowadays CE-CMR is the 'gold standard' for diagnosis,

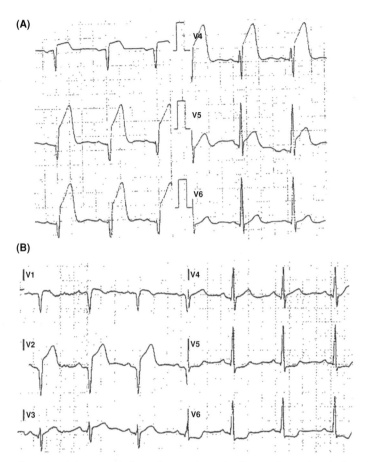

Figure 2.3   (A) ECG of a patient in hyperacute phase of ACS with great involvement of anterospetal zone. Observe ST-segment elevation from V1 to V5. (B) After 1 hour of fibrinolytic treatment the area at risk decreases significantly, being limited exclusively to septum (ST-segment elevation from V1 to V2 with ST-segment depression in V5–V6). In a chronic phase the patient presented a large septal infarction (see Figure 5.11) but without evident anterior involvement, because the treatment has limited the infarction to the area perfused by the septal branches.

location and transmurality identification in cases of MI (Figure 1.5). Later (p. 139), we explain the most frequent patterns of Q-wave infarction according to this correlation (Bayés de Luna, Batchvarov, Malik, 2006; Bayés de Luna et al., 2006a,b,c).

In the acute phase of an STE-ACS, the most important thing is to recognise, **through ST-segment deviations** (**elevations and depressions**), **the site of coronary artery occlusion**, correlating with a **myocardial area at risk** of larger or smaller size, and according to this information, a proper therapeutic decision will be made.

To perform these correlations, and bearing in mind the perfusion of the heart (Figure 1.13), it is worthwhile, as stated earlier (p. 18), **in order to better correlate ECG patterns and the affected zones to divide the LV into two zones: anteroseptal** with a certain lateral wall involvement and, frequently, inferior extension (**LAD occlusion**) **and inferolateral** (**RCA** or **LCX**).

In the past, in patients without reperfusion treatment, usually exists a clear relationship between the site of artery occlusion, myocardial area at risk and final infarcted area. However, the area at risk with the modern treatment in general diminishes considerably in size. Furthermore, sometimes, even if the culprit artery was reperfused, this has not been sufficient to avoid an extensive infarction (Figure 2.3).

This explains why **the ECG in the chronic phase is more useful to detect the infarcted area than to predict the site of occlusion that gave rise to this infarction.** On the other hand, **in the acute phase a good correlation exists between ST-segment elevations and depressions, the area at risk and the site of coronary artery occlusion,** although often the same patient during the evolution of ACS may have variable ST-segment deviations, this being a sign that the occlusion of the artery has changed usually with treatment. In general, the degree of occlusion decreases in the case of successful reperfusion, so consequently the myocardial area at risk will be smaller (see p. 23 and Figure 2.3).

Later on in this book (see p. 69 and 137) we will explain all these correlations in greater detail, and we will look at the areas at risk (Table 4.1) and the areas of infarct (Figure 5.9). Due to reperfusion treatment the correlation of the ST-segment changes during an ACS with the occluded artery and the area at risk (Table 4.1) are usually different than the presence of Q waves of infarction in the chronic phase (Figure 5.9). Therefore, usually it is not possible to quantify, based on the area at risk, how large the MI will be.

Therefore, we use **two different classifications, one for STE-ACS (see p. 70, Table 4.1) and the other for the Q-wave MI (see p. 137,** Figure 5.9). However in the case of Q-wave infarction we do not know how the coronary artery is after the treatment, but we can presume how was the occlusion that generated the infarct (see Figure 5.9). **In the clinical practice, we will do the opposite exercise: from the ECG patterns (ST-segment deviations) to the occluded artery in the acute phase** (see 'STE-ACS: From the ECG to the occluded artery and area at risk', and Figures 4.43 and 4.45) **and from the ECG pattern (Q wave) to the chronic area in the chronic phase** (see 'Location of Q-wave MI' and Figure 5.9). These two approaches will be discussed extensively later on in this book.

CHAPTER 3

Electrocardiographic pattern of ischaemia: T-wave abnormalities

Normal limits of the T wave

We will remind here (Bayés de Luna, 1999) the characteristics of a normal T wave with respect to its morphology and voltage, including situations as vagal overdrive, where a higher-than-normal T wave may be recorded, as well as the leads where the T wave may be observed in normal conditions, flattened or negative.

Morphology and voltage: In general the ascending part of T wave is slower, starting at ST-segment level, which is isoelectric (Figure 3.1A) or presents slight depression (sympathetic overdrive) (Figure 3.1C) or slight elevation. This latter morphology is frequently seen in right precordial leads, with ST-segment convex with respect to the isoelectric line (Figure 3.1B) and in vagal overdrive and/or early repolarisation also in leads with dominant R wave (Figure 3.1D). Sometimes, a usually tall T wave in V1 follows an rSr' with tiny r' that is followed by small ST-segment elevation (see Figure 3.1G). Sometimes in the cases of elderly persons or in women with hormonal insufficiency, the positive T wave may be symmetric and follow a rectified ST segment (Figure 3.1F). In such cases it is mandatory to carry out a differential diagnosis with other causes, such as the early phase of left-ventricular enlargement (LVE) or even of IHD. This symmetric positive T-wave morphology can be recorded in the absence of heart disease and may be seen in other conditions, such as chronic alcoholism, although in this case the T wave usually shows a higher voltage (Figure 3.16) (Bayés de Luna, 1999). Later (see 'Clinical point of view' p. 35) we will comment that in the early phase of STE-ACS and in coronary spasm it may be seen transiently, especially in V1–V3, a symmetric and positive T wave usually preceded by rectified or even olightly de pressed ST segment (see Figures 3.8B and 8.6). In children it is normal to

observe a negative T wave in right precordial leads with a particular morphology (infantile repolarisation pattern) (Figure 3.1E). The normal T wave is correlated with the morphology of a normal T loop recorded in the vectorcardiogram (VCG), presenting a slower and frequently irregular initial inscription part (Figure 3.2A,B).

It is difficult to define the limits of a normal T-wave voltage even though it tends neither to be lower than 2–3 mm in the HP and 1–2 mm in the FP, nor higher, under normal conditions, than 6 mm in an FP and 10 mm in HP, especially in men. In women it tends to be a little lower. The T wave may sometimes be very tall, without any pathological explanation, as occurs in cases of vagal overdrive or in very thin subjects (T wave in precordial leads of over 15 mm in height). Sometimes a positive T wave may have a low voltage, without any apparent explanation, which may have, according to some authors, prognostic implications in the long term. Epidemiological studies have demonstrated that a low-voltage T wave in lead I is a marker of poor prognosis in the follow-up (McFarlane and Coleman, 2004).

Location: The T wave in adults should be positive in all leads except in VR, where it must be negative (as the T loop falls in the negative hemifield of this lead). Frequently, it is also negative but of low voltage or flattened in V1 and, on occasion, especially in women and in blacks, may also be so in V2 or even in V3. In V1 the T wave is never tall but it may be tall but asymmetric in V2 (Figure 3.1B), with the ascending slope of a slower inscription and convex with respect to the isoelectric line. In leads III and VF, and even in II, the T wave (even in the presence of tall R wave) may be flattened or negative but asymmetric and of low voltage. Also, the VL lead may record a flattened or slightly negative T wave but only in persons with a vertical heart, generally presenting rS or QS morphology and a negative P wave.

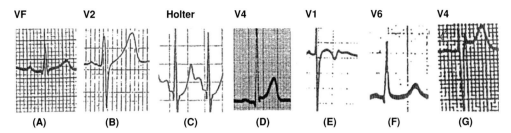

VF	V2	Holter	V4	V1	V6	V4
(A)	(B)	(C)	(D)	(E)	(F)	(G)

Figure 3.1 (A) and (B) show normal ST segment and T wave. (B) shows ECG with a certain ST-segment elevation but convex in respect to the isoelectric line. (C) is an example of a repolarisation pattern in case of sympathetic overdrive. (D) shows early repolarisation. (E) shows repolarisation of child's heart. (F) is rectified ST segment in an elderly person (70 years) with no heart disease. (G) shows the ST-segment elevation, convex in respect to the isoelectric line following a tiny r wave. This morphology may be observed in subjects with thoracic anomalies and should be distinguished from atypical Brugada's syndrome (see Figure 4.52).

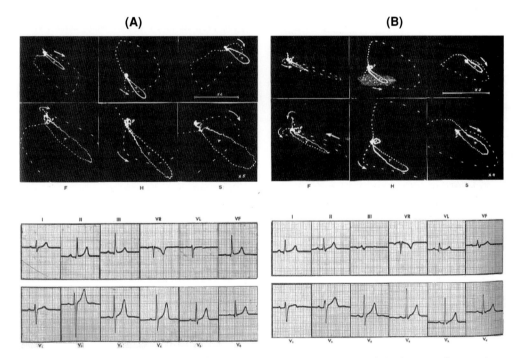

Figure 3.2 (A) shows normal electrocardiogram and vectorcardiogram of a man with vertical heart. Observe the clockwise rotation of the QRS loop in the frontal plane, as it occurs in 65% of normal individuals. In the horizontal plane, QRS loop turns counter-clockwise, while in right sagittal plane in clockwise direction, as it happens normally. See the T loop with the first part of slower recording as happens with the first part of a normal T wave. (B) shows normal electrocardiogram and vectorcardiogram of a man with semihorizontal heart. Observe the narrow, counter-clockwise loop in the frontal plane. In the horizontal (H) and right sagittal plane (S), the loop direction is counter-clockwise and clockwise, respectively.

The electrocardiographic pattern of ischaemia

This pattern is recorded when a **delay in cellular repolarisation** exists in a certain area of myocardium related with a diminished blood perfusion to this area less important than that necessary to generate an ECG pattern of injury, or other non-related ischaemic causes. **This delay of repolarisation gives rise to a more prolonged transmembrane action potential (TAP) in this area (Figure 2.1(2)), which is seen in the ECG as a flattened/negative T wave**

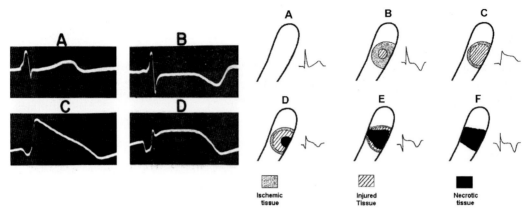

Ischemic tissue   Injured Tissue   Necrotic tissue

Figure 3.3 Left: Recordings in case of **experimental** occlusion of LAD coronary artery in a dog with open heart. (A) Control. (B) ECG pattern of ischaemia (negative T wave). (C) ECG pattern of injury (ST-segment elevation). (D) Appearance of ECG pattern of necrosis (Q wave). Right: (A) Control. (B) The ischaemic area reaches the epicardial surface and negative T wave appears. (C) The injured area reaches the epicardial surface and elevation of ST segment appears. (D) The Q wave of infarction appears when the necrotic area reaches the epicardial surface, but still remains important injury area that explains the ST-segment elevation. (E) Healing process. The ischaemic and injury areas are reduced. The ST segment nearly disappears, but negative T wave appears again and is even more visible in chronic phase (F) when only necrotic area exists. Therefore, this negative T wave is related to presence of necrosis, not to active 'ischaemia'. See in Figures 3.4 and 8.5 how the sequence of ECG changes are different, in clinical cases and in experimental occlusion in a conscious dog with closed thorax. (Adapted from Bayley (1944) and Sodi (1956)).

(**ECG pattern for subepicardial ischaemia**) or symmetric and usually taller-than-normal T wave with QTc prolongation (**ECG pattern of subendocardial ischaemia**) located in different leads according to the corresponding affected zone – anteroseptal or inferolateral (see 'Experimental point of view' – below – and Figure 3.5).

The ECG pattern of subepicardial ischaemia, is more consequence of previous ischaemia than due to the presence of 'active' ischaemia. On the contrary, the ECG pattern of predominant subendocardial ischaemia (symmetric and usually taller-than-normal positive T wave accompanied by rectified ST segment and prolongation of QTc interval) represents the first ECG change induced by 'active' ischaemia (Figure 3.7).

In the VCG the T wave of subepicardial ischaemia, which is the only one that is usually recorded because the T wave of subendocardial ischaemia is very transient, presents a T loop of homogeneous inscription and frequently small and more or less rounded, although it may be very narrow in some planes (Figure 3.17).

Firstly, we will refer to cases presenting with a narrow QRS. Thereafter (see 'Electrocardiographic

pattern of ischaemia in patients with ventricular hypertrophy and/or wide QRS' p. 54) we will briefly comment on the ECG pattern of ischaemia in the presence of a wide QRS or other confounding factors (LVH).

Electrophysiological mechanisms of the ECG pattern of ischaemia

Experimental point of view

The experimental study of ECG changes induced by ischaemia has been done along the time using different methodologies. In the 1940s it was demonstrated (Bayley, 1944a,b) that the experimental occlusion of the coronary artery in animals with open thorax (see 'The concept of ECG patterns of ischaemia, injury and necrosis' p. 20) induced three sequential ECG patterns: ischaemia (negative T wave), injury (ST-segment deviations) and necrosis (Q wave) (Sodi Pallares and Calder 1956; Cabrera 1958) (Figure 3.3). During the experimental acute occlusion, a Q wave of necrosis is recorded in the area with necrotic tissue. This area is surrounded, during certain period of time, by areas of injured and ischaemic tissue where the ECG

Experimentally, the delay in repolarisation induced by ischaemia in case of coronary occlusion first is predominantly subendocardial. This delay is responsible for the prolongation of QTc interval and for the recording of symmetric T wave usually of higher voltage (taller T wave) (see Figure 3.5). If the delay is subepicardial or even transmural (see 'The concept of ECG patterns of ischaemia, injury and necrosis') (p. 20). this delay of repolarisation without change of shape of TAP generates a flattened or negative T wave.

morphologies of injury (ST-segment elevation) and ischaemia (negative T waves) are recorded (Figure 3.3). However in chronic phase usually the area and ECG pattern of injury disappear, and the ECG pattern of ischaemia that often exists does not represent the presence of 'active' ischaemia. This latter ECG pattern is more due to repolarisation changes induced by necrosis.

In isolated perfused heart of different animals Janse (1982) demonstrated that ischaemia induced by the occlusion of a coronary artery produces a shortening of repolarisation in the ischaemic area during a very early and brief phase (expressed by a shortening of the TAP in this area). Nevertheless, after this very early phase, a delay in repolarisation (TAP) can be observed in the same area (Cinca et al.1980; Surawicz, 1996). Other authors have demonstrated that, when the myocardium is cooled down – equivalent to an ischaemia – the affected area (subendocardium or subepicardium) shows from the beginning a lengthening of the TAP in the cooled area (Burnes et al., 2001).

When acute coronary occlusion is carried out in experimental animals with closed thorax,* it gives rise, during the initial phase of ischaemia, to a delay in repolarisation (TAP) in the subendocardium, which is the area that first suffers ischaemia (Lengyel et al., 1957). This subendocardial ischaemia is evidenced by a tall and peaked T wave immediately followed by ST-segment elevation (injury pattern) if the occlusion persists and the ischaemia becomes severe and transmural (see 'ECG pattern of injury' p. 55). This pattern may be self-limited if the occlusion is temporary, as in coronary spasm (Prinzmetal angina) (Bayés de Luna et al., 1985). Nevertheless, if the occlusion remains, it generates abnormal Q wave accompanied by the progressive normalisation of ST segment and the appearance of a negative T wave that, as we have said previously, does not represent 'active' ischaemia (Figure 3.4). Figure 3.7 shows all these changes appearing in clinical occlusion of epicardial artery. Recently, Mahrholdt et al. (2005a, b) have shown by CE-CMR the progressive appearance of transmural MI starting also from the initial subendocardial involvement (Figure 8.6). Thirty years ago (Reimer, 1977) also demonstrated by pathological studies that after irreversible ischaemia the necrosis first appears in the subendocardium.

The electrophysiological explanation of how this delay in repolarisation in the ischaemic area generates the experimental electrocardiographic pattern of ischaemia, a taller-than-normal T wave if the ischaemia is subendocardial or a flattened or negative T wave when it is subepicardial may be done by two theories (Bayés de Luna, 1978; Coksey, Massie and Walsh, 1960).

1. Theory of the sum of TAPs: This theory, which explains the origin of the normal ECG as the sum of subendocardial TAP plus the subepicardial TAP (Figure 3.5A), is also useful for understanding how the symmetric and usually taller-than-normal T wave is generated in subendocardial ischaemia and how a flattened or negative T wave is recorded in case of subepicardial ischaemia. In Figures 3.5B–D we can observe how the sum of TAPs from the ischaemic area, which is more prolonged due to the existence of a repolarisation delay in that area, plus the TAP in the other normal area produces the aforementioned T-wave changes.

2. Theory of the vector of ischaemia: The area with subendocardial (Figure 3.6A) or subepicardial (Figure 3.6B) ischaemia is not yet fully repolarised, due

---

*A ligation is made when the animal is awake after having being operated on in order to apply an occluder band. This is similar to what happens in the human in the case of coronary spasm.

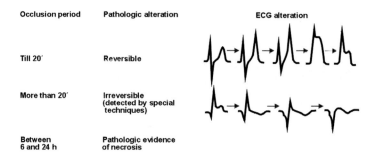

Occlusion period	Pathologic alteration	ECG alteration
Till 20′	Reversible	
More than 20′	Irreversible (detected by special techniques)	
Between 6 and 24 h	Pathologic evidence of necrosis	

Figure 3.4 Electrocardiographic – pathological correlations after the occlusion of a coronary artery in an experimental animal with its thorax closed. It changes from a subendocardial ischemia pattern (tall and peaked T wave) to a pattern of a subepicardial injury, transmural in clinical practice, (ST segment elevation) when the acute clinical ischemia is more severe. Finally, the "q" wave of necrosis develops, accompanied as time passes by an increasingly evident pattern of subepicardial ischemia (it is transmural after the occlusion of a coronary artery, though it is expressed as subepicardial in the ECG). In the chronic phase the pattern of negative T wave is related more to changes that necrosis has induced in the repolarization, then to a presence of clinical "active" ischemia (see p. 38).

to the delay in the TAP and, therefore, carries a negative charge (Figure 3.6). Similar to what occurs in the normal heart, repolarisation begins in the area that is less ischaemic and thus the direction of the repolarisation phenomenon (〰➤) goes from the less ischaemic area to the more ischaemic area. Due to the fact that the ischaemic area suffers a delay in repolarisation, a flow of current having a vectorial expression is generated going from the more ischaemic (negative) to the less ischaemic area (positive) (Yan and Antzelevitch, 1998). Therefore this vector is directed from the ischaemic area, which is not yet fully repolarised and carrying a negative charge, to the normal area, which has already completed its repolarisation and has a positive charge. This vector of ischaemia has a positive charge (vector head) that points to normal area. **Therefore, the vector of ischaemia moves away from the**

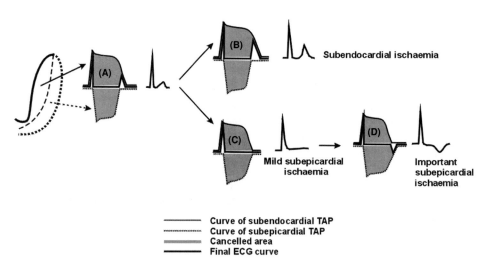

(A)
(B) Subendocardial ischaemia
(C) Mild subepicardial ischaemia
(D) Important subepicardial ischaemia

——— Curve of subendocardial TAP
·············· Curve of subepicardial TAP
═══ Cancelled area
━━━ Final ECG curve

Figure 3.5 Explanation of how the sum of the TAP from the subepicardium and the subendocardium explain the ECG, both in the normal situation (A), as in the case of subendocardial ischaemia (B) (tall and peaked T wave) and in mild (C) and severe (D) subepicardial ischaemia (flattened or negative T waves). This is the consequence of the repolarisation delay in ischaemic areas and the more prolonged TAP.

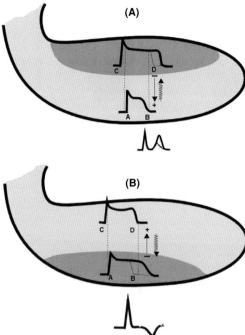

Figure 3.6 (A) Subendocardial ischaemia. Subepicardial repolarisation is complete, but the TAP in the subendocardium still presents negative charges and is longer than normal (TAP prolongation further beyond the dotted line) because the subendocardium is not completely repolarised yet. Thus, the vector of ischaemia that is generated between the already-polarised area in the subepicardium with positive charges and the subendocardial area still with an incomplete repolarisation (with negative charges) due to the ischaemia in that area is directed from the subendocardium to the subepicardium, with the head of vector coinciding with the positive charge of dipole of repolarisation. The direction of the head of vector of ischaemia is opposed to the repolarisation phenomenon, because the direction of this phenomenon (〰➤) goes from the less ischaemic area (subepicardium) to the more ischaemic area (subendocardium). Therefore, the subepicardium is faced with the vector head (positive charge of the dipole), which explains why the T wave is more positive than normal. In subepicardial ischaemia, a similar but inverse phenomenon (B) occurs, which explains the development of flattened or negative T waves (see also Figure 3.5).

ischaemic area.* This is the reason why, despite the fact that the repolarisation phenomenon goes

---

*It should be noted that the infarction vector also moves away from the infarction area (p. 133), while the injury vector is directed towards the injured area (p. 58).

from the less to the more ischaemic area, the vector of ischaemia faces the subepicardium when **the ischaemia is of the subendocardi al type** and generates a **taller-than-normal T wave**, and vice versa, faces the subendocardium and generates a **flattened or negative T wave when the ischaemia is subepicardial** (Figure 3.6). In the case that the experimental ischaemia is transmural, it is expressed from the epicardial or precordial leads as subepicardial (negative T wave) (Figure 3.7D).

Clinical point of view

The electrophysiological mechanism that explains the patterns of clinical ischaemia is different in cases of subendocardial and subepicardial (transmural) ischaemia.

(a) The electrophysiological mechanism of subendocardial ischaemic pattern: symmetric and usually taller T wave with rectified ST segment and accompanied by QTc prolongation. It is well known since the 1940s (Dressler, 1947) that in the hyperacute phase of a total coronary artery occlusion, especially in the heart without any previous significant ischaemia (coronary spasm or in some STE-ACS evolving Q-wave infarction), a tall and peaked T wave may be the first manifestation of ischaemia (Figure 3.7B). This morphology is probably due to an increase in extracellular potassium related to a hyperpolarisation of myocytes as a consequence of opening of ATP-dependent K^+ channels due to an acute ischaemia. This hyperpolarisation of myocites is more evident in the endocardium and prolongs the repolarisation in this area (prolonged QTc) (Wang et al., 1996). This tall, peaked and symmetric P wave is generated during the second phase of repolarisation (Figure 3.6A). This explains that usually an ST segment often rectified is recorded.

This pattern of positive T wave is followed if the ischaemia persists, as occurs in the case of experimental coronary artery occlusion (Figure 3.4) or of STE-ACS or Prinzmetal angina (Figure 3.8A) **by the electrocardiographic pattern of subepicardial injury (ST-segment elevation)** (Table 2.1, and Figures 3.7C and 8.7). Usually, this occurs rarely during PCI. Recently, Kenigsberg (2007) has demonstrated that during PCI the first manifestation of ischaemia is prolongation of QTc that is present in all cases, and due to the short duration of ischaemia it is only followed by clear changes in morphology of T wave

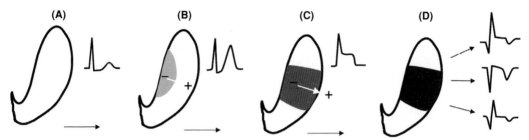

Figure 3.7 Observe how different degrees of ischaemia that appear sequentially after coronary occlusion in a heart without previous ischaemia (A) explain the ECG morphologies. (B) Ischaemia predominant in the subendocardial area (T wave symmetric and usually taller than normal with longer QT interval). (C) In the presence of more severe ischaemia evolving to transmural injury, ST-segment elevation is present. (D) If the ischaemia persists, transmural necrosis expressed as Q wave of necrosis and a negative T wave appears.

or ST-segment deviations in small number of cases (see p. 270). The reason is that, after a short period of predominant subendocardial involvement (subendocardial ischaemia), the ischaemia, if it is important and persistent, generates a severe transmural and homogeneous involvement of all ventricular wall, with the formation of 'low-quality' TAP in the entire wall. Thus, the pattern of positive T wave (sudden, hyperacute, predominant subendocardial ischaemia) changes to a pattern of ST-segment elevation (more important, persistent and homogeneously transmural ischaemia) that may evolve into a Q-wave infarction (Table 2.1 and Figure 3.7D).

In some cases of coronary artery spasm of just a few seconds' duration, the reversible subendocardial ischaemia pattern may be the unique electrocardiographic change recorded. Sometimes, while passing from one pattern to another (from a positive T with rectified ST segment to an ST-segment elevation), intermediate patterns can be observed, such as a wide positive T wave without ST-segment elevation (Figures 3.8A and C). In this case, opposite to what happens in normal individuals (Figure 3.1B), the ascendent slope of a T wave tends to rise suddenly and is not clearly convex with respect to the isoelectric line (compare Figures 3.1B and 3.8C).

(b) The electrophysiological mechanism of subepicardial ischaemic pattern: flattened or negative T wave.

In clinical practice an exclusively subepicardial area of ischaemia does not exist, but in case of transmural ischaemia, the onset of repolarisation is delayed longer in the epicardium than in the endocardium with the result that the endocardial muscle is the first to recover. Repolarisation then occurs in the involved wall in an endocardial-to-epicardial

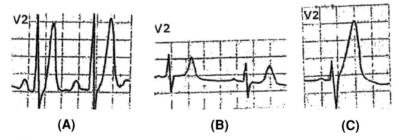

Figure 3.8 Morphologies of taller than normal T wave in patients with ischaemic heart disease. (A) T wave very tall not preceded by rectified ST segment: This morphology is frequently observed in a transitory form in case of Prinzmetal angina (Figure 8.44). (B) A tall T wave, very symmetric and with previous rectified ST segment completely abnormal for V2 lead, which may be frequently observed in a hyperacute phase of an ACS with ST-segment elevation (see Figures 8.5 and 8.7). (C) V2 lead: T wave with very wide base and straight ascendent slope of T wave that can be seen in a patient with an acute myocardial infarction. This pattern is transition between the typical pattern of subendocardial ischaemia (B) and the pattern of STEMI (Figure 8.7) that is clearly different from the mild ST-segment elevation and tall T wave that may be seen as a variant in normal individuals (Figure 3.1B).

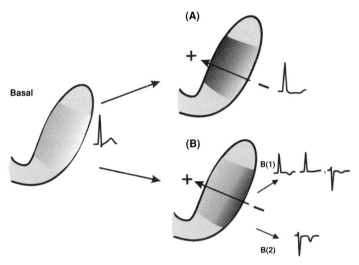

Figure 3.9 In case that in basal state a certain degree of ischaemia with subendocardial predominance exists too mild to produce clear ECG changes, an increase of 'active' ischaemia still with subendocardial predominance will produce an ST-segment depression (subendocardial injury pattern) (A). If as a consequence of ischaemia there is a delay in repolarisation predominating in subepicardium or being transmural, a flattened or negative T wave appears in leads with, but also without, predominant R wave (B-1) (subepicardial ischaemia pattern). The latter pattern is probably more consequence of ischaemia (post-ischaemic pattern) that due to active ischaemia. Especially when the negative T wave is deep as seen in V1–V4 it may be considered a reperfusion pattern (B-2). In (A) the injury vector moves towards the injured area, and in (B) the ischaemia vector moves away from the ischaemic area (see Figures 3.6 and 4.8). Remember that if the ischaemia is transmural, it is expressed from the epicardium or precordial leads as subepicardial. Therefore the vector of ischaemia moves away also from subepicardium.

direction, the reverse of normal, and it is expressed in the ECG as a negative T wave, as happens in case of experimental subepicardial ischaemia (Figure 3.6B). This happens because the ischaemic vector is going from epicardium to endocardium (Figure 3.9B). The proximity of precordial leads to subepicardial area may also contribute to it (Hellertein and Katz, 1948). Different morphologies with or without Q wave and ST-segment deviations, and with more or less important negative T wave, are recorded in relation with presence of associated injury and necrosis areas, the side of recording and the electrode location.

A flat or negative T wave may be present in different clinical settings of IHD and may be explained by different, but not always well understood, mechanisms.

1. Acute coronary syndromes: A new flattened or negative T wave in ACS may be recorded in two different clinical situations (Table 8.1):

(a) **As a part of clinical syndrome of NSTE-ACS, new flattened or negative T wave usually non-deep** is one of the classical ECG patterns of NSTE-ACS (Table 8.1). This pattern may be recorded in right precordial leads and more frequently in leads with a dominant R wave (Figure 3.9B(1)). In general it corresponds to a non-proximal subocclusion of any of the coronary arteries, often two, when the pattern is seen in leads with dominant R wave (Figure 3.23), or to LAD occlusion sometimes proximal when the pattern is present in V1–V3 (Figure 8.23). **The negative T wave may be due to 'active' ischaemia,** when the changes are dynamic and/or appear during angina pain. If the negative T wave is present in the absence of anginal pain, it may probably be considered a **reperfusion pattern.** However it is clear that we need to know more about the mechanism that explains the delay of repolarisation responsible for the presence of flattened or negative T wave during NSTE-ACS or in chronic state. In any case, if in the presence of flattened or mildly negative T wave ST-segment depression appears on exertion, 'active' ischaemia exists with subendocardial predominance (Figure 4.64 and Table 2.1B(1)).

(b) As a part of clinical syndrome of STE-ACS, the negative T wave appears **in the subacute phase of STE-ACS** and may also correspond to an **atypical pattern recorded in the dynamic process of STE-ACS.**

–**Negative T wave in the subacute phase of STE-ACS**: In STE evolving Q-wave MI a transmural and homogeneous involvement of the entire ventricular wall exists. A negative T wave appears shortly after the Q wave develops and coincides with the decrease in the ST-segment elevation (Figures 3.7D, 3.18 and 3.19). When this occurs clinical ischaemia is decreasing and part of the injured myocardium (ST-segment elevation) converts into infarcted tissue (Q wave of infarction). Classically, it was considered that residual ischaemia that exists in the ventricular wall myocardial area surrounding the infarction and injury tissue (Figure 3.3) may explain the presence of flattened or negative T wave. However, as happens in the chronic phase of Q-wave MI, **in the origin of the pattern of subepicardial ischaemia that appears in the evolutive phase of STE-ACS, the changes induced in ventricular repolarisation by the ACS probably are most important than 'active' ischaemia.**

–**Deep negative T wave in precordials (V1–V2 to V4–V5) as an atypical pattern of STE-ACS:** It corresponds to a critical proximal subocclusion of the LAD that has been **spontaneously, and partially, reperfused** or even complete LAD occlusion but with great number of collaterals (De Zwan, Bär and Wellens, 1982) (Figures 3.9B(2) and 3.21, and Table 8.1). This is an ECG dynamic pattern that may evolve without treatment to STE-ACS, with homogeneous and global cardiac wall involvement. In this case, the T wave will first pseudonormalise (Figure 3.21) and then, if ischaemia persists, an ST-segment elevation would appear (Figure 8.3B), even evolving to a Q-wave infarction (Table 2.1A). However currently in the majority of cases the treatment aborts the appearance of MI. It is necessary to perform a coronary angiography as soon as possible to check the grade and exact location of stenosis in LAD but, in absence of symptoms or dynamic changes of ST, not as an emergency. Really, in this case, the presence of negative T wave in the evolution of ACS is not a marker of cell death but is caused by changes in ion channels in areas of the heart that are still viable after severe ischaemia (post-ischaemic changes).

If this pattern (very deep negative T wave from V1–V4–V5) appears after reperfusion (fibrinolysis or PCI) treatment in a patient with STE-ACS, it is considered as a sign that the treatment of revascularisation has been effective (**reperfusion pattern**). In these cases there is usually no need for PCI, although the patients have to be carefully watched because on some occasion a new coronary event may evolve, if for instance an intratent thrombosis appears (Figure 8.9).

2. Chronic phase of IHD (Figures 3.18, 3.19 and 4.64): The negative T wave may be present in patients with and without previous Q-wave MI. In the first case usually the negative T waves are recorded in leads with Q wave. In this case this **ECG pattern is clearly explained more by the changes produced by infarction in ventricular repolarisation than by the presence of residual 'active' ischaemia (post-necrosis changes).** In other cases, if active ischaemia exists, ECG changes are usually present on exercise test, usually in a form of ST-segment depression (Figure 4.64, p. 124).

The ischaemia that occurs clinically secondary to an acute total coronary artery occlusion is first predominantly subendocardial (symmetric and usually taller T wave) and then transmural and homogeneous (ST-segment elevation), and later, in general, a Q wave of necrosis appears, accompanied by a negative T wave (pattern of subepicardial ischaemia). The latter, in this context, is more a post-ischaemic or postnecrosis change than the expression of 'active' ischaemia (Table 2.1 and Figure 3.7).

Table 3.1 Causes of taller-than-normal T wave (aside from ischæmic heart disease; Figure 3.8).

1. **Normal variants** (vagotonia, sportsmen, etc.; Figure 3.11)
2. **Acute pericarditis.** (Usually with mild ST elevation; Figure 4.48A)
3. **Alcoholism** (Figure 3.16)
4. **Hyperkalaemia** (Figure 3.15)
5. **Not long-standing left-ventricular hypertrophy** (especially in cases of diastolic overload, such as aortic regurgitation; (Figure 3.12)
6. **Stroke** (Figure 3.14)
7. **In V1–V2 as a mirror pattern of lateral ischaemia or ischaemia secondary to left-ventricle hypertrophy** (Figures 3.10 and 7.4)
8. **Congenital AV block** (Figure 3.13)

Electrocardiographic pattern of subendocardial ischaemia: diagnosis and differential diagnosis

The ECG pattern of subendocardial ischaemia – a T wave more symmetric and often taller preceded by rectified ST segment and accompanied by QTc prolongation (T wave of subendocardial ischaemia) – is observed in the acute phase of IHD (Table 2.1A) but may also be seen in other situations (Table 3.1).

T wave of subendocardial ischaemia

The T wave of subendocardial ischaemia is a temporary pattern that **may be recorded during a brief time in the hyperacute phase of STE-ACS (Figure 8.7) and during a coronary spasm (Figure 8.46)** (Table 2.1A). It is difficult to record in a surface ECG due to the short duration of its appearance.

This positive T wave usually presenting typically an appreciable voltage, although sometimes not exceeding 5 mm, is symmetric and appears often after a rectified or even slightly descendent ST segment (Figure 8.7) as it arises in the second phase of repolarisation (Figures 3.5 and 3.6). It is very difficult to be sure whether the T wave is really taller than normal if no sequential ECGs allowing for the comparison of T-wave voltage are available. It has been demonstrated that, on occasion, a transitory increase in the 'pointing up' of the T wave with only a slight increase in its voltage, sometimes difficult to

evaluate even with sequential ECG recordings, may be the only expression of ischaemia. Nevertheless, on other occasions, a T wave of significant voltage may be observed. In this case the T wave often has a wide base and is not preceded by a rectified ST segment (Figures 3.8A and C and 8.46), because in reality, it is the first sign that a positive T wave is converting into an ST-segment elevation (Figure 8.8). This morphology is recorded, above all, in the right precordial leads (V1–V4) (Figures 3.8B and C) as an expression of initial subendocardium involvement during a hyperacute occlusion of an epicardial artery, in this case the LAD, although it may also be observed in inferior leads in case of an RCA or LCX occlusion. The cases of cardiac spasm (Prinzmetal angina) are usually recorded during Holter monitoring (Figure ?? and 8.46).

We should remember that in some chronic coronary patients, those who present a transmural infarction classically named inferoposterior but with the new classification we define as inferolateral MI (Figure 5.9B(3)), a tall, frequently peaked, and in this case persistent, T wave may be recorded in V1–V3 as a consequence of the changes that the transmural infarction produced in repolarization (mirror pattern of inferobasal and lateral subepicardial ischaemia) (Figure 3.10).

Taller-than-normal T wave in other situations

Table 3.1 presents the most frequent causes of more positive than normal T waves, different from IHD. Some examples, including variants of normality (vagal overdrive) (Figure 3.11), are shown in Figures 3.11–3.16. Sometimes the morphologies are very characteristic, as the tall symmetric T wave with relatively narrow base in left-ventricular diastolic overload, as in important aortic regurgitation (Figure 3.12) and in a congenital AV block (Figure 3.13), or the T wave with wide base and irregular morphology that may be observed in some patients due to the toxic effects of some drugs and in some cerebrovascular accidents (Figure 3.14). Additionally, very tall and peaked T waves may be recorded in some cases of moderate hyperkalaemia due to renal failure (Figure 3.15) and at times in chronic alcoholism without heart failure (Figure 3.16).

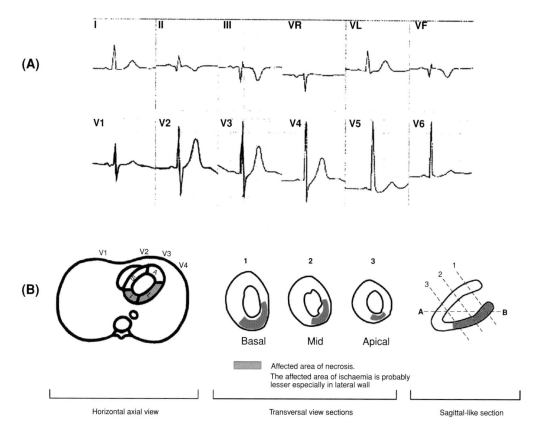

Figure 3.10 (A) ECG with a typical pattern of chronic subepicardial ischaemia in the leads facing the inferior wall (negative T wave in II, III and VF) and the lateral wall (positive peaked T wave in V1–V2). There is a necrosis in the same area in which a QR complex in II, III and VF and an RS complex in V1 are recorded. (B) Horizontal axial vision of the heart, transverse vision of the heart at basal, mid and apical area and sagittal-like vision of the heart (CMR) (see Figures 1.8 and 1.11). Segments involved are 4, 5, 10 and 11 and perhaps 3, 9, 15 and 16. The RS pattern in V1 is explained especially by the involvement of segments 5 and 11.

Electrocardiographic pattern of subepicardial ischaemia (transmural): diagnosis and differential diagnosis

The ECG pattern of subepicardial ischaemia – flattened or negative T wave – is observed in IHD (Table 2.1), but it may also appear in other situations (see Table 3.2). We have to remember that the ECG pattern of subepicardial ischaemia (negative T wave) although may probably be due to real 'active' ischaemia (ACS), more often appear in the dynamic changes of some ACS as a reperfusion pattern or is explained by the changes that MI has induced in ventricular repolarisation (chronic Q-wave MI) (p. 37 and Table 8.1).

Flattened or negative T wave in IHD
(Figures 3.17–3.27)
We will discuss the diagnostic and location criteria. The clinical presentation and prognostic implications of the ECG pattern of subepicardial ischaemia in different clinical settings of IHD will be discussed in Part II of this book (p. 289).

Diagnostic criteria: morphology and voltage

The normal T wave (see 'Normal limits of the T wave' p. 30) is recorded as positive in almost all leads except VR and often V1, and, on occasion, III, VF and rarely II and even in VL in cases of a vertical heart with rS or QS morphology and usually

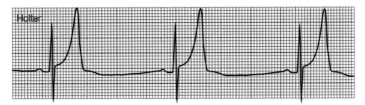

Figure 3.11 Tall and peaked T wave not secondary to ischaemic heart disease recorded at night (Holter) in a sportsman with vagal overdrive. Note the significant bradycardia, the asymmetric T wave and the slight ST-segment elevation (early repolarisation). There is a significant right vagal overdrive (quite significant sinus bradycardia), but hardly any left vagal overdrive (PR interval: 0.20 s). In sportsmen with left vagal overdrive, a second-degree Mobitz type I atrioventricular block (Wenckebach type) can be seen at night.

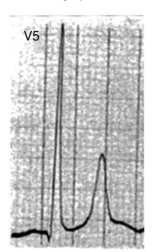

Figure 3.12 Male, 42 years old, with severe but not long-standing aortic regurgitation. Note the evident q wave in V5, the intrinsic deflection time (IDT) ≥0.07 s, the height of the R wave is >30 mm and the T wave is tall and peaked (14 mm). There is also a negative U wave.

negative P wave. When the normal T wave is negative, it is of low voltage (except in VR) and asymmetric. Therefore, the appearance of a flattened or negative T wave in the other leads (T-wave voltage lower than 2–3 mm in the HP – V2–V6 and than 1–2 mm in the FP – I, II and VL) is probably abnormal (see 'Flattened or negative T wave in other clinical settings' p. 49) and should be considered as an ECG pattern of subepicardial ischaemia.

In Figure 3.17 different examples of T waves of subepicardial ischaemia together with their corresponding VCG loops are presented. It is of particular interest to observe the homogeneous inscription of ischaemic T loop as compared to a normal T loop, which presents a slower first part of inscription, whether closed or opened (Figure 3.2).

The negative T wave is usually symmetric and of variable voltage, but in general it does not exceed 8–10 mm. Its base is usually not very wide, as it

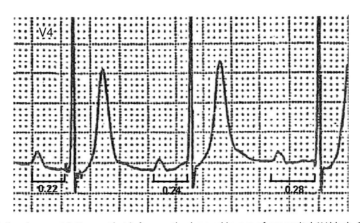

Figure 3.13 Very tall and symmetric T wave that is frequently observed in case of congenital AV block. Observe the changes of PR interval due to the presence of dissociated P waves.

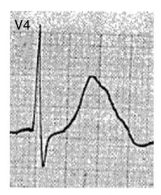

Figure 3.14 Very wide and tall T wave in a patient with a severe stroke. The QT interval is very long (640 ms).

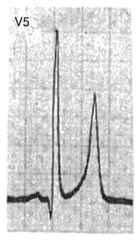

Figure 3.15 Tall, narrow and quite peaked T wave with a slight ST-segment elevation in a patient with hyperkalaemia secondary to renal failure.

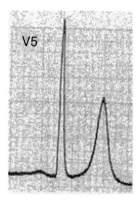

Figure 3.16 Male, 38 years old, moderate drinker for over the last 20 years. He presents palpitations, but not heart failure. In the leads facing the left ventricle, a symmetric and peaked T wave of 13 mm in height was recorded.

Table 3.2 Causes of negative or flattened T waves (aside from ischaemic heart disease).

1. **Normal variants**: Children, pertaining to black race and hyperventilation, women (right precordial leads), etc. May sometimes be diffuse (global T-wave inversion of unknown origin). More frequently observed in women.
2. **Pericarditis**: In this condition, the pattern is usually extensive, but generally the negativity of T wave is not very important (Figures 3.28 and 4.48 above C).
3. *Cor pulmonale* **and pulmonary embolism**. (Figure 3.30)
4. **Myocarditis (perimyocarditis)** (Figure 3.29) and **cardiomyopathies** (Figure 3.31)
5. **Alcoholism** (Figure 3.38)
6. **Stroke** (Figure 3.32): Not frequent.
7. **Myxoedema**: (Figure 3.37)
8. **Sportsmen** (Figure 3.33): With or without ST-segment elevation. Hypertrophic cardiomyopathy, especially apical type, must be ruled out.
9. After the administration of certain **drugs** (prenylamine and amiodarone) (flattened T wave) (Figure 3.39).
10. **Hypokalaemia**: The T wave can be flattened but usually the ST-segment depression is more evident.
11. **Post-tachycardia** (Figure 3.36)
12. **Abnormalities secondary** to left ventricular hypertrophy or to left bundle branch block.
13. **Intermittent left bundle branch block** (Figure 3.34) and other situations of intermittent abnormal activation [pacemakers (Figure 3.35), Wolf–Parkinson–White syndrome].

starts in the second part of systole, which explains the well-defined ST-segment generally observed.

Figures 3.18 and 3.19 show the evolution of two MIs from the acute phase with a huge ST-segment elevation until the appearance of Q wave of necrosis and negative T wave of subepicardial ischaemia. In Figure 3.20, a patient with chronic MI of inferior wall presents in the same ECG a different grade of ECG pattern of subepicardial ischaemia (negative and deep T wave in inferior leads, tall and positive T wave in right precordial leads as a mirror pattern and flat T wave in V6).

The deep negative T wave that may be seen in V1–V4–V5 is explained by LAD proximal occlusion that has been totally or partially opened spontaneously or after treatment (see 'Typical and atypical patterns of STE-ACS and NSTE-ACS' p. 210 and Figure 3.21).

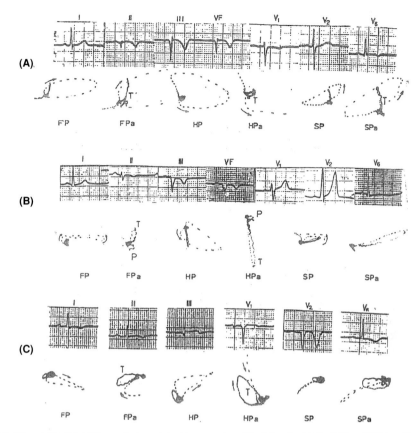

Figure 3.17 (A) and (B) ECG–VCG correlation of the T wave and the T loop of subepicardial ischaemia in two patients with myocardial infarction: (A) of the inferior wall and (B) of the inferior and lateral walls. Observe that a T loop in both cases shows homogeneous inscription and is directed upwards (see FPa) in the first case and upwards and forward in the second case (see HPa). The QRS loop of (A) rotates only clockwise and of (B) rotates first clockwise and later counter-clockwise. In the first case inferior MI is isolated and in the second, associated to superoanterior hemiblock (no final 'r' in II, III and VF) (see Figures 5.54 and 5.62). QRS loops in both cases are directed upwards and in case of inferolateral infarction also forward.
(C) ECG–VCG correlation of the T wave and T loop in case of subepicardial ischaemia of anteroseptal zone. Observe how the T loop with homogeneous inscription (symmetric negative T wave in ECG) and a QRS loop that is directed backwards and to the left with counter-clockwise direction and the T loop backwards and to the right (see HPa).

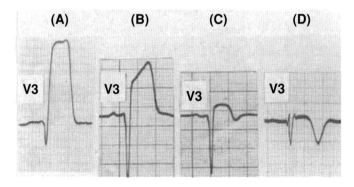

Figure 3.18 Acute infarction of anteroseptal zone with ST-segment elevation in the prefibrinolytic era. Evolutionary phases: (A) at 30 min, (B) 1 day later, (C) 1 week later and (D) 2 weeks later.

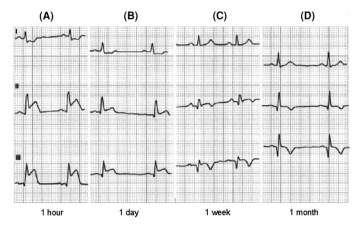

Figure 3.19 Evolution of inferior wall infarction due to RCA occlusion after RV branches treated with fibrinolysis. Observe the ST-segment deviations: depression in lead I, elevation in II, III and VF with III > II. Along the time can be seen the disappearance of the ST-segment elevation and appearance of Q wave of necrosis and negative T wave.

Sometimes T-wave morphology may be ±. This is consequence that the ECG pattern of ischaemia is generated especially in the second part of the systole (Figure 3.6). This morphology specially appears in V1–V4 as a post-ischaemic pattern due to spontaneous, or induced by treatment, reperfusion in case of LAD occlusion (Figure 3.21) (atypical pattern of STE-ACS) (see Figure 8.3B and p. 210). Figures 3.22 and 3.23 show two patients, one in stable phase and the other in the presence of ACS that presents flat or mildly negative T wave in only some leads (regional involvement).

On the other hand, an evident U wave (Figures 3.24 and 3.25) or even a less obvious one (Figure 3.26) in the presence of a positive T wave is equivalent to subepicardial ischaemia (Reinig, Harizi and Spodick, 2005).

Subepicardial ischaemia (primary repolarisation alteration) is frequently associated with LVE or LBBB (secondary repolarisation alteration), whereby mixed patterns are generated (Figure 3.27).

Location criteria

The negative T wave of subepicardial ischaemia is recorded in different leads, depending on the myocardial area affected by the occluded coronary artery (inferolateral or anteroseptal). In general, in case of single-vessel disease ischaemia is regional; therefore, a mirror pattern may be observed in the FP (Figures 3.10 and 3.20). Much probably, ischaemia at rest is usually explained by only a culprit artery, even may be stenosis in other arteries (multivessel disease).

In case of involvement of the inferolateral zone (RCA and/or LCX) negative T wave in II, III and VF with often mirror image in V1–V3 (positive T wave in V1–V3) appears. An example of a negative T wave of subepicardial ischaemia in the inferolateral zone with its corresponding VCG pattern can be observed in Figure 3.17A, B. This figure shows the T loop with homogeneous and narrow inscription directed upwards (inferior involvement) and also forwards (lateral involvement),

It is difficult to define the strict diagnostic criteria that will assure that we are in front of a T wave with an ECG pattern of **subepicardial ischaemia.** Nevertheless, we consider that **this diagnosis may be done** in the following circumstances:
• **Negative or flattened T wave (positive voltage less than 2–3 mm in an HP and 1–3 mm in an FP) in I, VL, II and in V2–V3 to V6,** especially if the changes are dynamic.
• We should remember that the T wave should always be negative in VR and may be flattened or even slightly negative in III, VF and V1 and sometimes in VL, V2 and II (see 'Normal limits of the T wave') p. 30.

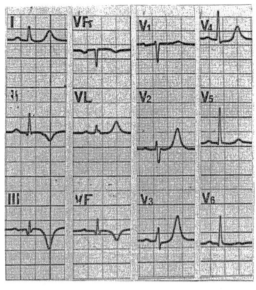

Figure 3.20 Old inferior infarction with lateral ischaemia (positive and symmetric T wave in V1–V3), with TV3 > TV1. The presence of flat T wave in V6 suggests that low lateral wall is also affected. Observe the negative T wave in II, III and VF (inferior ischaemia) and the positive T wave in I and VL that appears as a mirror pattern.

(A)　　　　　　　　　　　　　　　**(B)**

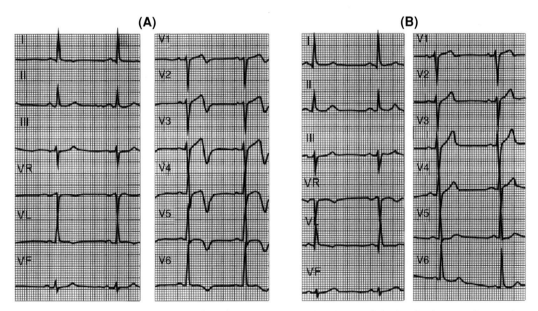

Figure 3.21 (A) ECG with a quite negative T wave in V1–V2 to V5, with extension to I and VL corresponding to a critical lesion in the proximal part of left anterior descending coronary artery that practically normalises during a chest pain crisis (B). This corresponds to an atypical pattern of STE-ACS (see Figure 8.3B). The normalisation of this pattern is an intermediate situation between the negative T wave and the ST-segment elevation that would appear if the chest pain were more intense and prolonged. It is quite important to bear this in mind and perform sequential ECGs, as the normal ECG during the angina crisis can provide quite confusing and dangerous information.

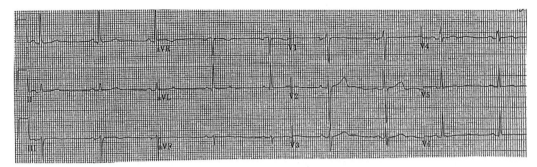

Figure 3.22 A patient with chronic non-proximal multivessel disease. Observe the basal ECG with the flattened T waves in various leads, especially in FP and V5–V6. The presence of this pattern in a chronic phase is usually due to post-ischaemic changes.

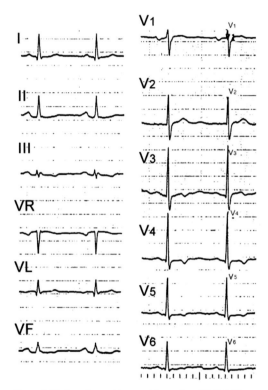

Figure 3.23 A patient with unstable angina (NSTE-ACS) with new, flattened or slightly negative T wave in various leads.

corresponding to a symmetric and negative T wave in II, III and VF (A and B) and a symmetric and positive T wave in V1 and V2 (B). Isolated lateral ischaemia may explain positive T wave in V1–V2, and theoretically if inferior involvement also exists,

in cases of very lean individuals with true posterior wall (Figure 1.13C) the T wave would be more positive in V2–V3 than in V1. If all inferior wall is flat, the vector of ischaemia will be directed only upwards. It is likely that the T wave will be more negative in III than in II lead if the inferior wall involvement is due to RCA occlusion. The opposite may occur in some cases of an occlusion of a dominant LCX.

In occlusion of OM branch (isolated involvement of the lateral wall), a flattened or negative T wave may be observed in V5-V6, and frequently in I and VL. In case of **occlusion of first diagonal (involvement of mid-anterior and lateral wall)**, the negative T wave is usually seen in VL and I and sometimes in II, III and VF, but usually is not evident in V5-V6.

In case of proximal LAD occlusion, the ECG changes (flattened or negative T waves) are observed in V1–V6 and in I and VL (Figure 3.21). Figure 3.17C shows the open T loop of homogeneous inscription directed to the right and backwards, corresponding to the negative T wave recorded from V1 to V6 in case of an extensive anterior involvement.

On the other hand, at times, especially in the presence of multivessel coronary disease, negative, flattened or very low voltage positive T waves may be recorded in various leads due to delay in repolarization without subendocardial predominance that is usually consequence of post-ischaemic changes (reperfusion) (see p. 32, Figures 3.22 and 3.23). The differential diagnosis of this pattern from the ECG pattern found in some cases of pericarditis may be

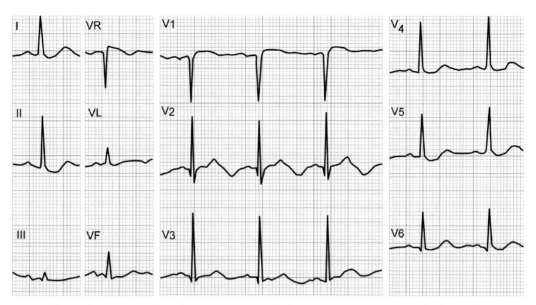

Figure 3.24 A patient with unstable angina who presents slight ST-segment depression in various leads, especially in II, III, V4–V6 and significantly marked negative U wave in V2–V3. This patient presents an important LAD occlusion.

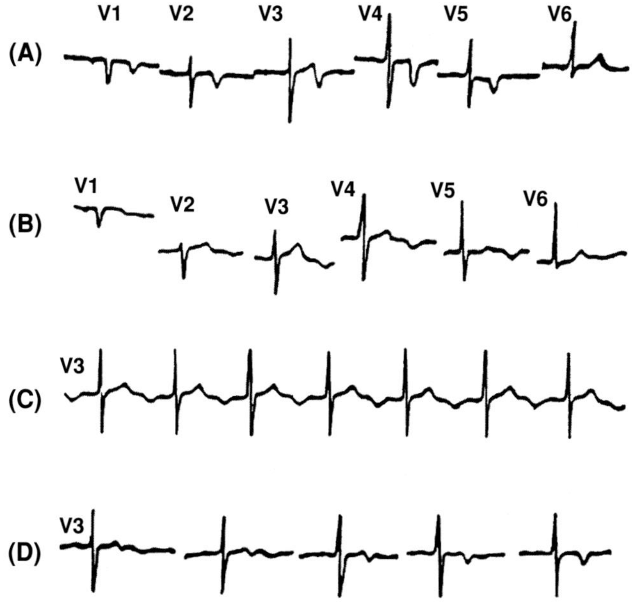

Figure 3.25 (A) Basal ECG (V1–V6) with ECG pattern of important subepicardial ischaemia in a 65-year-old patient with daily crisis of variant angina that always appeared at the same hour. During a crisis (B,C), there is pseudonormalisation of the ST segment with an evident negative U wave. A few seconds later, the ECG returns to the original situation (D). The five morphologies in the fourth strip are samples taken minute by minute, with a total duration of pain of 6 min that shows the changes in V3 from positive, T-negative U wave during pain to negative T wave after the crises.

(A)   **(B)**

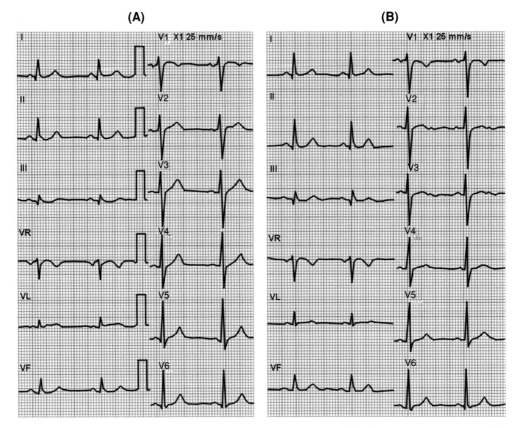

Figure 3.26 A 46-year-old patient with dubious precordial pain. The ECG (B) presented very discrete changes in V2–V3 leads (slightly negative U wave with somehow positive T wave). These small changes are significant when compared with previous ECG (A). The exercise stress test was positive and the coronary angiography showed proximal LAD stenosis resolved by PCI. The following ECG was equal to initial one (A).

(A)   **(B)**   **(C)**

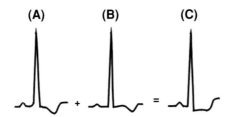

Figure 3.27 The mixed repolarisation changes (C) are explained by the combination of the primary changes due to ischaemia (A) and the changes secondary to the depolarisation abnormalities (e.g. LVH) (B).

We should remember that while **the vector of injury moves towards the injured area** (see Figure 4.8), **the vectors of ischaemia and infarction move away from the ischaemic and infarcted areas**, respectively (Figures 3.6, 3.10 and 5.3). (p. 35, 54, 131).

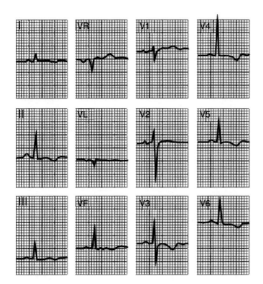

Figure 3.28 A patient with chronic constrictive pericarditis. The T wave is negative in many leads, but not quite deep, without the 'mirror' pattern in the frontal plane. The T wave is only positive in VR and V1 because as this is a diffuse subepicardial ischaemia, they are the only two leads in which the ischaemia vector that is directed away from the ischaemic area is approaching the exploring electrode.

very difficult. The clinical history, the result of an exercise stress test and the presence of Q waves of necrosis may be helpful in the differential diagnosis between multivessel coronary artery disease and pericarditis.

Flattened or negative T wave in other clinical situations

Table 3.2 shows the most frequent causes, apart from IHD, of a negative or flattened T wave. Figures

3.28–3.39 summarise different examples of these patterns, with their sometimes very characteristic corresponding morphologies.

In case of a negative or flattened T wave we should always keep in mind chronic pericarditis as a differential diagnosis. Apart from different characteristics of the clinical history and the character of pain, the type of subepicardial ischaemic ECG pattern observed in pericarditis following the hyperacute phase may be of help in the differentiating process. The myocardial involvement is usually more extensive in pericarditis than in IHD (there is no mirror pattern in the FP in pericarditis) and also the negativity of T wave is generally smaller (Figure 3.28), except in some cases with associated myocarditis (Figure 3.29). The evolution of the patient's clinical condition and the presence of Q wave are useful in the differential diagnosis. Nevertheless if two- or more vessel disease exists, alterations in repolarisation in the IHD are also diffuse and are sometimes not accompanied by Q waves. On the other hand, as previously said, if myopericarditis is present, quite evident negative T waves that are impossible to distinguish from those of IHD may be recorded (Figure 3.29). In the acute phase of pericarditis ST-segment elevation, usually mild and sometimes with tall T wave, (Figure 4.48) and PR-interval alterations (elevation in VR and depression in II) are frequently observed because of atrial injury, while no Q waves of infarction are present (Figures 4.48 and 4.49).

Other examples of flattened or negative T wave (Table 3.2) are as follows: very negative and transitory T waves in V1–V4 that appear in acute overload of RV due to a decompensation of cor pulmonale

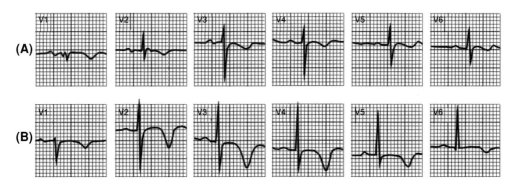

Figure 3.29 (A) ECG of a patient with chronic ischaemic heart disease. (B) ECG of a patient with myopericarditis. The ECG does not aid in this case in establishing the differential diagnosis. Even, the patient with myopericarditis shows more negative and deeper T waves.

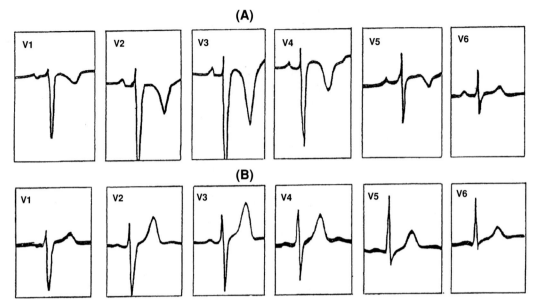

Figure 3.30 A 60-year-old patient with chronic 'cor pulmonale' who during respiratory infection presented ECG pattern of acute overload of right cavities (A) that disappeared some days later (B).

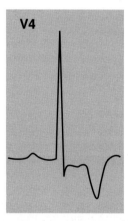

Figure 3.31 Typical pattern of repolarisation (deep negative and rather symmetrical and narrow T wave) frequently seen in patients with hypertrophic cardiomyopathy of apical type. The absence of septal q wave is explained by the presence of septal fibrosis (CE-CMR) and the deep negative T wave by craniocaudal asymmetry of septum (Dumont, 2006). A tall R wave is usually seen from V2–V3 to V5–V6 without Q wave.

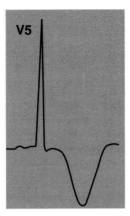

Figure 3.32 Female, 75 years old, with stroke. Note the large negative T wave with a quite wide base nearly without ST segment and a quite long QT interval (>500 ms). The patient died a few hours later.

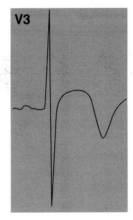

Figure 3.33 Negative T wave with an ST-segment elevation in an apparently healthy sportsman (normal echocardiogram and coronary angiography). Pattern not modified during 20 years that corresponds to the type D described by Plas (Figure 1.109; Plas, 1976). However, most sportsmen who die suddenly show similar patterns, generally with normal coronary arteries, but some of them with evidence of hypertrophic cardiomyopathy.

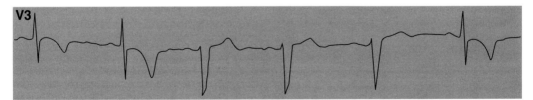

Figure 3.34 Patient with an advanced but intermittent left bundle branch block. A negative T wave is observed in the complexes that do not present left bundle branch block pattern. It is explained by 'cardiac memory' phenomenon due to the disappearance of the pattern of left bundle branch block. The repolarisation changes persist for a certain period of time as the consequence of the lack of the adequacy of the refractory periods of left ventricle to the new situation of normal intraventricular conduction.

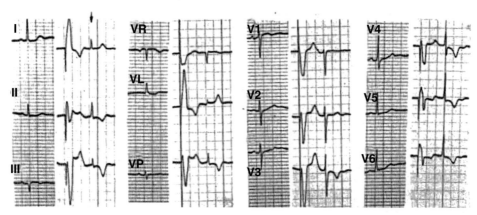

Figure 3.35 Four sets of leads with basal ECG (left) and after pacemaker implantation in the RV (right) in a patient without ischaemic heart disease. Note the negative T wave in sinus rhythm complexes after implantation due to 'cardiac memory' phenomenon. Characteristically, in case of 'cardiac memory' repolarisation abnormalities in patients without ischaemic heart disease, as happens in this case, the T wave is positive in I and VL, in the presence of inverted T waves in precordial leads.

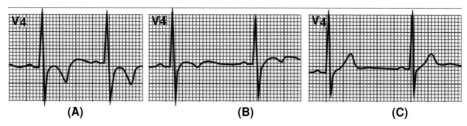

(A)   **(B)**   **(C)**

Figure 3.36 A 54-year-old man with paroxysmal arrhythmias and no structural heart disease. After a crisis of paroxysmal atrial fibrillation with an average ventricular rate response of 170 beats/min that lasted 6 hours, an evident negative T wave with a slight ST-segment depression was present and slowly disappeared over the next few days. (A) Recording immediately after the crisis. (B) Two days later, the pattern markedly decreased. (C) At 7 days, the ECG was normal. The need to perform complementary tests, or not to, to rule out ischaemia depends on the clinical characteristics in each case and the duration and depth of the pattern. In this case, coronary angiography was normal.

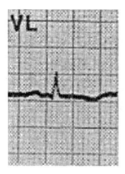

Figure 3.37 Low QRS complex and T-wave voltage in all the ECG leads. This pattern, especially if it is accompanied by bradycardia, must lead one to suspect myxedema. Generalised low-voltage patterns can be seen in many other processes, in which there is a border factor that decreases the voltage secondary to cardiac causes (e.g. myocardial fibrosis in myxedema, as in this case, or pericarditis) or extracardiac causes (emphysema, pleural effusion, ascites, etc.).

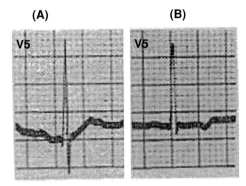

Figure 3.38 Flattened and split (A) or slightly negative T wave (B) in two patients with myocardial involvement secondary to alcohol abuse, without heart failure. Similar patterns can be recorded in other circumstances (administration of drugs).

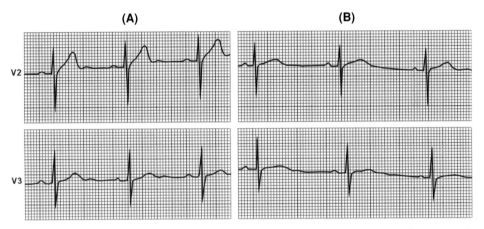

Figure 3.39 A 47-year-old man, who refers a history of paroxysmal arrhythmias, with a normal ECG. After 2 months of treatment with amiodarone, repolarisation, which was normal (A), showed a flattened and dome-like T wave (sometimes it is bimodal) (B). The QT interval lengthened but it is difficult to measure exactly how much it lengthened due to the flattening of the T wave.

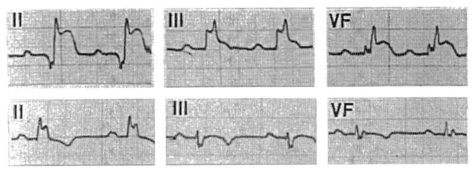

Figure 3.40 (A) Acute phase of an infarction in a patient with complete left bundle branch block. Note the clear ST-segment elevation. In the chronic phase (B), the symmetrical T wave in III (mixed pattern of repolarisation abnormality) leads to the suspicion of associated ischaemia.

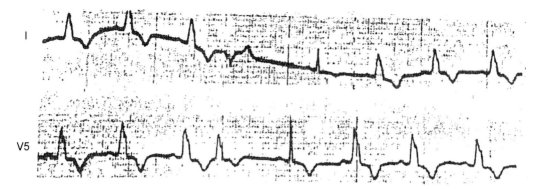

Figure 3.41   Symmetric negative T wave (see leads I and V5) in a patient with hypertension and intermittent complete left bundle branch block, who presents symmetric T wave when the LBBB disappears after a ventricular extrasystole. This is a mixed pattern (ischaemia + LVH). Also the T wave of complexes with LBBB presents more symmetric morphology than in cases of isolated LBBB.

(Figure 3.30), deep and narrow T wave in apical hypertrophic cardiomyopathy (Figure 3.31), wide and very negative T wave in some cerebrovascular accidents (Figure 3.32), repolarisation alteration – ST-segment elevation and negative T wave – observed in some athletes with no apparent heart disease (Figure 3.33), negative and sometimes deep T wave due to 'cardiac memory' (Rosenbaum et al., 1982; Denes et al., 1978) (Figures 3.34 and 3.35), negative T wave occasionally seen after a paroxysmal tachycardia (Figure 3.36), flattened T waves in myxedema (Figure 3.37) and alcoholics (Figure 3.38), and flattened, and sometimes bimodal, T wave due to amiodarone treatment (Figure 3.39). In the case of negative T wave due to 'cardiac memory' in patients with pacemaker, it has been described that in the absence of IHD, the T wave is positive in I and VL, even in the presence of deeply negative T wave in precordial leads (Figure 3.35).

Diagnosis of electrocardiographic pattern of ischaemia in patients with ventricular hypertrophy and/or wide QRS

The electrocardiographic pattern of subepicardial ischaemia is a primary alteration of repolarisation and if it occurs in individuals that already present secondary alteration of repolarisation, such as ventricular hypertrophy (especially LVH with strain) or wide QRS especially complete LBBB, the pattern of subepicardial ischaemia modifies the secondary alteration of repolarisation due to ventricular enlargement or LBBB, producing so-called mixed patterns (Figure 3.27). In these cases, frequently, the negative T wave secondary to ventricular enlargement and/or LBBB appears more symmetric (Figures 3.40 and 3.41).

CHAPTER 4

Electrocardiographic pattern of injury: ST-segment abnormalities

Normal limits of the ST segment

The ST segment should be, under normal conditions, isoelectric or present only a slight (less than 0.5 mm) upward or downward deviation. A slight ST-segment elevation (1–1.5 mm) with normal morphological characteristics, slightly convex with respect to the isoelectric line, may be recorded in normal subjects, above all in the right precordial leads (Figure 3.1B).

Non-pathological ST-segment depression tends to present a rapid ascent quickly crossing the isoelectric line (Figures 3.1C and 4.1C). This ST-segment depression observed during exercise or sympathetic overdrive forms part of a circumferential arch, involving the depressed ST and PR segments (Figures 4.1C and 4.2B). On the other hand, vagal overdrive and early repolarisation may present an ST-segment elevation of 1–3 mm, convex with respect to the isoelectric line that is recorded mainly in the intermediate precordial leads (Figures 3.1D and 4.1A).

Lastly, we should remember that TP (or UP) intervals, prior to and following the ST segment being evaluated, form the points of reference for assessing ST-segment depression and elevation (Figure 4.2B, C). If these intervals are not located at the same level (at the isoelectric line) or are not visible well, the PR interval of the cardiac cycle in question should be used as the reference. If the latter is descendent, the ECG recording at the onset of the QRS complex may be used as the reference to measure the ST-segment depression at 60 milliseconds of J point (Figure 4.2C, D). On the other hand, it is advisable to record the ECG with adequate amplified measuring systems to assure the correct measurement of ST changes (Figure 4.3).

The electrocardiographic pattern of injury

The electrocardiographic pattern of injury is recorded from the myocardial area in which, as a consequence of diminished blood supply (more important than the one that generates the ECG pattern of ischaemia) or other non-ischaemic causes, an **evident diastolic cellular depolarisation exists** (Figure 2.1(3)). **This leads to the formation of a 'low-quality' TAP in the injury area which is expressed in the ECG as ST-segment depression or elevation** (see 'Experimental point of view' – below – and Figure 4.5). This ECG pattern usually represents especially in the setting of ACS and especially, when the changes are dynamic, the existence of 'active' ischaemia.

As can be observed in the VCG, the final part of QRS loop (2 in Figure 4.14) is displaced from the beginning (1 in Figure 4.14), the free space being the expression of the injury vector (see distance 1–2 in Figure 4.14).

We will firstly refer to cases with normal QRS complex and later on we will briefly comment on how the presence of an ECG pattern of injury may be suspected in patients with wide QRS.

Electrophysiologic mechanism of the electrocardiographic pattern of injury

Experimental point of view

Many aspects of the mechanism of ischaemia-induced ST-segment changes lack solid biophysical underpinning, although it has been recently demonstrated (Hopenfeld, Stinstra and Macleod, 2004) that the electrocardiologic response to

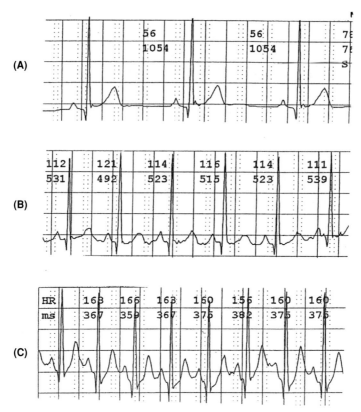

Figure 4.1 Holter recording of a very young patient with early repolarisation pattern recorded at night (A) that disappeared at daytime (B). During tachycardia the repolarisation presents changes typical of sympathetic overdrive (C).

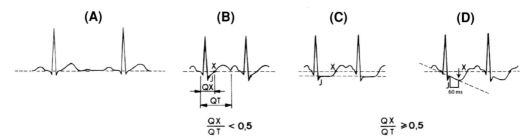

Figure 4.2 Normal resting ECG (A) and the normal electrocardiographic response to the exercise (B). Although the J point is depressed, it reaches rapidly the point X so that QX/QT <0.5. The response is abnormal when QX/QT ≥0.5 (C). In (D) in the absence of an evident TP interval and in the presence of descending PR segment, the initial part of QRS complex is taken as the reference point to measure the ST-segment depression at 60 ms of the J point.

ischaemia depends strongly on the anisotropic conductivity of the myocardium. In this book we will not go very much inside all these new types of experimental bases of ischaemia-induced ST changes, because they are not completely known. As an example in animal models, progressive epicardial coronary blood flow reduction fails to produce ST-segment depression at normal heart rates (De Chantal et al., 2006).

According to the membrane response curve (Singer and Ten Eick, 1971) (Figure 4.4), **the area with significant and persistent ischaemia shows**

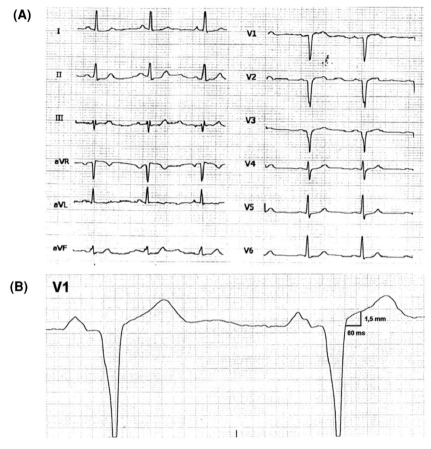

Figure 4.3 Observe how an amplified ECG (4x) allows the proper assessment of ST-segment deviation. (A) Post-myocardial-infarction patient with slight ST-segment elevation in right precordial leads. When amplified ECG was applied, at 60 ms of J point one may observe an ST-segment elevation of 6 mm that corresponds to 1.5 mm in normal ECG (B).

an evident **diastolic depolarisation, which produces a 'low-quality' TAP in this area (slower upstroke, lower voltage, smaller area, etc.)** (Figure 2.1(3)). When diastolic depolarisation occurs in the subendocardium, an ST-segment depression is recorded in the ECG (**electrocardiographic pattern of subendocardial injury**), and when the injury occurs in the subepicardium (or is transmural), an ST-segment elevation is generated (**electrocardiographic pattern of subepicardial injury**). The electrophysiologic explanation for these electrocardiographic patterns may be based on the following two theories (Bayés de Luna, 1978; Coksey, Massie and Walsh, 1960; Cabrera, 1958; Sodi Pallares, 1956).

1. Theory of the TAP summation (Figure 4.5): The normal ECG may be explained as summing up of the subendocardium TAP plus the subepicardium TAP (Bayés de Luna, 1999). This theory is also useful in explaining the origin of the ST-segment elevation and depression in case of subepicardial and subendocardial injury, respectively. Figure 4.5 shows how the summing up of 'poor-quality' TAP of the injured area (subendocardium in the subendocardial injury and subepicardium in the subepicardial injury – clinically transmural) plus TAP of the rest of the LV only cancels out some part of the TAP of the injury-free area. Consequently, this allows for the recording of an ST-segment depression in case of subendocardial injury (Figure 4.5B) or ST-segment elevation in case of subepicardial injury (Figure 4.5C). The ST-segment elevation or depression will be more or less significant, according to

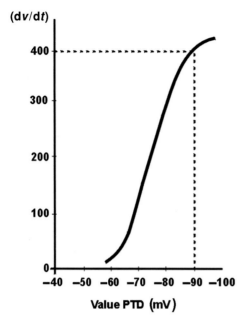

Figure 4.4 Note the relationship between the value of DTP in mV and the velocity of response (response dv/dt).

'poor-quality' TAP that exists in the injured area (Figure 4.5).

2. Theory of the injury vector (Figures 4.6–4.8): The electrocardiographic pattern of suben-

docardium or subepicardial injury can also be explained if we consider that an injury current exists between the injured area (less electrically charged) and the normal area (more electrically changed). One hypothesis considers that the electrocardiographic pattern of injury is explained by an injury current in diastole and the other by an injury current in systole (Bayés de Luna, 1978, 1999; Janse, 1982; Mirvis and Goldberger, 2001).

It has been shown in the experimental setting that both currents intervene in the genesis of ST-segment elevation and depression (Hellerstein and Katz, 1948; Janse, 1982) (Figures 4.6 and 4.7). However, **only the hypothesis of the systolic injury current will be discussed because this current is the one expressed in clinical practice, since the ECG equipments are adjusted by AC amplifiers to maintain a stable isoelectric baseline during diastole.** Consequently, the original changes in the TQ interval secondary to diastolic depolarisation are not recorded during the diastole, but their effects on the systolic period are expressed as changes in the TAP morphology (Figures 4.6 and 4.7). Indeed, during the systolic depolarisation phase, even though all the cells are depolarised, the normal cells because of their greater previous polarisation –

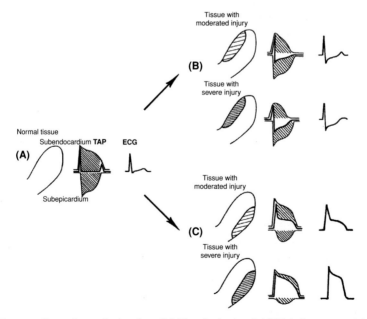

Figure 4.5 How the respective patterns of subendocardial (B) and subepicardial (C) injuries are generated according to the theory that the normal ECG pattern (A) is the result of the sum of subendocardial and subepicardial PATs.

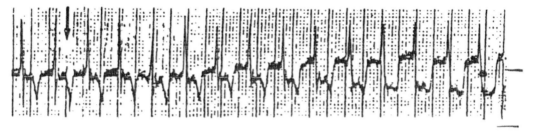

Figure 4.6 The electrode located in the epicardium of anterior cardiac wall records a simultaneous ST-segment depression and T-QRS elevation after subepicardial ischaemia of posterior wall (arrow) is produced. (Adapted from Hellerstein and Katz, 1948.)

more polarised during diastole – preserve a normal transmembrane resting action potential and are more electrically charged than are the injured cells. Thus, during systolic depolarisation they are more negative than the injured cells (Figure 4.8). This could explain the existence of a systolic injury current that would go from the normal cells (more negative) towards the injured cells (less negative means that they are comparatively relatively positive) (Figure 4.8(1A)).

This systolic injury current can express itself in the form of an **injury vector**, considering that the current flow runs from the more negative area (less ischaemic or normal) to the less negative or relatively positive area (injured). The injury vector is expressed by ST-segment elevation or depression (Figure 4.8(1A)). **If the experimental injury has developed in the subendocardium, the injury vector** that **is directed towards the injured area** (p. 60, Figure 4.8(1A)) generates an ST-segment

depression during the systole in precordial electrodes, immediately following the QRS complex. The slope of this ST segment will decrease during the second part of systole as the myocardial cells will be repolarised. **In case of subepicardial experimental injury**, the injury vector generates an ST-segment elevation by the same phenomenon (Figure 4.8(1B)), and the slope of ST segment also decreases during the second part of systole.

Clinical viewpoint

In human beings, the electrocardiographic injury pattern is seen in the presence of evident and persistent clinical ischaemia. When we extrapolate the findings in the experimental field to clinical practice, it could be considered that when the ischaemia is important, persistent and predominant in a certain area (subendocardium or subepicardium), an evident diastolic depolarisation in that area generates a 'low-quality' TAP (slower

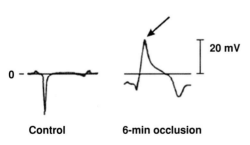

Control 6-min occlusion

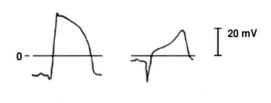

8-min occlusion 33-min occlusion

Figure 4.7 Local DC extracellular electrocardiograms from the left ventricular subepicardium of an isolated pig heart before (control) and 6, 8 and 33 min after coronary artery occlusion. Horizontal lines indicate zero potential. Note decrease in resting potential (TQ-segment depression in extracellular complex) and reduction in action potential upstroke velocity with the appearance of ST-segment elevation. After 8 min of occlusion the ECG shows monophasic morphology. (There is a TQ depression and huge ST-segment elevation.) Surprisingly, 33 min after occlusion there is a temporary reappearance of electrical activity, but after 1 h the ischaemic zone becomes permanently unexcitable. Characteristically, some time before the ischaemic cells become unresponsive they presented electrical alternance of amplitude and duration of action potential. (Adapted from Janse, 1982.)

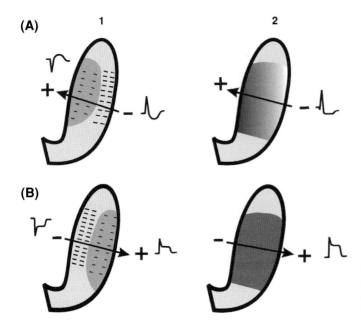

Figure 4.8 Subendocardial (A) and subepicardial (B) injury vectors in case of experimental (1) or clinical (transmural) injury (2).

upstroke). The development of an ST-segment elevation or depression (injury pattern) therefore could also be explained. However, from the clinical point of view, an exclusively subendocardium or subepicardium involvement does not exist. In fact, two different situations of distribution of a significant ischaemia in the LV occur, which generate the ST-segment elevation and depression patterns, as well as the reciprocal patterns.

(a) The electrophysiological mechanism of subendocardial injury pattern: ST-segment depression: If significant and persistent ischaemia occurs predominantly in the subendocardium, although subepicardium areas with less ischaemia are usually found (fewer grey areas and with more negative electrical charges in Figure 4.8(2A)), a subendocardial injury pattern is recorded in the ECG (ST-segment depression). This is explained by the predominance of subendocardium involvement, as compared to that of the subepicardium. We should remember that under normal conditions, during systole, the subendocardium arteries of a lesser calibre are more vulnerable to compression than are the subepicardial arteries and, consequently, coronary flow towards the subendocardium decreases (Bell and Fox, 1974). Visner et al. (1985) demonstrate that this decrease in subendocardium coronary flow is accompanied by an increase in LV end diastolic

pressure. This reduced endocardial-to-epicardial flow ratio is even more evident: (a) in situations such as exercise and stress, which decrease even more the already smaller flow distribution towards the subendocardium that is observed under normal conditions; (b) in NSTE-ACS (unstable angina and non-Q-wave MI), because of an incomplete occlusion of a coronary artery that generates an increase in the impairment of perfusion of subendocardium area of myocardium that already presented subendocardial ischaemia. All these situations favour the development of an ST-segment depression (Figure 4.8(2A)).

Both the clinical ST-segment depression pattern and the experimental subendocardial injury pattern have a common explanation: the sum of subendocardium TAP, which is of worse quality than in the subepicardium (Figure 4.5), or the generation of an injury vector (Figure 4.8). In NSTE-ACS the presence of new ST-segment depression is related with the presence of evident 'active' ischaemia predominantly in the subendocardium. On the other hand, the presence of flat or negative T wave is related with previous ischaemia (often is a reperfusion pattern) without subendocardial predominance (Table 2.1 and Figure 3.9).

One question that needs to be understood is why during exercise testing an increase in the height of T wave as the expression of subendocardial is-chaemia is not recorded, but an ST-segment de-pression is. The explanation may be the following: the electrocardiographic pattern of subendocardial ischaemia (tall and peaked T wave), which is of-ten transiently recorded in the initial phase of the complete occlusion of an epicardial artery, occurs in a myocardium that has usually not presented ev-ident previous ischaemia. This tall T wave is the ex-pression of the sudden decrease in subendocardium flow after total occlusion, which is followed by the ST-segment elevation because of significant, trans-mural and homogeneous ischaemia. Therefore, it is a transition pattern from the normal positive but less tall T wave and the ST-segment eleva-tion (Figure 3.7B).* However, during a pathological exercise test there is, in general, an increase of ischaemia in a certain area where the subendo-cardium is already suffering from poor perfusion because of an evident but incomplete previous coro-nary stenosis. As we have already discussed, phys-ical exercise decreases subendocardial perfusion because during the exercise test the subendocardial arteries have less vasodilatory capacity than that of the subepicardial ones (see before). Consequently, an inadequate redistribution of coronary flow oc-curs, with a significant increase in clinical ischaemia that predominates at the subendocardium level, al-though sometimes affects all the wall but without homogeneous transmural involvement. This phe-nomenon is the consequence that the occlusion of the artery is not total and that the coronary blood flow to subendocardium is severely im-paired. Consequently, the electrocardiographic pat-tern that is recorded is ST-segment depression (Figure 4.8(2A)). However, if during an exercise test, a coronary spasm occurs, the important transmural and homogeneous involvement that this produces due to total coronary occlusion would explain the occurrence of ST-segment elevation (Figure 11.3).

There is a reasonable correlation between the in-jured subendocardium area and the leads show-ing ST-segment depression, though it is less ev-ident than in case of areas with ECG pattern of subepicardial injury (see 'ECG pattern of subepi-cardial (transmural) injury in patients with narrow QRS') (p. 63). When a large left-ventricular area is involved, as in the ACS due to left main incom-plete occlusion (**circumferential involvement**), ST-segment depression is virtually seen in all the leads, with the exception of VR and, sometimes, V1 and III. In these leads, ST-segment elevation is seen as a mirror pattern, since the injury vector is di-rected from the subepicardium towards the suben-docardium in an upward, backward and rightward direction and therefore is recorded as a negative deflection from the majority of leads (Figure 4.9). When the presence of ST-segment depression is seen in less number of leads (usually <6), the exten-sion of injury is considered regional and usually in-volves especially leads with RS or dominant R wave (V4–V6, I and/or VL) (Sclarovsky, 1999) (see 'ST-segment depression in ishaemic heart disease' p. 111 and Table 8.1).

(b) The electrophysiological mechanism of ST-segment elevation:
Generally, this ECG pattern is related to acute and total occlusion of an epicardial coronary artery in a patient without important previous ischaemia. In this case the presence of significant and persis-tent ischaemia generates a transmural and homo-geneous involvement of all ventricular wall and an ST-segment elevation, as in case of exclusive subepi-cardial experimental injury, is recorded. This pat-tern is recorded probably because there is more injury in the epicardial area and also because the electrodes located closer to epicardium are record-ing more subepicardial involvement. In fact, due to proximity of the recording electrode to the subepicardium, the injury vector head faces the epicardium, as happens in the experimental subepi-cardial injury, and consequently, an ST-segment elevation is recorded (Figure 4.8B(2)).

Since the injury pattern develops at the end of depolarisation, at the end of the generation of the QRS complex and the beginning of repolarisation, the electrocardiographic expression starts during the first part of ST segment and last during all ST segment and T wave in cases of very important in-jury. It should be recalled that in the ECG pattern of ischaemia, the T-wave changes occur during the

---

*It should be reminded (Bayes de Luna, 1999) that the T wave in the normal ECG is positive because the surface ECG leads face the head of the vector of repolarisation. That goes from the area with less physiological flow (theoretically is-chaemic), the subendocardium, to the area with more physi-ological flow, the subepicardium.

(A)

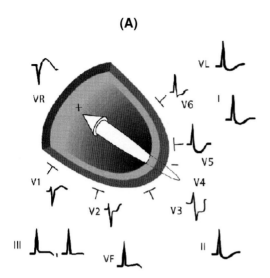

(B)

Figure 4.9 (A) In case of diffuse subendocardial circumferential injury due to incomplete occlusion of left main trunk (LMT) in a heart with previous important subendocardial ischaemia, the injury vector that points circumferential subendocardial area is directed from the apex towards the base, from forward to backwards and from left to right. This explains the typical morphology of

ST-segment depression in all the leads except VR and V1, with maximal ST-segment depression in V3–V5. As the injury vector faces more VR than V1 the ST-segment elevation in VR > V1. (B) Typical ECG of LMT critical subocclusion. The ST-segment depression is higher than 6 mm in V3–V5 and there is not evident final positive T wave in V4–V5.

second part of repolarisation – T wave – and for that the negative T wave is usually preceded by the evident existence of ST segment. When the ischaemia is clinically very important, as in the course of some STE-ACS, electrocardiographic changes in the final portion of the QRS complex, as a decrease in the S-wave voltage in case of rS morphology, may be seen (Figure 8.7). On the other hand, during an exercise test that is expressed by an ST-segment depression if there is an S wave, this wave may increase.

There is an equivalent to the ST-segment elevation pattern, the negative ST-segment depression in V1–V4 as a mirror image, greater than small ST-segment elevation in inferior/lateral leads. This pattern and some atypical patterns of STE-ACS as tall T wave in hyperacute phase of STE-ACS, and deep negative T wave in V1–V4–V5 as a sign of reperfused STE-ACS, will be discusses in detail in the second part of this book (p. 212) (Table 8.1) (Figure 8.3).
(c) Reciprocal patterns (ST-segment elevation and depression): In the course of an STE-ACS, an ST-segment depression is frequently recorded in opposing leads. This allows to understand which coronary artery is occluded but also to know the site of occlusion and the anatomical characteristics of the

artery. Figures 4.10–4.12 show that ST-segment deviations in reciprocal leads allow one to know
–whether the occlusion located in the LAD is proximal or distal to the first diagonal branch (Figure 4.10);
–whether the occlusion is located in the RCA or in the circumflex (LCX) (Figure 4.11);
–whether the occlusion is proximal or distal to the first septal branch (S1) (Figure 4.12) (see section 'Location criteria: from the occluded artery to the ECG and vice versa') (p. 66).

In theory the presence of subendocardial or transmural injury in completely opposite areas of the heart may decrease or even conceal the two injury vectors (Madias, 2006). However, in practice, this does not occur usually, because the ischaemia is usually due to occlusion of only one vessel and this does not generate equal and opposed injured areas (Rautaharju, 2006). Furthermore, with the same amount of injury in two opposite areas, it is more visible in the surface ECG of the injury area that is more close to subepicardium. In the chronic phase it is more often seen that a new vector of infarction in opposed area may cancel the Q-wave pattern of a previous infarction (see Figure 5.38).

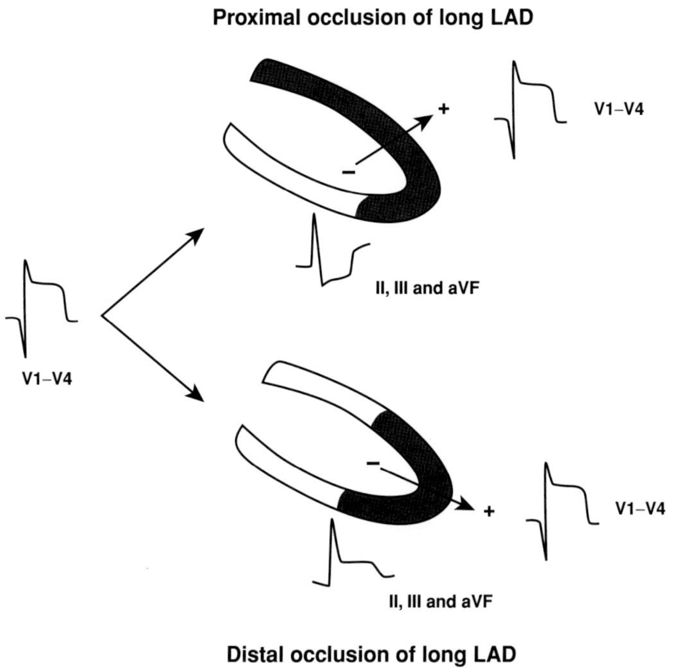

Proximal occlusion of long LAD

Distal occlusion of long LAD

Figure 4.10 In an acute coronary syndrome with ST-segment elevation in V1–V2 to V4–V6 as the most striking pattern, the occluded artery is the left anterior descending coronary artery (LAD). The correlation of the ST-segment elevation in V1–V2 to V4–V5 with the ST morphology in II, III and VF allows us to know if it is an occlusion proximal or distal to D1 (see Figure 4.43). If it is proximal, the involved muscular mass in the anterior wall is large and the injury vector is directed not only forward but also upward, even though there can be a certain inferior wall compromise because of long LAD. This explains the negativity recorded in II, III and VF. On the contrary, when the involved myocardial mass in the anterior wall is smaller, because the occlusion is distal to D1, if the LAD is long, as usually occurs, the injury vector in this U-shaped infarction (inferoanterior) is of course directed forward, but often somewhat downwards instead of upwards, and so it generally produces a slight ST-segment elevation in II, III and VF.

Electrocardiographic pattern of subepicardial injury in patients with narrow QRS: diagnosis and differential diagnosis

The ECG pattern of ST-segment elevation (subepicardial injury) is found in IHD, but also in other situations as well. In the second part we will comment that the presence of clinical signs of ischaemia (precordial pain, etc.) and the presence of ST-segment elevation of the characteristics explained here (typical and atypical patterns – see Table 8.1) constitute the clinical syndrome known as ACS with ST-segment elevation (STE-ACS), which has different clinical and ECG characteristics (Tables 8.1 and 8.2) than ACS without ST-segment elevation (NSTE-ACS). However, in both clinical syndromes (STE-ACS and NSTE-ACS), there are leads with ST-segment elevation and ST depression, but we make the diagnosis of one or other syndrome depending upon the predominant pattern (see p. 62). We will now discuss the diagnostic and location criteria of typical STE-ACS. In the second part we will comment the specific characteristics of these ECG patterns in different clinical settings of IHD specially related to prognosis.

ST-segment elevation in IHD

Diagnostic criteria: morphology and voltage

The typical morphology of subepicardial injury seen in STE-ACS is an evident ST-segment elevation, generally concave with respect to the isoelectric line that is persistent for more than 30 minutes

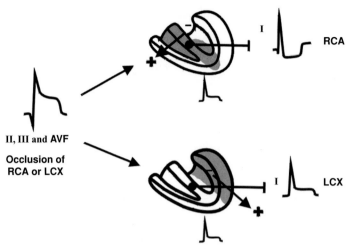

Figure 4.11 In an acute coronary syndrome with ST-segment elevation in II, III and VF as the most striking abnormality, the study of the ST-segment elevation and depression in different leads will allow us to assure if the occluded artery is RCA or LCX and even the site of the occlusion and its anatomical characteristics (dominance, etc.). This figure shows that the presence of ST-segment depression in lead I means that this lead is facing the injury vector tail that is directed to the right and, therefore, the occlusion is located in the RCA. On the contrary, when the occlusion is located in the LCX, lead I faces the injury vector head and, in this case, it is directed somewhat to the left and will be recorded as an ST-segment elevation in lead I. To check the type of ST-segment deviation in lead I is the first step of the algorithm for identification of the occluded artery (RCA or LCX) in case of ACS with ST-segment elevation predominantly in inferior leads (see Figure 4.45).

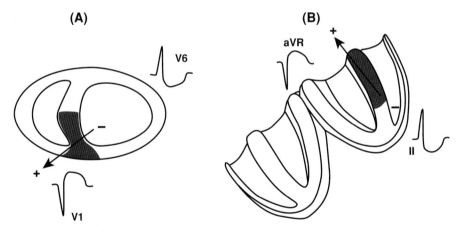

Figure 4.12 In case of high septal involvement due to LAD occlusion proximal to S1 branch, the injured area produces a vector of injury directed upwards, to the right and forwards. Vector of injury in HP (A) and FP (B). This explains the presence of ST-segment elevation in VR and V1 and ST-segment depression in II, III, VF and V6.

(Figure 4.13A). According to the Minnesota Code (Blackburn et al., 1960), **the ST-segment elevation must be of new onset, ≥1 mm in one or more of the following leads: I, II, III, VL, VF or V5–V6, or ≥2 mm in one or more of the leads V1 through V4**, to be considered diagnostic of ACS. In most of the recent clinical studies on fibrinolytic agents, an **ST-segment elevation ≥1 mm in two or more adjacent leads is required** to diagnose ACS (Cannon, 2000).

Recently, Menown, McKenzie and Adgey (2000) have demonstrated that, using the criteria of the Minnesota code, 85% of all cases are correctly

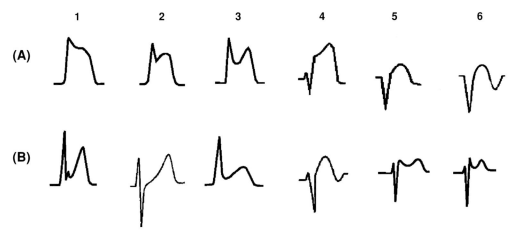

Figure 4.13 More characteristic ST-segment elevation morphologies observed in patients with ischaemic heart disease (A) and other processes (B). Type A(1) to A(6) morphologies are suggestive of acute coronary syndrome; type B: ST-segment elevation in other processes: B(1) early repolarisation; B(2) normal variant in V1; B(3) pericarditis; B(4) and B(5) Brugada's syndrome (B(4) is similar to A(6) but in the latter the QRS presents QS morphology); B(6) thoracic abnormalities (Figure 4.52C). Some patterns may be seen also in other processes. For example, the patterns B(3) and B(4) in acute coronary syndromes. Therefore, it is very important to correlate the ECG pattern with the clinical findings.

diagnosed with high specificity ($\cong$95%) and intermediate sensitivity (<60%). The specificity of ST-segment deviations (elevations and depressions) has been shown to increase when the number of leads evidencing this change increases and when the changes are dynamic or of new onset. It has also been demonstrated that even when other variables of the QRS-T are added, the diagnostic power of the ECG is not increased.

It is necessary to correlate these changes with the clinical setting of the patient. To use these criteria without clinical judgement would probably lead to overdiagnose the STE-ACS. Therefore, it is convenient to improve our ability to differentiate ischaemic than non-ischaemic ST-segment elevation pattern (Birnbaum, 2007) (see 'ST-segment elevation in other clinical settings') p. 107.

In the VCG, the final part of the ventricular depolarisation moving away from the initial part may be more or less evident, according to the grade of injury (2 with respect to 1 in Figure 4.14). Also, it is followed usually by a frequently rounded loop that is slowly recorded with homogeneous speed. The changes of ST segment detected by VCG loop have been used to monitorise ST-segment resolution in patients under fibrinolytic treatment (Dellborg et al., 1991).

The cases with transient ST-segment elevation usually correspond to a variant (Prinzmetal) angina due to coronary spasm, which is one of the atypical types of ACS (see p. 271). On the other hand, in some ACS, there are in the beginning ST shifts (ups and downs). Usually, these cases finally belong to the group of ACS without ST-segment elevation. In the hyperacute phase of an ACS, as well as in Prinzmetal angina (especially when the R wave is tall), the ST-segment elevation may be convex with respect to the isoelectric baseline (Figure 4.13A(3)). However, mild ST-segment elevation convex with respect to the isoelectric baseline is more frequently seen in normal individuals or in other situations outside IHD (early repolarisation, pericarditis, etc.) (see 'ST-segment elevation in other clinical settings'). On the other hand, it should be borne in mind that the pattern may change and therefore it is convenient to record sequential ECGs.

When the subepicardial injury occurs in the inferior and lateral wall (LCX or RCA occlusion), the direct pattern of the ST-segment elevation is seen in inferior leads and in the leads recorded in the back (posterior thoracic leads). In these cases, often an ST-segment depression is recorded in V1–V3 leads, as a 'mirror' pattern of ST-segment elevation recorded in the back (Figure 4.15).

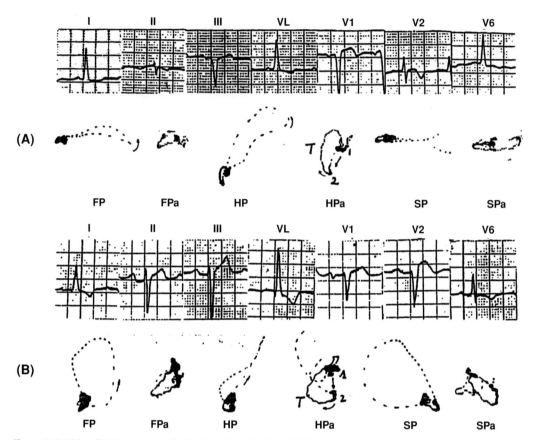

Figure 4.14 ECG and VCG in two cases (A, B) of anterior subepicardial injury. See the injury vector (arrows between 1 and 2).

Typical examples of the ST-segment elevation more frequently seen in IHD are shown in Figure 4.13A, compared to normal variants and other situations, which may present ST-segment elevation, such as pericarditis Figure 4.13B. Figures 3.18 and 3.19 show the typical sequential changes of STE-ACS evolving to Q-wave MI (see 'Evolving ECG patterns in STE-ACS') p. 216.

Location criteria: from the occluded artery to the ECG and vice versa

In the classical ECG assessment of an STE-ACS, the leads with electrocardiographic changes give to us an approximate diagnosis of the location of the injury (anteroseptal vs inferolateral zone). However not much information was given regarding what the occluded artery was, where the occlusion was located and how large the area at risk was. Therefore, for example, the classical interpretation of

the ECG recording shown in Figure 4.16 would be STE-ACS due to LAD occlusion involving the anteroseptal zone, but without making any mention about the location of occlusion and the exact area at risk. On the other hand, the ECG in Figure 4.17 could correspond, according the classical interpretation, to an STE-ACS that affected the inferior and posterior wall but without making any mention about the culprit artery (RCA vs LCX) and the location of occlusion. However, in the first case with the current knowledge, we may locate the place of occlusion between the first septal (S1) and the first diagonal (D1) (ST-segment elevation in V2–V5 with ST-segment depression in II, III and VF and without ST-segment elevation in VR and V1 and/or ST-segment depression in V6). Therefore we may know very approximately the myocardial area at risk (inferior and lateral walls) (see p. 72, and Figures 4.20 and 4.21).

ACS: diagnostic criteria and morphological characteristics of ST-segment elevation in patients with a narrow QRS complex (measured at 60 ms from the J point)*:

- ↑ST ≥ 1 mm in two or more leads from V4 to V6, I, AVL, II, III and AVF.
- ↑ST ≥ 2 mm in two or more adjacent leads from V1 to V3 in the absence of LVE with evident systolic overload. In this situation a false pattern of ST-segment elevation as a mirror image of V6 may be recorded (see Figure 7.4).
- It should be either of new onset or dynamic.
- The ST-segment elevation of ischaemic origin is more often concave in respect to the isoelectric line. However it may also present convex morphology with respect to isoelectric line (see Figures 4.13 and 8.44).

- There are normal variants and many others clinical situations without ischaemia that present ST-segment elevation even evident (see 'ST-segment elevation in other clinical settings') (p. 107). The differential diagnosis is usually easy when the elevation is evident but may be difficult when it is small (see 'ST-segment elevation in other clinical settings'). (p. 107)

* We have demonstrated that these were not significant differences in the measurements performed of 20, 40 and 60 milliseconds from the J point.

In the second case we now know that this ECG corresponds to an occlusion of very dominant RCA after RV marginal branches (ST-segment elevation in III > II, ST-segment depression in I, and V1–V3 and ST-segment elevation in V6 ≥ 2 mm) (see p. 89, and Figures 4.35 and 4.36).

We will comment on the following pages about how we may obtain all this information through the adequate and careful study of the correlations between the coronary angiography and the deviations of ST and their projection in the positive and negative hemifields of different leads. All this information will permit us to better know what the area at risk due to the occluded artery is and will help to decide on the need for and even the urgency of performing a primary PCI (Bayés de Luna, Fiol and Antman, 2006; Fiol et al., 2004b; Gallik et al., 1995; Gorgels and Engelen, 2003; Sclarovsky, 1999). We will focus on the ACS of patients with ischaemia due to only one critical artery occlusion, although it may exists in other arteries in other non-critical lesions. Later on (see 'ST-segment changes in patients with active ischaemia due to multivessel disease') we will comment on the ST-segment deviations in patients with ischaemia due to critical multiple-vessel occlusion.

Now we will discuss two different aspects of these correlations: (1) **how to know the area at risk and the corresponding ECG based on the location of the occluded artery, and 2) performing the oppo-**

site exercise about how to know the area at risk and the occlusion site based on the ECG findings. In one previous publication (Bayés de Luna, Fiol and Antman, 2006) we commented all the aspects that we are explaining now in the following pages The clinicians receiving the patient with chest pain in the emergency department should obviously carry out this second exercise at a first glance for diagnosing and taking the best decision to salvage as much as possible the myocardial muscle, because the ECG changes appear much earlier than enzymes elevation.

STE-ACS: from the occluded artery to the area at risk and the corresponding electrocardiographic abnormality. (see Table 4.1; Bayés de Luna, Fiol and Antman, 2006)

The **correlation between the occluded artery and the electrocardiographic signs** that develop during the acute phase has been possible due to revascularisation-therapy-related coronary angiograms. The deviations in the ST segment that are seen in leads other than those used for the diagnosis of the STE-ACS (precordial leads for the LAD occlusion and inferior leads for the LCX or RCA occlusion) are useful for (a) better identifying the anatomical characteristics of the LAD occlusion, in case that the ST-segment elevation is more striking in the precordial leads, and (b) determining which the occluded artery is (RCA or LCX) in case

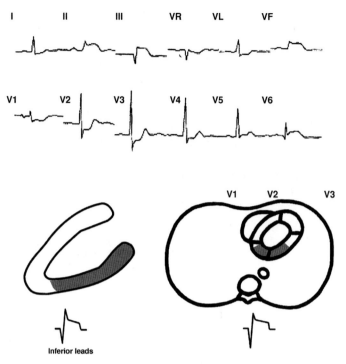

Figure 4.15 Subacute phase of inferolateral infarction. The ECG shows Q in II, III, VF, RS in V1 and tall R wave in V2, with ST-segment depression in V1–V3 and ST-segment elevation in II, III and VF. The inferolateral subepicardial injury vector is directed towards the injured zone (downwards and backwards) and therefore produces ST-segment depression in V1–V3, as well as ST-segment elevation in II, III and VF. The presence of ST-segment depression in lead I, ST-segment elevation in III > II and the lateral involvement (ST-segment elevation in V6) is due to non-proximal occlusion (ST-segment depression in V1–V3) of a very dominant (ST-segment elevation in V6) right coronary artery. The local vector of lateral injury (see Figure 4.35) explains the ST-segment elevation in V6.

the most striking ST-segment elevation is recorded in II, III and/or VF.

All that which is of great interest for the best therapeutic decision (e.g. an urgent PCI) is based on the concept that the injury vector is approaching the injured area and generates an ST-segment elevation in the leads facing the vector head and an ST-segment depression in the leads facing the vector tail (opposed leads) (Figures 4.10–4.12). Therefore, **the injury vector direction** is conditioned by the myocardial area at risk, which will be different according to the occluded artery and the site of the occlusion.

Thus, based on the leads showing ST-segment changes, including reciprocal changes, it is possible to know (a) the **involved artery and the occlusion site**, and (b)**the myocardial area at risk** (area with acute infarction or at risk of infarction). This area and the risk for infarction in the absence of successful reperfusion therapy could be quantified by determining the number of leads with ST-segment elevation (Aldrich et al., 1988) (see p. 224) (Table 4.1). In Figure 1.14 the segments of the LV perfused by the LAD, RCA and LCX that may be compromised in case of their occlusion at different levels are shown in a 'bull's-eye' pattern and in Figures 1.8 and 1.9, the same segments in different perspectives. In **STE-ACS** such ST-segment patterns will be used to show the correlation: LAD, RCA or LCX occlusion at different levels with involved myocardial area.

In the presence of an STE-ACS, the coronary angiography – area at risk – and the surface ECG correlation presents high specificity and acceptable sensibility. The cases with lower correlation

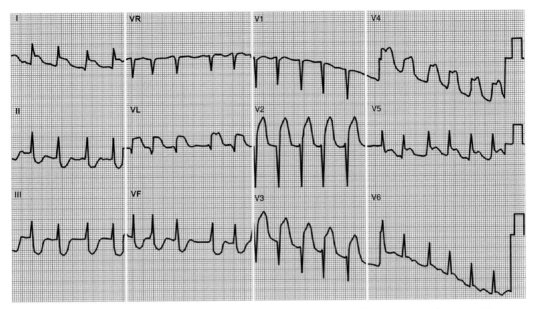

Figure 4.16 Acute myocardial infarction in a patient with rapid atrial fibrillation. The ECG shows ST-segment elevation in V2–V5, I and VL. Leads II, III, and VF present an evident ST-segment depression as a mirror pattern of ST-segment elevation in precordial leads. This is a pattern of acute coronary syndrome with ST-segment elevation of the anterior wall according to the classical classification. Nowadays, we would say that it corresponds to STE-ACS due to LAD occlusion proximal to D1, but distal to S1. The absence of evident ST-segment elevation in VR and V1 and of ST-segment depression in V6 and the ST-segment depression in III > II (see Figure 4.21) are in favour of this location.

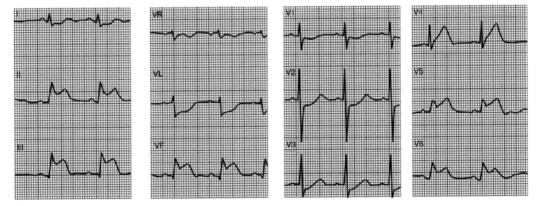

Figure 4.17 Acute myocardial infarction with ST-segment elevation in II, III and VF and ST-segment depression in V1–V3. This pattern corresponds classically to an infarction involving inferior and posterior walls. Nowadays, this is the pattern of STE-ACS of inferolateral zone evolving to inferolateral infarction due to distal occlusion of a dominant RCA (ST-segment depression in I and V1–V3, ST-segment elevation in III > II with ST-segment elevation in V6), without the right ventricle involvement (slight, but evident ST-segment depression in V1–V3). Therefore, the presence of ST-segment elevation in III > II and ST-segment depression in lead I instead of elevation assure that RCA and not LCX is the occluded artery.

Table 4.1 STE-ACS. From the altered ECG (ST-segment elevation and reciprocal changes) to the injured myocardial area and the occluded artery.

A Most prominent pattern of ST elevation in precordial leads and VL* Anteroseptal zone			B Most prominent pattern of ST elevation in inferior wall and/or lateral leads† Inferolateral zone		
Occluded artery	**Injured myocardial area** (see Figure 1.8)	**Leads with ST changes**	**Occluded artery RCA vs LCX**	**Injured myocardial area** (see Figure 1.8)	**Leads with ST changes**
1. LAD occlusion proximal to D1 and S1	Extensive anteroseptal zone (especially 1, 2, 3, 7, 8, 9 13,14, 16 and 17 segments)	• ↑ V1 to V4–V5 and aVR • ↓ ST in II, III, aAVF and sometimes V5–V6	7. RCA occlusion proximal to the RV branches	Same as type 8 plus injury of RV	• ↑ II, III and aVF with III > II • ↓ S in I and aVL • ↑ V4R with T+ • ST isoelectric or elevated in V1
2. LAD occlusion proximal to D I but distal to S I	Antero-septal or extensive anterior (especially 1,7, 8, 13,14, 16 and 17 segments)	• ↑ V2 to V5–V6, I, VL • ↓ ST in II, III and aVF	8. RCA occlusion distal to the RV branches	Inferior wall and/or the posterior part of the *septum* (especially 3,4,9,10, 14 and 15 segments)	• ↑ II, III and aVF with III > II • ↓ in I and aVL • ↓ ST in V1–V3 but if affected zone is very small, almost no ↓ ST in V1–V2
3. LAD occlusion distal to DI and SI	Apical (especially 13,14, 15, 16,17 and part of 7 and 8 segments)	• ↑ V2 to V4–V5 • ST ↑ or = in II, III and aVF If LAD is short, less evident changes	9. Very dominant RCA occlusion	Great part of inferolateral zone (especially 3,4,5,9,10,11, 14, 15, 16 and 17 segments) injury of RV if is proximally occluded	• ↑ ST in II, III, aVF (III > II) • ↓ ST in V1–V3 < ST in II, III and aVF. If the RCA is proximally occluded, ST in V1–V3 = or ↑ • ↓ ST in I and aVL – VL > V1 • ↑ ST in V5–V6 ≥ 2 mm
4. LAD occlusion proximal to SI but distal to DI	Anteroseptal (especially 2, 8, 13, 14, 15, 16 and 17 segments)	• ↑ V1 to V4–V5 and aVR • ST ↑ or = in II, III and aAVR • ↓ ST in V6	10. LCX occlusion proximal to first obtuse marginal (OM) branch	Lateral wall and inferior wall, especially the inferobasal segment (especially 4,5,6,10, 11,12 and part of 16 segments)	• ↓ ST in V1–V3 (mirror image) often greater than ↑ ST in inferior leads • ↑ ST in II, III and aVF (II > III) • Sometimes, ↑ ST in V5–V6 • ↑ ST in I and VL

(Continued)

Table 4.1 (*Cont.*)

	A			B	
	Most prominent pattern of			*Most prominent pattern of*	
	ST elevation in precordial leads and VL*			*ST elevation in inferior wall and/or lateral leads†*	
	Anteroseptal zone			*Inferolateral zone*	
5. LAD subocclusion including D1 but not S1, or selective D1 occlusion	Mid-anterior (especially 7,13,12 and part of 1 and 16 segments)	• ↑ I, aVL, and sometimes V2 to V5–6 • ↓ II, III and aAVF (III > II)	11. First OM occlusion	Part of lateral wall (especially 5, 6, 11, 12 and 16 segments).	• Often ↑ ST I, VL, V5–V6 and/or in II, III and aVF usually slight. • Often slight ↓ ST in V1–V3
6. LAD subocclusion including S1 but not D1, or selective S1 occlusion	Septal (especially 2, 8 and sometimes part of 1, 3, 9 and 14 segments)	• ↑ V1–V2 and aVR • ↓ I, II, III, aVF and V6	12. Very dominant LCX occlusion	Great part of inferolateral zone (especially 3,4,5,6,9,10,11, 12,15 and 16 segments)	• ↑ ST in II, III and aVF (II ≥ III) often greater than ST ↓ in V1–V3. • The ST may be ↓ in aVL but usually not in I. • ST elevation in V5–V6 sometimes very evident

LAD, left anterior descending; RV, right ventricle; LCX, circumflex artery; RCA, right coronary artery; LV, left ventricle.
* See algorithm in Figure 4.43.
† See algorithm Figure 4.45.

present coronary anomalies, confounding factors as ventricular enlargement or coronary occlusion in LCX (OM) (Figure 4.40). However, the cases with wide QRS and LVH with strain pattern are not included here and will be discussed later (see 'ECG pattern of injury in patients with ventricular hypertrophy and/or wide QRS'). Other limitation of this approach is the transient nature of some ST-segment deviations. Sometimes the ST-segment changes that are important for the diagnosis (e.g. the elevation of ST in V4R lead in case of occlusion of the proximal RCA) do not last long. On other occasions, on the contrary, as occurs in V1–V2 in cases with a proximal occlusion of the LAD, there is quite a long delay until the ST-segment changes appear or, at times, they do not even appear if the ACS is aborted. Therefore, just one ECG recording is sometimes not enough to arrive at the presumptive diagnosis.

These correlations in the most frequent STE-ACS due to the occlusion of a coronary artery at different levels **will be discussed as follows**: in each case, the schematic representation with the occlu-sion site, the involved myocardial segments and the spatial location of the injury vector are shown. **The correlation of the injury vector with the positive and negative hemifields of the different leads explains the ST-segment elevations or depressions that are seen in different situations** (Table 4.1).

The correlations that will be presented are based on the segmentation of the LV into two zones: the anteroseptal and the inferolateral (Figure 1.14 and p. 17). The **involvement of the anteroseptal zone** corresponds to cases with occlusion of the LAD **and its branches (Table 4.1A), while the involvement of the inferolateral zone corresponds to the occlusion of the RCA and the LCX** (Table 4.1B). We will study 12 different locations of coronary occlusions that define 12 areas at risk, 6 in the anteroseptal zone (Table 4.1A) and 6 in the inferolateral zone (Table 4.1B). The ECG patterns that match with these different areas will be commented and discussed in all cases.

(a) **Anteroseptal zone: occlusion of the LAD and its branches** (Table 4.1A(1–6); Arbane and Goy, 2000; Fiol et al., 2007; Martinez-Doltz et al.,

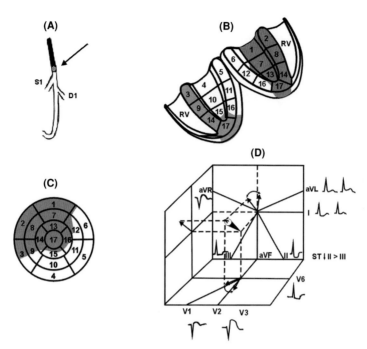

Figure 4.18 STE-ACS due to LAD occlusion proximal to D1 and S1. (A) Site of occlusion; (B) myocardial area at risk; (C) involved segments are marked in gray in 'bull's-eye' projection; (D) vector of injury and its projection in three planes: frontal, horizontal and sagittal. The injury vector is directed somewhat to the right because the occlusion is proximal not only to D1 but also to S1.

2002; Prieto et al., 2002; Sclarovsky, 1999; Wellens, Gorgels and Doevendans, 2003).

The LAD perfuses the anterior wall and the anterior portion of the septum and great part of the inferior part of the septum and portion of the mid-low anterior part of the lateral wall (see p. 17). If, as frequently occurs (≈80%), it is a long artery that wraps the apex and perfuses part of the inferior wall (Figures 1.2 and 1.14), the first diagonal branch (D1) and the first septal branch (S1) take off from the proximal portion of the LAD. Generally, the first diagonal branch (D1) is located below the first septal branch (S1). It is the opposite in almost 10% of the cases.

The LAD occlusion may be located (a) above the first diagonal (D1) and the first septal (S1) branches, (b) proximal to D1 but not to S1 branches, (c) distal to both the S1 and D1 branches, (d) proximal to S1 but not to D1 branch, (e) LAD occlusion encompassing the diagonal branches but not the septal branches or just a selective D1–D2 occlusion and (f) LAD occlusion encompassing the septal branches but not the diagonal branches or rarely a selective S1–S2 occlusion.

All these cases will be commented on, considering the correlation between the ST-segment elevations and depressions in the acute phase with the myocardial area at risk. In Part II of the book (see 'ST-segment elevation on admission' p. 221), we will comment about all the parameters that are markers of prognosis. These include the study of ST-segment deviations that we will now explain in detail and other factors as the summation of ST-segment deviations and the ST-segment morphology as a predictor of the grade of ischaemia.

1. **Occlusion proximal to D1 and S1 branches*** (Figures 4.18 and 4.19, and Table 4.1A(1)): When the occlusion is located above the D1 and S1

---

*From the practical point of view, this has to be considered above the first big diagonal and septal branches. Sometimes these are the second septal or diagonal, because often the anatomically first diagonal and especially the first septal are very short.

(A)

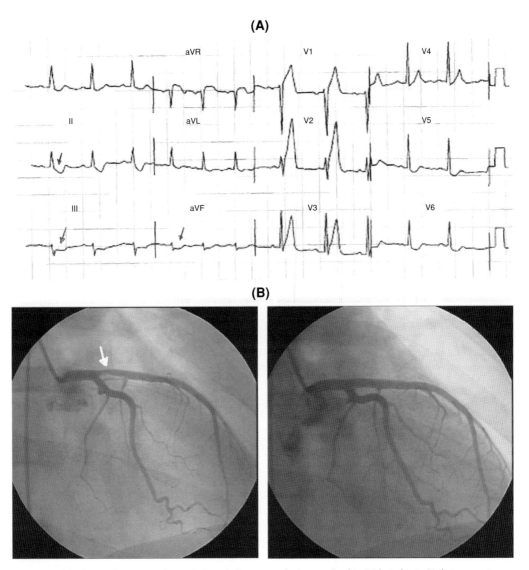

(B)

Figure 4.19 (A) The ECG in STE-ACS due to LAD occlusion proximal to D1 and S1 in a hyperacute phase. An evident ST-segment elevation from V1–V3 and VR is recorded. Also ST-segment depression in II, III, VF (more evident in II) and in V5–V6 is present. This may be explained by LAD occlusion proximal to D1 but also to S1 that generates a injury vector directed upwards, to the right and forwards. (B) Coronary angiography before (left) and after (right) reperfusion therapy. The arrow indicates the place of occlusion.

branches (Figure 4.18A), **the area at risk** is large and without treatment could lead to an extensive anterior infarction. However, with the initiation of an urgent therapy, its size could be greatly limited, and the infarction not so extensive. The area affected by the occlusion may be seen in Figure 4.18B, and its projection onto a polar map is shown in Figure 4.18C. The more affected segments are 1, 2, 7, 8, 13, 14 and 17, and part of segments 12, 16, 3, 9 and 15.

In this case, the **vector of injury** is directed anteriorly and upwards, and somewhat to the right or the left, depending on whether septal, the most frequent, or lateral involvement predominates (Figure 4.18D). The projection of this vector in the positive and negative hemifields of different leads explains the ST-segment elevation from V1 to V4 and in VR (Ben-Gal et al., 1998). When the involvement of anterolateral area is predominant, the ST-segment elevation is also seen in VL because the vector of injury falls in the positive hemifield of VL (around −90°). The larger the ST-segment elevation in VL (anterolateral involvement), the lesser the changes in VR (anteroseptal involvement) and vice versa.

An ST-segment depression occurs in the inferior leads because the injury vector is directed upwards. Usually, it is more evident in II than in III since lead II is more opposed to VR (anteroseptal compromise is usually predominant over the anterolateral compromise) and therefore the injury vector fails more in the negative hemifield of lead II. Generally, there is ST-segment depression in V5–V6 also because the anteroseptal compromise is usually predominant over the anterolateral compromise and the injury vector is directed somewhat to the right and upwards (Tamura et al., 1995a, b) (Figures 4.18D and 4.19). In our experience (Fiol et al., 2007), ST-segment depression in the inferior wall (III plus VF ≥ 2.5 mm) is quite suggestive of a proximal occlusion of LAD above D1, while ST-segment depression in V6 with ST-segment elevation in VR, and/or V1 is quite specific of the occlusion above the S1 branch (Σ of ST deviations in VR + V1−V6 ≥ 0, see Figure 4.43 in the lower right side). Different authors (Birnbaum et al., 1996b) have considered that ST-segment elevation in VL ≥ 1 mm is a good sign to diagnose occlusion before D1. However, in our experience, the ST-segment depression in III + VF ≥ 2.5 mm presents a higher specificity.

However the presence of ST-segment elevation in V5–V6 also depends on the relative importance of the arteries perfusing the low-lateral wall, second-third diagonal versus obtuse marginal. In case of great diagonal branches the occlusion will encompass the low-lateral wall and ST-segment elevation in V5–V6 may be seen. On the contrary, in case of very dominant obtuse marginal branch, LAD occlusion proximal to D1 and S1 will present usually only ST-segment elevation in V1–V4 because the low-lateral wall is perfused by obtuse marginal (Figure 4.19). Also it has been demonstrated (Ben-Gal et al., 1998) that the lack of ST-segment elevation in V1 in some cases

of high septal involvement (occlusion above S1) may be explained by the fact that the superoseptal portion is perfused specially not only by LAD but also by the RCA (double perfusion). Therefore the anatomy of coronary branches has a great influence in the explanation of ST-segment deviations.

A typical electrocardiographic example of this type of STE-ACS is shown in Figure 4.19A, along with its correlation with the coronary angiogram (Figure 4.19B) before and after fibrinolytic therapy. There is a great obtuse marginal that perfuses the low-lateral wall and may at least partially explain that ST-segment elevation is only seen in V1–V3 (see above).

2. Occlusion proximal to D1 branch, but distal to the S1 branch (Figures 4.20 and 4.21, and Table 4.1A(2)): When the occlusion is above the D1 but not S1 branch (Figure 4.20A), **the area at risk** could also lead to an anterior wall infarction, with extension to mid-low part of septal and lateral anterior wall (due to the proximal occlusion above the D1 branch). Remember that the upper anterior part of lateral wall is perfused by the LCX. When the S1 branch is small, the area of the septal wall involved will be larger. Without the initiation of urgent and appropriate therapy, the necrosis of the septal wall could be large (all the septal branches distal to S1) and consequently could lead to an extensive infarction (Figure 4.20B). The area involved by the occlusion and its projection onto a polar map is shown in Figure 4.20C. The more affected segments are 1, 7, 8, 13, 14, 16 and 17, but also part of segment 12, and sometimes part of segments 2, 8, 15 and 16.

In this case, the **injury vector** is directed anteriorly, upwards and somewhat to the left (Figure 4.20D). The projection of the injury vector in different positive and negative hemifields of different leads of FP and HP explains the ST-segment elevation from V2–V3 to V5–V6. However it does not usually explain the ST-segment elevation in V1 because the projection of this vector in the HP falls often a little to the left in the limit of negative hemifield of V1 or close to it. Also, these correlations explain the ST-segment elevation in lead I, especially in VL, and the ST-segment depression in the inferior leads (III + VF ≥ 2.5 mm)

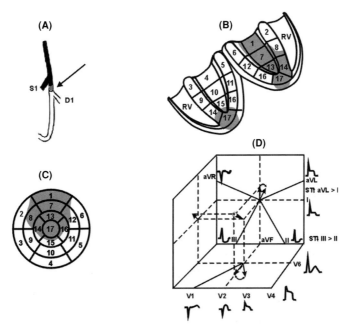

Figure 4.20 STE-ACS due to LAD occlusion proximal to D1 but distal to S1. (A) Site of occlusion; (B) myocardial area at risk; (C) 'bull's-eye' polar map with involved segments. Very often, the apex is involved because the LAD is frequently long. (D) Injury vector in the acute phase is directed somewhat to the left, as the high part of septum is not involved.

(Figures 4.20 and 4.21). Usually, more ST-segment depression is seen in III than in II, since lead III is opposed to VL, and therefore the injury vector falls more in the negative hemifield of III and more directly this lead faces the injury vector tail (Figure 4.21).

A typical example of this type of STE-ACS is shown in Figure 4.21A, along with its correlation with the coronary angiogram (Figure 4.21B) before and after fibrinolytic therapy.

3. **Occlusion distal to S1 and D1 branches** (Figures 4.22–4.24, and Table 4.1A(3)): When the occlusion is located below the S1 and D1 (Figure 4.22A), **the area at risk** involves the inferior third of the left ventricular, with almost invariably some inferior involvement and only low-lateral involvement (apical involvement). In Figure 4.22B the area affected can be observed, and in Figure 4.22C a polar map of that area is shown. The more affected segments are 13, 14, 15, 16 and 17, and sometimes part of segments 7, 8, 9, 12 and 16.

In this case, **the injury vector** is also directed anteriorly and often rather to the left and usu-ally downwards, because the injury vector is directed to the apex which presents a downward and leftward position in the thorax. When the LAD is long, as occurs in 90% of cases, it perfuses a portion of the inferior wall, and then the vector of injury is clearly directed downwards (Figure 4.22D). The projection of this vector in the FP and HP explains the ST-segment elevation from V2–V3 to V4–V6 but not in V1 and/or VR because usually the vector of injury falls in the limit of positive and negative hemifield of V1 and clearly in the negative hemifield of VR. Due to downward and leftward direction of this vector, there is usually slightly ST-segment elevation in II, III and VF (II > III). When the LAD is short, the infarction distal to S1 and D1 is small, and no changes are typically seen in the FP, or if they occur, they consist of just a slight ST-segment elevation or depression.

A typical electrocardiographic examples of this STE-ACS are shown in Figures 4.23A and Figure 4.24A, with its coronariographic correlation before and after fibrinolytic therapy (Figure 4.23B and 4.24B.

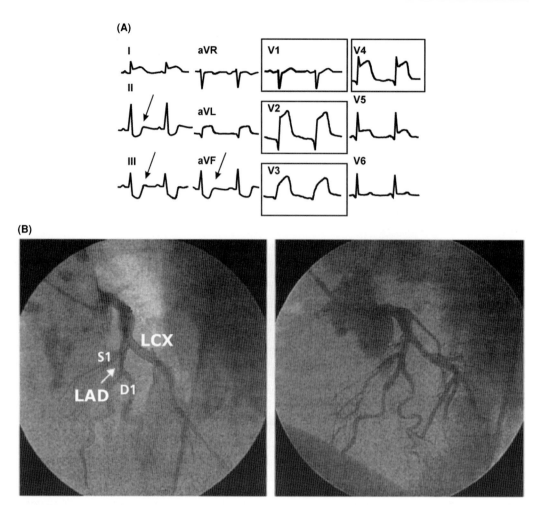

Figure 4.21 (A) The ECG in STE-ACS due to LAD occlusion, proximal to D1, but distal to S1. Observe the ST-segment elevation from V2 to V5, with ST-segment depression in II, III, and VF more evident usually in III than II due to the direction of injury vector. There is neither ST-segment elevation in V1 and VR nor ST-segment depression in V6. (B) Coronary angiography before (left) and after (right) reperfusion therapy. The arrow indicates the place of occlusion.

Also, the ST-segment elevation is seen in the precordial and inferior leads in the presence of an STE-ACS due to the very proximal occlusion of the RCA before the RV marginal branches. In this case usually the ST-segment elevation in V1 > V3–V4, while in an STE-ACS due to the distal occlusion of the LAD, the contrary occurs (i.e. the ST-segment elevation is V1 < V3). Table 4.2 shows the ECG criteria that allow differentiating the culprit artery (proximal RCA or distal LAD) in the case of ST-segment elevation in precordial leads and inferior leads.

4. Occlusion proximal to the S1 branch but distal the D1 branch (Figure 4.25 and Table 4.1A(4)): When the occlusion is located above, the S1 but not the D1 (Figure 4.25), which rarely occurs (<15% of the STE-ACS), the **area at risk** could lead to a relatively extensive anterior infarction when the D1 branch is quite small and the D2 branch is large. However, usually more septal and anterior than lateral involvement is seen (Figure 4.25B,C). Currently, with the new treatments employed in the acute phase, most of these cases end up being just an apical infarction

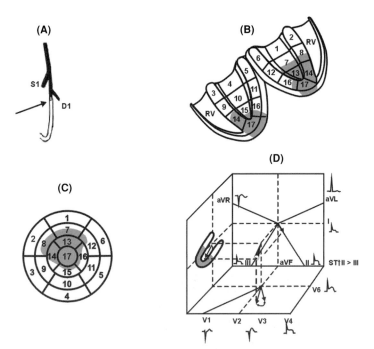

Figure 4.22 STE-ACS due to occlusion of long LAD, distal to D1 and S1. (A) Site of occlusion; (B) myocardial area at risk; (C) involved segments in 'bull's-eye' projection; (D) injury vector directed forward but somewhat downwards and to the left, resulting in ST-segment elevations in frontal and horizontal plane leads (V2–V6) and with ST-segment elevation in II > III.

or even a septal infarction if the distal occlusion disappears and only remains the involvement of septal branches. The area more usually involved by the occlusion may be seen in Figure 4.25B, and its projection onto a polar map is shown in Figure 4.25C. The more affected segments are 2, 8, 13, 14, 16 and 17, and generally part of segments 3, 7, 9 and 15. Usually, segment 1 and great part of segment 7 are spared because they are protected by the occlusion of the LAD distal to D1.

The **injury vector** is directed anteriorly and to the right because the injury vector faces the anteroseptal area and often downwards (occlusion distal to D1), especially if the LAD is long and wraps the apex, affecting part of the inferior wall. Then, if the anterior wall is not greatly affected because the occlusion occurs below a big D1, the involvement of the inferior wall can turn out to be more important than the involvement of the anterior wall. The projection of this injury vector in the positive and negative hemifields of different leads of FP and HP explains the ST-segment elevation from V1 to V4 and

that the elevated or isoelectric ST segment in the inferior leads is more evident in III than in II. An ST-segment depression is seen in V5–V6 and VL and often an ST-segment elevation in VR because the occlusion is proximal to S1 (Figure 4.25D).

A typical electrocardiographic example of this STE-ACS is shown in Figure 4.25.

5. **LAD incomplete occlusion involving the diagonal branches, but not the septal branches, or selective occlusion of the first diagonal branch (D1)** (Figures 4.26–4.28, and Table 4.1A(5)) (Birnbaum et al., 1996a): In this case (Figure 4.26A) **the area at risk** usually involves the mid-anterior wall and part of the mid-low-lateral wall, but not the basal portion of lateral wall that is perfused by LCX. In Figure 4.26B,C the involved myocardial area and the polar map of that area are shown. The more affected segments are 7 and 13 and, generally, part of segments 12 and 16.

The **injury vector** is directed upwards, leftwards and forwards (Figure 4.26D). According

(A)

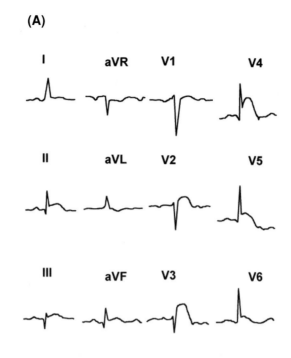

(B)

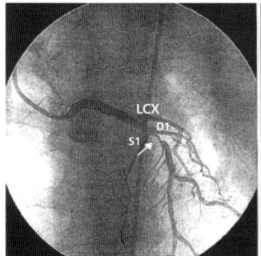

Figure 4.23 (A) The ECG in STE-ACS due to LAD occlusion distal to D1 and S1. Observe the ST-segment elevation from V2 to V5–V6 with somewhat ST-segment elevation in II, III, VF (II > III). (B) Coronary angiography before (left) and after (right) reperfusion therapy. The arrow indicates the place of occlusion.

to the correlations, injury vector – projection in positive and negative hemifields of different leads – explains the ST-segment elevation in I and VL and, sometimes, in the precordial leads, especially from V2–V3 to V5–V6, and the ST-segment depression in II, III and VF (III > II). The presence of slight ST-segment depression in V2–V3 may be seen in some cases of multiple-vessel occlusion (D1 + LCX especially). Classically, it was considered that VL lead faces the high-lateral wall. However, the presence of ST-segment elevation in VL is explained by the involvement of

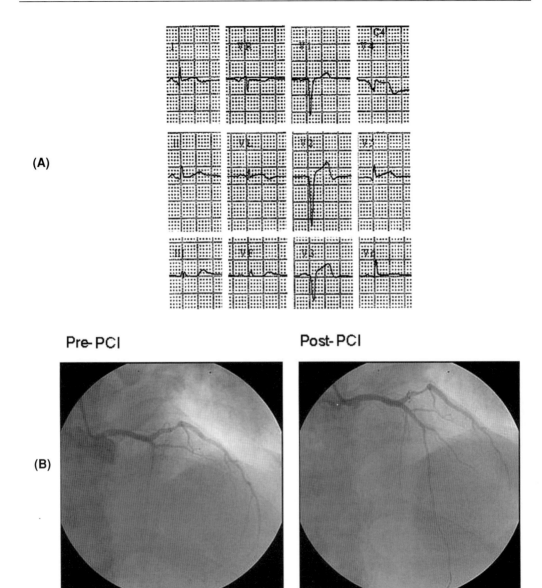

(A)

(B)

Pre- PCI

Post- PCI

Figure 4.24 (A) STE-ACS in subacute phase with evident ST-segment elevation in V2–V4 with isoelectric ST segment in inferior leads and ST-segment depression in VR with ST isoelectric in V1 and V6. All these ST-segment deviations favour LAD occlusion distal to S1 and D1 (see p. XX). (B) The coronary angiography confirms the distal LAD occlusion.

mid-anterior and mid-lateral wall perfused by D1 and not by the high-lateral-wall involvement that is perfused by LCX. In case of occlusion of first obtuse marginal branch the injury vector is often directed slightly downwards and in some cases if the injury vector points more downwards, the ST may be flat or even depressed in VL but not in I (located between +60° and +90°) (Figure 4.40) (p. 95).

An electrocardiographic example of this type of STE-ACS with QS in VL in the chronic phase is shown in Figures 4.27 and 4.28. The QS morphology in VL without Q in V5–V6 is due to mid-anterior-wall infarction and not to high-lateral infarction (see p. 139).

6. **LAD incomplete occlusion involving the septal branches but not the diagonal branches or, more rarely, selective occlusion of the**

Table 4.2 The ST segment elevation in precordial leads (especially V1- V3-V4)* and inferior leads (II, III and VF).

Leads	RCA (Proximal RCA)	LAD (Distal occlusion of long LAD *or* distal occlusion of the LAD + total occlusion of the RCA with collateral vessels)
V1–V3–V4	Usually ST ↑ (V1 > V3–V4)	Usually ST ↑ (V3–V4 > V1)
Inferior leads	Usually ST ↑ greater than in precordial leads, if not (Figure 10.4) there is ST ↑in V1 that is not seen in LAD distal occlusion	ST ↑ usually smaller than in precordial leads
I and aVL	The ST segment depression (usually the sum ≥ 5 mm)	Usually non-ST-segment depression, especially in I

* In exceptional cases of proximal occlusion of very dominant RCA, the ST-segment elevation may be seen in all precordial leads, in V1 to V3–V4 due to proximal occlusion and in V5–V6 due to very dominant RCA (local injury vector) (see Figure 8.39).

S1–S2 branches (Figures 4.28 and 4.29, and Table 4.1A(6)): In this case the **area at risk** involves more or less extensively, according to the number of septal branches involved, the septal wall. Often the involvement is especially of mid-apical septal part because the LAD incomplete occlusion is distal and also with certain extension towards the anterior wall. This occlusion is rarely located in the S1 or S2 branches. In Figure 4.29B, C the involved area and the polar map are shown. The most affected segments are 2 and 8 and, sometimes, part of segments 3, 9 and 14.

The **injury vector** is directed anteriorly, upwards and to the right (Figure 4.28D) and, therefore, its projection in the positive and negative hemifields of different leads of the FP and HP explains the ST-segment elevation in V1, V2 and VR, with ST-segment depression in II, III VF (II > III) and V6, and lack of ST-segment elevation in VL.

In Figure 4.29 an example of an STE-ACS secondary to occlusion of a large S1 branch during a PCI procedure is shown (Tamura, Kataoka and Mikuriya, 1991). Figure 2.3 shows an STE-ACS that in (a) before the fibrinolytic treatment suggests LAD occlusion above D1 and S1 (ST-segment elevation from V1 to V5 and isoelectric in V6). After 20 minutes of the treatment

---

STE-ACS: the ST-segment elevation in the precordial leads

1. Occlusion of the LAD proximal to D1: ST-segment elevation in V2 to V4–V6, and frequently VL and sometimes VR. ST-segment depression is recorded in at least two inferior leads (III + VF ≥ 2.5 mm), which in general is less important than the ST-segment elevation seen in the precordial leads.

2. Occlusion of LAD distal to D1 branch: ST-segment elevation also in V2 to V4–V6. Regardless of its relation to S1, no ST-segment depression is usually seen in II, III and VF. In turn, an isoelectric or not significantly elevated ST segment is recorded.

3. Occlusion of LAD proximal to S1: Regardless of where D1 is, there is an ST-segment elevation in VR and V1 to V4–V5 and an ST-segment

depression in V6 because the injury vector is directed upwards and rightwards.

4. Occlusion of LAD located below the S1 and D1 (distal occlusion): ST-segment elevation in V2 to V4–V6. A generally slight ST-segment elevation is seen in leads II, III and VF.

5. Incomplete occlusion of LAD involving diagonal but not septal branches or selective occlusion of D1: Often ST-segment elevation in I, VL and V5–V6 and sometimes even in more precordial leads, and ST-segment depression in II, III and VF (III > II).

6. Incomplete occlusion of LAD involving septal branches but not diagonal branches: Rarely selective occlusion of S1–S2. ST-segment elevation in V1–V2 and VR, and ST-segment depression in V6 and II > III.

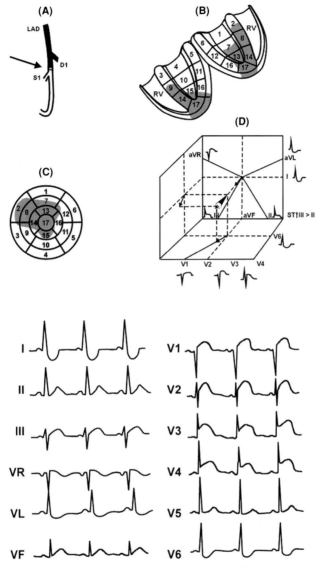

Figure 4.25 Above: (A) STE-ACS due to LAD occlusion proximal to S1 but distal to D1. (A) The site of occlusion. (B) Myocardial area at risk. (C) 'Bull's-eye' polar map with involved segments. (D) Injury vector directed to the right and forwards due to occlusion proximal to S1. In case of a long LAD involving also inferior wall, the vector can be directed somewhat downwards due to relatively small myocardial area of anterior wall involved in case of occlusion distal to D1. The occlusion distal to D1 explains the ST-segment elevation from V1 to V3–V4 and ST-segment elevation in II, III and VF (III > II) and the occlusion proximal to S1 – the ST-segment elevation in VR, and ST-segment depression in V6, I and VL due to injury vector directed somewhat to the right. Below: Typical example of ECG in ACS with LAD occlusion proximal to S1 and distal to D1. Observe ST-segment elevation in II, III and VF (III > II) due to occlusion distal to D1 and ST-segment elevation in VR and V1 with ST-segment depression in V6 due to occlusion proximal to S1.

the patient presents and ECG is suggestive of non-complete occlusion of LAD involving septal branches but not diagonal branches (ST-segment depression in V5–V6). As a matter of fact this patient finally presented an ECG pattern of huge but exclusive septal infarction, although the LAD was open with the treatment (Figure 2.3).

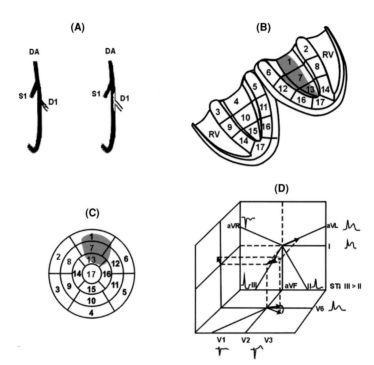

Figure 4.26 STE-ACS due to occlusion of D1 or incomplete occlusion of LAD involving D1. (A) Site of occlusion. (B) Myocardial area at risk. (C) 'Bull's-eye' polar map with involved segments. (D) Injury vector with its projection in frontal and horizontal planes and the corresponding ECG patterns.

(b) Inferolateral zone: RCA or circumflex occlusion (Table 4.1B(7–12); Bairey et al., 1987; Birnbaum et al., 1994; Fiol et al., 2004b; Herz et al., 1997; Kosuge et al., 1998; Lew et al., 1987; Tamura et al., 1995a,b): The RCA perfuses a portion of the inferior septal wall and the inferior wall, including, generally, segment 4 (inferobasal), which was classically named posterior wall, and sometimes the apex. It may also perfuses the inferior (apical) part of lateral wall if it is quite dominant. When the occlusion is proximal and compromises the right marginal branches that perfuse the RV, the infarction also affects most of that ventricle. Along its final course it divides into two branches, the posteroseptal (directed towards the inferior part of the septal wall) and the posterolateral, towards the inferior wall and, when it is quite dominant, to the inferior part of the lateral wall especially its apical part (Figures 1.1 and 1.14).

The LCX, after a certain course, curves backwards and gives rise to one or several OM branches (Figures 1.2 and 1.13). The LCX perfuses a great portion of the inferior part of the lateral wall, great portion of the anterior part especially the basal segment and sometimes part of the inferior wall, especially segment 4 (inferobasal – former posterior segment). When it is quite dominant, it also perfuses the inferior part of that wall and even a portion of the inferior part of the septal wall.

7. **RCA occlusion proximal to the RV branches** (Figures 4.30–4.32 and Table 4.1B(7)): When the RCA occlusion is proximal to the RV branches (Figure 4.30A), **the area at risk** involves the RV and part of inferolateral zone, more or less extensive according to the dominance of RCA. In Figure 4.30B, C the involved myocardial area is shown, as well as the polar map in case of balanced dominance. The more affected segments are 3, 4, 9 and 10, and part of segments 14 and 15.

The **vector of injury** in cases of infarction due to non-proximal occlusion of the RCA is directed downwards posteriorly and to the right. Due to the RV extension in case of very proximal RCA occlusion, the injury vector is directed more to the right than posteriorly (compare Figures 4.30D

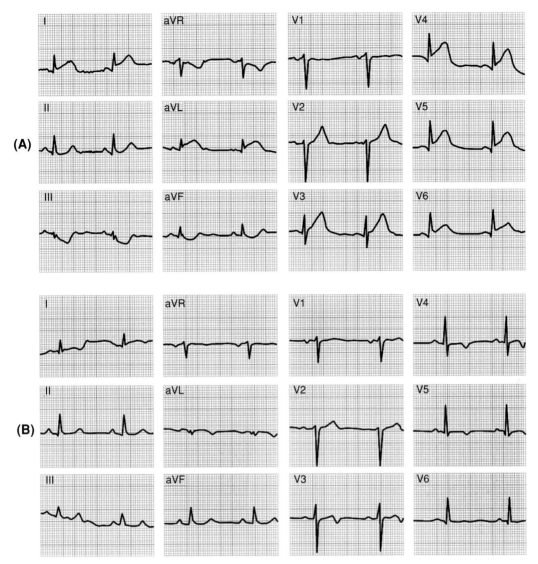

Figure 4.27 (A) Typical ECG pattern of STE-ACS due to D1 occlusion. Observe the ST-segment elevation in I, VL and also V2 to V5 and ST-segment depression in II, III and VF (III > II). (B) See the same case in chronic phase with QS in VL and low-voltage R in lead I as isolated abnormalities without abnormal QRS pattern in V5–V6.

and 4.33D). The projection of the injury vector in the positive and negative hemifields of different leads of the FP and HP explains the ST-segment elevation in II, III and VF (III > II), and the ST-segment depression in I and VL (VL > I). It also explains why an ST-segment elevation may be recorded in V1–V2 (Fiol et al., 2004c). (It is shown in Figure 4.30D how the projection of injury vector in HP may fall between approximately +110° to +200°–210°). For the same rea-

son, an ST-segment elevation may be recorded in V3R and V4R. Lead V4R is useful during the hyperacute phase to distinguish between an occlusion of the RCA proximal to the RV artery and an occlusion of the RCA distal to the RV artery and an occlusion of the LCX (Wellens, 1999; Wellens, Gorgels and Doevendans, 2003) (Figure 4.31). However, ST-segment changes in this lead are quite transient and, also, are generally not recorded. Therefore, lead V1 (isoelectric or

(A)

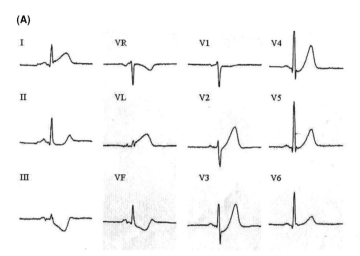

(B)

Pre-PCI	Post-PCI

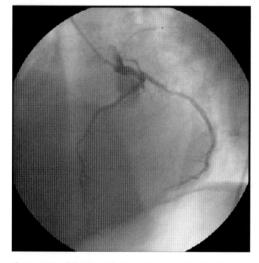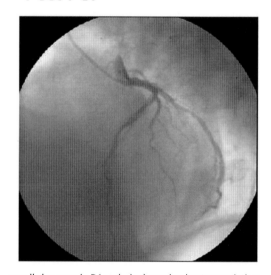

Figure 4.28   (A) ACS with clear ST-segment elelvation in I and VL, and ST-segment depression in II, III and VF. This strongly supports D1 occlusion (see p. 80). The presence of mild-ST-segment depression in V2–V3 (the contrary that usually happens in D1 occlusion) may be due to association of RCA or LCX occlusion, as is in this case (70% distal RCA occlusion) (see text). (B) Coronary angiography before and after PCI.

elevated ST segment) has been shown to be equally useful (Fiol et al., 2004) for detecting that the occlusion is proximal to the RV branches. It also has the advantage of not requiring the recording of additional leads. Figure 4.32 shows the similar morphology of ST in V1 and V3R.

In case of RCA occlusion proximal to RV branches, sometimes if the RCA is very short with just involvement of the RV (Finn and Antman, 2003), an ST-segment elevation may be seen not only in inferior leads but also in leads from V1 to V3–V4, even with greater ST-segment elevation in V1–V3, but the ST-segment elevation in V1 is usually greater than that in V3–V4 (V1 > V3 or V4) (Figure 10.4), the opposite that occurs in LAD occlusion distal to the S1 and D1 branches. In these latter cases, ST-segment elevation may also be seen in the precordial and inferior leads, but with ST-segment elevation in V3–V4 > V1 (Sadanandan et al., 2003) (see Table 4.2).

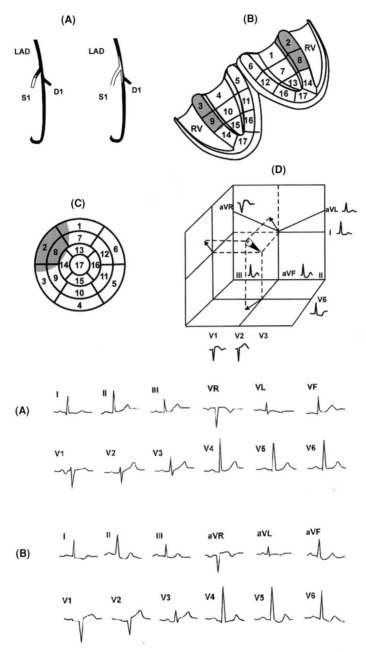

Figure 4.29 Above: STE-ACS due to incomplete occlusion of LAD involving the septal branches but not the diagonal branches. In exceptional cases only S1 or S2 occlusion may be found. (A) Site of the occlusion. (B) Myocardial area at risk. (C) Involved segments in a bull's-eye projection. (D) Injury vector projected on frontal, horizontal and sagittal planes and the corresponding ECG patterns. Below: (A) Control ECG. (B) Typical ECG pattern in case of occlusion of a large S1 artery during PCI procedure with involvement of the basal and probably also mid-septal part. Observe the ST-segment depression in inferior leads (II > III) and V6, and ST-segment elevation in VR and V1.

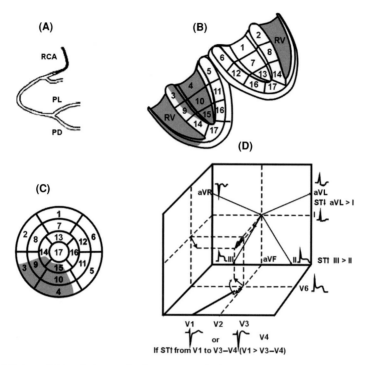

Figure 4.30 STE-ACS due to RCA occlusion proximal to right ventricle branches (arrow). (A) Site of occlusion. (B) Myocardial area at risk. (C) Polar map in 'bull's-eye' projection with the most involved segments marked in gray. (D) Injury vector projected on frontal, horizontal and sagittal planes with corresponding ECG patterns. Observe that the injury vector due to RV involvement is directed more forwards usually in the positive hemifield of V1 than in case of RCA occlusion distal to RV branches (see Figures 4.32 and 4.34).

The lack of apparent ST-segment depression in V1–V3 may also be observed in the STE-ACS due to a very distal occlusion of non-dominant RCA. In these cases, since the area at risk is small, the ST-segment elevation is not very apparent in II, III and VF. This is usually, on the contrary, in the STE-ACS due to an RCA occlusion proximal to the RV marginal branches.

A typical electrocardiographic example of this type of STE-ACS is shown in Figure 4.32A, along with its correlation with the coronary angiogram (Figure 4.32B) before and after a primary PCI.

8. RCA occlusion distal to the RV marginal branches (Figures 4.33 and 4.34, and Table 4.1B(8)): In case of balanced dominance the **area at risk** may involve, if the occlusion is just distal to RV branches, similar part of inferolateral zone of the LV than in the case of occlusion proximal to RV branches (see above and Figure 4.30).

In Figure 4.33B, C the involved myocardial area and the polar map of that area are shown. The involved segments are 3, 4, 9 and 10 and part of segments 14 and 15. These cases never evolve towards a right-ventricular infarction, since the branches perfusing the RV are proximal to the occlusion.

The injury vector is directed downwards, rightwards (though less so than when the occlusion is proximal to the RV branches) and posteriorly, even though usually it is directed more downwards than posteriorly. Due to that usually the ST-segment elevation in inferior leads is greater than ST-segment depression in V1–V3. Although the segmentary left-ventricular involvement may be equal or quite similar to the involvement seen when the occlusion is located proximal to the RV branches, the direction of the vector of injury is quite different in both cases, due to the RV involvement (see above). The

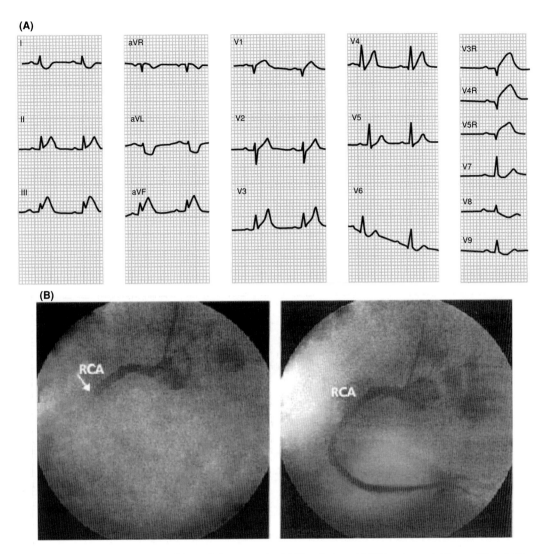

Figure 4.31 (A) Typical ECG in case of STE-ACS due to proximal RCA occlusion with RV involvement. Observe ST-segment elevation in II, III and VF with III > II, ST-segment depression in I and isoelectric or elevated in V1–V3 as well as in V3R–V4R leads with positive T wave. (B) Coronary angiography before (left) and after (right) reperfusion. The arrow indicates the place of occlusion.

projection of this vector in the positive and negative hemifields of different leads in the FP and HP explains why there is usually more ST-segment elevation in II, III and VF (III > II) than ST-segment depression in V1–V3 (projection vector in FP bigger than in HP) (see above) (Figure 4.33D). Because the injury vector is directed to rightwards and downwards, it is common that an ST-segment depression is recorded in lead I, and even more in VL because it falls in the negative

hemifield of both leads but more in the negative hemifield of VL.

A typical electrocardiographic example of this type of STE-ACS is shown in Figure 4.34A along with the correlation with coronary angiogram before and after a PCI (Figure 4.34B).

In the presence of occlusion of RCA even with involvement of inferobasal segment (classical posterior wall), but without involvement of lateral wall (pure inferior involvement), in the

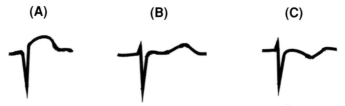

Figure 4.32 Usefulness of the ST/T changes in the extreme right precordial leads (V4R) to differentiate among the proximal RCA (A), distal RCA (B) and LCX involvement (C).

subacute phase, there are Q waves in inferior leads but the morphology in V1 is rS and not RS. The ST-segment depression in this case is usually bigger in V2–V3 than in V1 probably because both the vector of injury and the infarction that have the same direction but different senses are facing V2–V3 more than V1. In case of STE-ACS exclusively involving the lateral wall, in theory according the direction of the injury vector

the ST-segment depression in V1 > V3. However, the presence of ST-segment depression in V1 > V3 is not frequently seen, probably because cases of isolated injury of the lateral wall (non-dominant occlusion LCX) are much less frequent than the injury of inferior or inferolateral wall (RCA or dominant LCX occlusion) (ST↓ V3 > V1 in case of inferolateral injury – see Figure 4.15). The correlation between ST-segment changes in

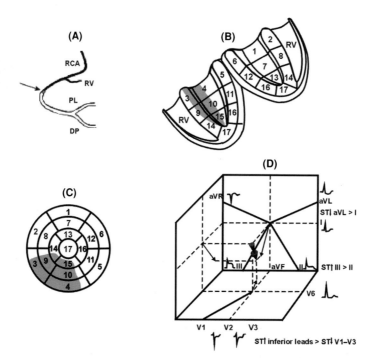

Figure 4.33 STE-ACS due to RCA occlusion after RV branches (arrow). At the same degree of dominance (RCA vs. LCX) the LV myocardial area at risk may be nearly the same as in case of occlusion proximal to RV branches if the occlusion is located just after these branches. (A) Site of occlusion. (B) Myocardial area at risk. (C) Polar map in 'bull's-eye' projection with the most involved segments marked in gray. (D) Injury vector projected in frontal, horizontal and sagittal planes is directed backwards and somewhat to the right but less than that in case of occlusion proximal to RV branches (see Figure 4.30), and the corresponding ECG patterns of ST-segment depression and elevation.

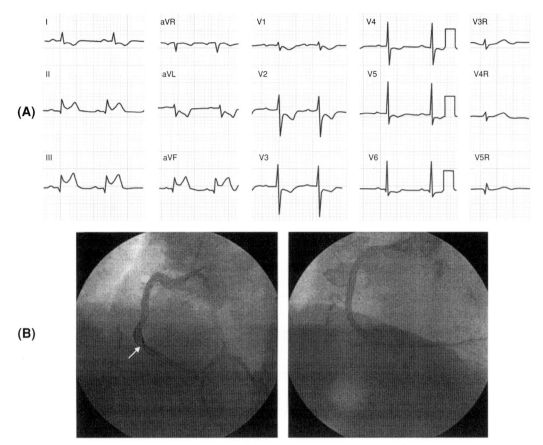

Figure 4.34   (A) Typical ECG in case of STE-ACS due to RCA occlusion distal to RV branches. Observe the ST-segment elevation in II, III and VF (III > II) with ST-segment depression in I. There exists ST-segment depression in right precordial leads (V1–V2). The right precordial leads also favour RCA occlusion after RV branches (see Figure 4.31). (B) Coronary angiography before (left) and after (right) reperfusion therapy. The arrow indicates the place of occlusion.

V1–V3 and deficits of perfusion detected by SPECT (nuclear medicine or other imaging techniques) will tell us if this hypothesis is correct.

9. Occlusion of a very dominant RCA (Figures 4.35 and 4.36, and Table 4.1B(9)): When the RCA is very dominant (Figure 4.35A), **the area at risk** involves a great part of inferolateral zone that includes great part of inferior septum, the inferior wall and even the apex if LAD is short, great portion of inferior and low-lateral wall. The involved segments are 3, 4, 5, 9, 10, 11, 14, 15 and 16 (Figure 4.35B, C).

The injury vector is directed downwards and posteriorly and a little rightwards. In the presence of occlusion proximal to RV branches, the injury vector will be more directed to the right

and even may fall in the positive hemifield of V1. This explains the ST isoelectric or even with slight elevation in V1. However, the presence of a local injury vector (Figure 4.35D) is necessary to explain the ST-segment elevation in V5–V6. This local vector may be visible in V5–V6 due to its proximity to precordial leads. The influence of this local vector is more evident when the occlusion is below RV branches. In this latter case, the injury vector is directed less rightwards and then counterbalance less the local injury vector. Therefore, the ST-segment elevation in V5–V6 is more visible in the absence of RV involvement.

Usually in these cases the presence of ST-segment elevation in II, III and VF is very

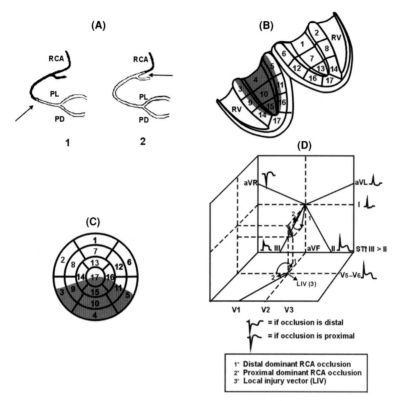

Figure 4.35 STE-ACS due to occlusion of very dominant RCA. (A) Site of occlusion that may be before or after the RV branches. (B) Myocardial area at risk. (C) Polar map in 'bull's-eye' projection with the most involved segments. (D) Injury vector projected in frontal and horizontal planes: (1) injury vector in case of distal occlusion; (2) injury vector in case of occlusion proximal to RV branches. Abbreviations: LIV, local injury vector that explains the ST-segment elevation in V5–V6 due to inferolateral involvement (very dominant RCA).

important and also if the occlusion is distal to RV branches the ST-segment depression is evident in V1–V3, although the ratio ($\Sigma \downarrow$ V1–V3)/($\Sigma \uparrow$ II, III, VF) < 1. The ST-segment may be isoelectric or even slightly positive in V1 or beyond if the occlusion is proximal to RV branches (see Table 4.2). **When the RCA is very dominant**, an ST-segment elevation ≥ 2 mm may be seen in V6 (Nikus et al., 2005) (apical inferolateral extension), but not in leads I and VL. In the latter leads an ST-segment depression is seen, while in case of a quite dominant LCX there may be ST-segment depression in VL but usually not in lead I (Figures 4.41 and 4.42). In exceptional cases of proximal occlusion of a very dominant RCA, due to typical ACS or dissecting aortic aneurysm type A affecting RCA (Figure 8.39), ST-segment elevation may be present in all precordial leads (V1–V4 due to proximal occlusion and V5–V6 due to very dominant RCA).

In the chronic phase in case of dominant RCA occlusion, there is involvement of inferior wall and some part of the lateral wall. This explains the Q wave in inferior leads and sometimes V5–V6 but not in lead I and aVL. Also, it explains the RS morphology in V1 because the vector of infarction of lateral wall points to V1 (see Figure 1.9). In case of occlusion of very dominant LCX, as all the lateral wall may be infarcted, we may find in chronic phase QR morphology in lead I and aVL, but usually not QS (see Figure 5.34), which is seen much more often in cases of occlusion of D1.

A typical ECG example of this type of STE-ACS along with its correlation with the coronary angiogram before and after a PCI is shown in Figure 4.36.

(A)

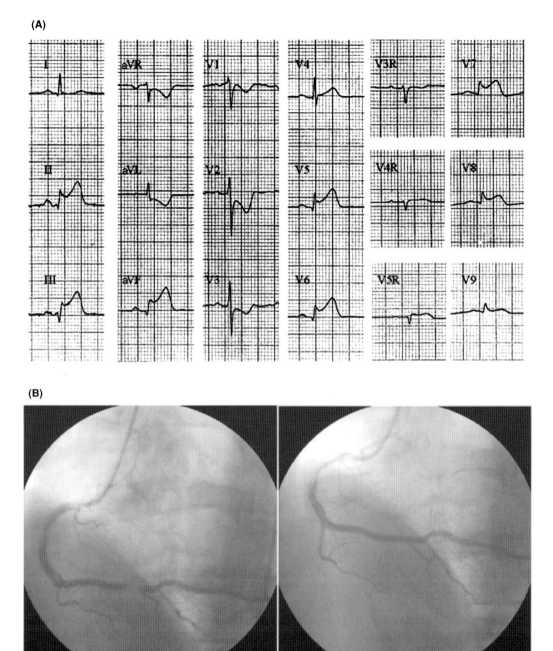

(B)

Figure 4.36 (A) Typical ECG in case of STE-ACS due to occlusion of very dominant RCA distal to RV branches. Observe the ST-segment elevation in inferior leads (III > II) and ST-segment depression the ST-segment depression in V1–V3 (occlusion distal to the take-off of RV branches). Furthermore, the ST-segment elevation in V6 is greater than 2 mm (occlusion of very dominant RCA). In extreme right precordial leads the ST is isoelectric in V3R and present slight elevation (<1 mm) in V4R. In this case the morphology of V1 was more useful than V4R to locate the place of occlusion. In this case the morphology of lead I (first step of algorithm in Figure 4.45) is not useful to diagnose RCA occlusion (isoelectric ST segment). (B) Coronary angiography before and after the reperfusion. The arrow shows the place of distal occlusion.

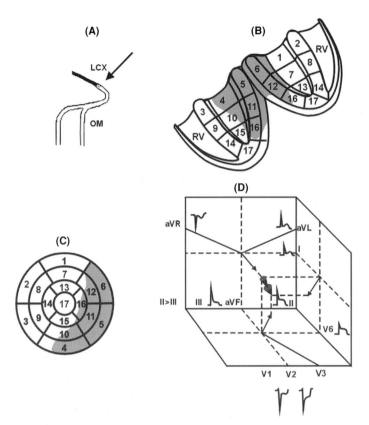

Figure 4.37 STE-ACS due to occlusion of LCX artery proximal to the obtuse marginal branch. (A) Site of occlusion. (B) Myocardial area at risk. (C) Polar map in 'bull's-eye' projection with the most involved segments marked in gray. (D) Injury vector directed backwards and somewhat to the left as projected in frontal, horizontal and sagittal planes, and the corresponding ECG patterns.

10. LCX occlusion proximal to the OM branch (Figures 4.37 and 4.38, and Table 4.1B(10)): In this case (Figure 4.37A) the **area at risk** encompasses the majority of lateral wall and may also compromise the inferior wall, especially the inferobasal segment. In Figure 4.37B, C the myocardial involved area along with the corresponding polar map in case of balanced dominance is shown. The most affected segments are 4, 5, 6, 10, 11 and 12, and part of 16.

The **injury vector** is directed leftwards and more posteriorly than downwards. The projection of this vector in the FP and HP (Figure 4.37) explains the ST-segment elevation often seen in lead I, the ST-segment elevation in II ≥ III and the ST-segment depression in V1–V3 equal to or of higher voltage than the ST-segment elevation in II, III and VF (Figures 4.37D and 4.38).

This is due to the fact that the non-dominant LCX perfuses the lateral wall and sometimes part of inferior wall especially the inferobasal segment, which explains, in case that this segment bends upwards, that ST-segment presents more depression in V1–V4 than elevation in II, III and VF. Sometimes the difference in voltage is striking (Figure 4.47). One hypothesis to explain that is related with a clear evidence that the inferobasal segment of inferior wall of the heart that is the part of inferior wall more perfused by LCX in these cases bends upwards and induces more ST-segment changes in the HP than in FP (Figure 4.45) (see p. 98 and 105).

A typical example of this type of STE-ACS is shown in Figure 4.38A, along with its correlation with the coronary angiogram (Figure 4.38B) before and after fibrinolytic therapy.

(A)

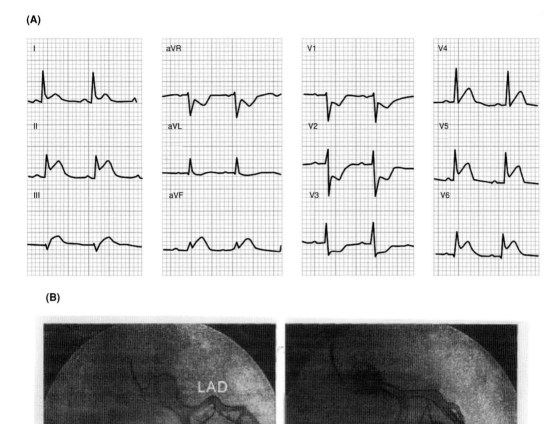

(B)

Figure 4.38 (A) Typical ECG in case of STE-ACS due to complete occlusion of LCX proximal to the obtuse marginal branch. Observe ST-segment elevation in II, III, VF (II > III), I and V5–V6, and ST-segment depression in V1–V3 more evident than the ST-segment elevation in V1–V3. (B) Coronary angiography before (left) and after (right) reperfusion. The arrow indicates the place of occlusion.

11. Occlusion of the OM branch (Figures 4.39 and 4.40, and Table 4.1B(11)): When the occlusion is located in the OM branch from the LCX (generally the first OM branch) (Figure 4.39A), the **area at risk** includes a great portion of both the inferior and especially the anterior part of the lateral wall (Figure 4.39B, C). The OM takes off from the LCX in the left-ventricular obtuse margin and, after perfusing the basal lateral wall (anterior and inferior part), is directed downwards along the border of lateral wall, often reaching the low portion of that wall. The most involved area is part of segments 5, 6, 11, 12 and 16. The perfusion of this area is shared with a ramus intermedius when present.

The vector of injury is directed leftwards and somewhat posteriorly and somewhat upwards or, more often, downwards (Figure 4.39D). The

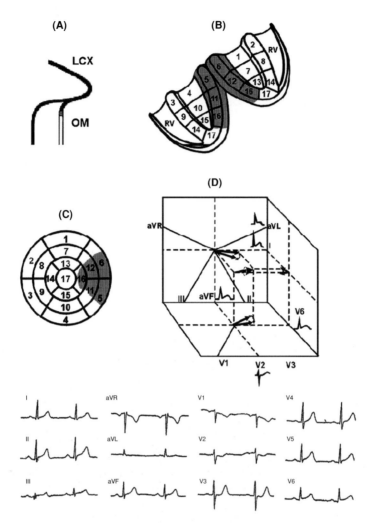

Figure 4.39 Above: STE-ACS due to occlusion of the obtuse marginal branch (OM). (A) Site of the occlusion. (B) Myocardial area at risk. (C) Polar map of the involved area. (D) Injury vector that is directed to the left (approximately 0° to +20° in the frontal plane) and somewhat backwards. Occasionally, if small, it hardly produces any ST-segment deviations. If they occur, the ST-segment elevation is observed in some lateral and inferior leads especially in I, II, VF and V6, with a usually slight ST-segment depression in V2–V3. In the case of STE-ACS secondary to the occlusion of the first diagonal (DI) in V2–V3, usually there is not ST-segment depression, and often ST-segment elevation is observed (Figure 4.27). Below: The ECG in case of STE-ACS due to incomplete occlusion of obtuse marginal artery (OM). Observe a slight ST-segment elevation in I, II and III; VF and V5–V6 with a slight depression in V1–V3 (compare with Figure 4.27 STE-ACS due to D1 occlusion).

projection of this vector in the positive and negative hemifields of different leads of the FP and HP explains the usually slight ST-segment elevation that is seen in the so-called lateral wall leads (I, VL and V5–V6) and sometimes also in the inferior leads, especially II and VF (Figure 4.39). In some rare cases the injury vector is directed more downwards and in this case the ST segment may be depressed in VL but not in lead I (located between +60° and +90°) (Figure 4.40). Since the injury vector is directed somewhat posteriorly, a usually slight ST-segment depression may be seen from V1 to V3 (Figures 4.39 and 4.40), rather than an ST-segment elevation that is frequently seen (usually V2–V4) in the STE-ACS due to a diagonal branch occlusion (Figure 4.27). This is

(A)

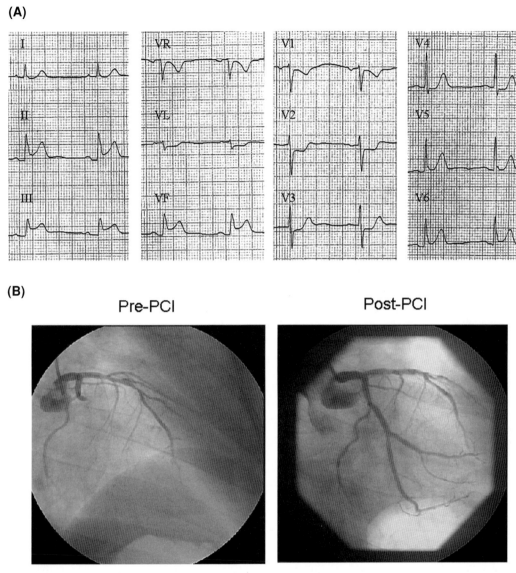

(B)

Pre-PCI   Post-PCI

Figure 4.40 (A) ECG of a 42-year-old man with ACS that presents slight elevation in II, III and VF, and ST-segment depression in V1–V3 with isodiphasic ST in lead I. It is not easy in this case to decide by the ECG if the occlusion is in RCA or LCX (OM). (B) The coronary angiography demonstrated that the occlusion was of a large OM. This case demonstrates that occasionally, especially when the changes of ST are not striking, may be difficult to identify through the ST-segment changes the culprit artery.

due to the fact that the injury vector in the diagonal occlusion is directed leftwards and upwards and somewhat anteriorly. Meanwhile, in the occlusion of the OM, it is usually directed also leftwards, but somewhat posteriorly and often a little downwards (Birnbaum et al., 1996a). Sometimes especially in case of LCX (OM) occlusion the ST-segment deviations do not present characteristic changes (Figure 4.40), and when the OM branch is small, the changes can be minimal, if they do. In fact, the ECG is often normal.

In subacute or chronic phase, 'qr' or 'r' morphology in 'lateral leads', I, VL and/or V5–V6, may be present frequently with RS (R) in V1, but

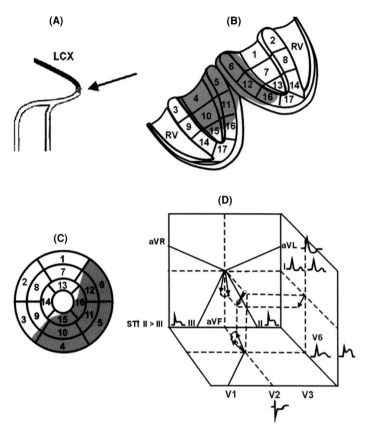

Figure 4.41 STE-ACS due to proximal occlusion of a very dominant LCX artery. (A) Site of occlusion. (B) Myocardial area at risk. (C) Polar map in 'bull's-eye' projection with the most involved segments marked in gray. (D) Important injury vector directed more backwards than downwards and less to the left or even a little to the right as projected in frontal, horizontal and sagittal planes, and the corresponding ECG patterns of ST-segment depression and elevation.

never QS in VL. On the contrary, in STE-ACS due to diagonal occlusion, QS morphology in VL may be present but without Q wave in V5–V6.

An example of this STE-ACS is shown in Figure 4.39, which in this case did not originate a Q-wave infarction in the chronic phase (normal ECG).

12.   Occlusion of a very dominant LCX (Figures 4.41 and 4.42, and Table 4.1B(12)): When the LCX is very dominant and the **occlusion is proximal** (Figure 4.41A), **the area at risk** involves a great part of inferolateral zone that includes the majority of the lateral and inferior wall and even some portion of inferior part of the septum. The involved segments are 3, 4, 5, 6, 9, 10, 11, 12, 15 and 16 (Figures 4.41B and C).

The **injury vector** due to very dominant LCX is important and less directed to the left because due to the dominance the LCX perfuses not only the lateral wall but also great part of the inferior wall. Its projection in FP and HP (Figure 4.41D) explains the following: (a) Sometimes there is ST-segment depression in lead VL but very rarely in lead I. (The injury vector is located usually between +60° and +90°.) This means that it usually falls in the negative hemifield of VL but still in the positive hemifield of lead I or just on the border between two hemifields. (b) ST-segment elevation in II, III and VF may be similar to the ST-segment depression in V1–V3, because the very dominant LCX perfuses not only the lateral wall but also great part of the inferior wall. However, in the cases that the ST-segment elevation in II, III and VF is superior to ST-segment depression in V1–V3, usually ST-segment elevation in II > III. In lead I there is no ST-segment

(A)

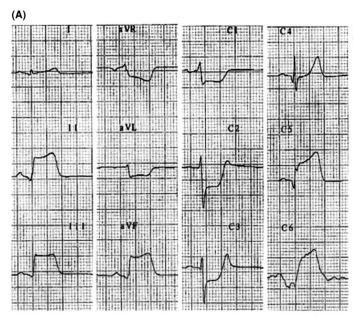

(B)

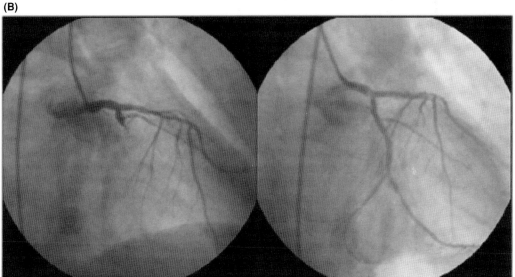

Figure 4.42 (A) The ECG in case of STE-ACS due to complete proximal occlusion of very dominant LCX artery. Observe the criteria of LCX occlusion. ST-segment elevation in II > III in the presence of isoelectric ST in I (second step of Figure 4.45). In VL there is ST-segment depression due to LCX dominance. In the normal cases of LCX occlusion there is not ST-segment depression in VL (isoelectric or elevated) (Figure 4.38). There is also a huge ST-segment elevation in V5–V6 more evident than in case of very dominant RCA (Figure 4.36). On the other hand, the sum of ST-segment deviations is much higher than in case of proximal occlusion of a non-dominant LCX (Figure 4.38). (B) Coronary angiography before (left) and after reperfusion.

depression, as usually happens in case of occlusion of very dominant RCA. Furthermore, the ST-segment elevation in V5–V6 is usually bigger than in case of a very dominant RCA (Figure 4.42).

In some cases of occlusion of dominant LCX, the ST-segment depression in V1–V3 is much evident than ST-segment elevation in inferior leads. In these cases usually the ST-segment depression in V3 is greater than that in V1. One possible hypothesis to explain that is that the injury area encompasses the lateral wall and also a great part of the inferior wall that is really posterior, as may happen in very lean individuals, and then the injury vector faces V3 more than V1 (see Figure 4.47 and p. 92 and 105). Also in some cases of non-proximal occlusion of dominant RCA may be seen that ST depression in V3 > V1. However the overall ST elevation in inferior leads is greater than in V1–V3 (see Figure 4.15).

If the occlusion of **dominant LCX is very distal**, the ECG characteristics are similar to the occlusion of non-dominant RCA, because in both cases the areas at risk are the same (part of the inferior wall).

A typical ECG example of STE-ACS due to very dominant LCX can be seen in Figure 4.42.

In the subacute or chronic phase due to involvement of the inferior and lateral walls, a Q wave in inferior leads sometimes with QII > QIII and lateral leads (V5–V6, I and VL) and RS morphology in V1 (even Rs) may be recorded (see Figure 5.34).

STE-ACS: from the ECG to the area at risk and the occluded artery. (Figures 4.43–4.47 and Table 4.1; Bayés de Luna, Fiol and Antman 2006; Fiol et al., 2004a–c, 2007; Sclarovsky, 1999; Wellens and Connover, 2003; Zimetbaum and Josephson, 2003).

From a clinical point of view, in the majority of cases, usually the most striking ECG abnormality found by the physician is ST-segment elevation located in the precordial leads (V1–V6) (anteroseptal zone) (Figure 4.43) or in inferior leads (inferolateral zone) (Figure 4.45). We will see how we can identify not only the culprit artery, but also the occlusion site.

1. Most striking ST-segment elevation is seen in precordial leads (V1–V2 to V4–V6) (Figure 4.43): This corresponds to LAD occlusion (Engelen et al., 1999; Haraphongse, Tanomsup and Jugdutt, 1984; Porter et al., 1998; Sapin et al., 1992; Tamura, Kataoka and Mikuriya, 1991, 1995a,b).

The rationale to know the characteristics of the occluded artery and the site of occlusion is shown in Figure 4.43. The positive predictive value of this approach is very high. The ST segment has to be first assessed in II, III and VF (to check for its depression or not), and later on the deviations of ST segment in VR, V1 and V6 have to be assessed. According to the ST-segment changes in these leads, the occlusion may be localised as proximal or distal to the first diagonal (D1) and/or the first septal (S1) branch (Fiol et al., 2007).

(a) When the ST segment is depressed (≥ 2.5 mm in III + VF), the occlusion is proximal to the first diagonal (D1) (90%). When the ST segment is also elevated in V1 and/or VR, or depressed in V6 (Σ of deviations of ST in VR + V1– V6 $\geq$ 0), the occlusion is probably also proximal to the first septal (S1) (Fig. 4.43). When this so-called septal formula involvement is <0 (Fiol et al., 2007), the occlusion is probably between first septal (S1) and first diagonal (D1) (Figures 4.20 and 4.21).

Some cases with LMT critical occlusion that do not have previous important subendocardial ischaemia and usually no important collateral circulation **may present an STE-ACS with ST-segment elevation in precordials and ST-segment depression in III and VF $\geq$ 2.5 mm**. A group of patients of these characteristics corresponds to STE-ACS due to coronary dissection affecting the LMT (see 'Coronary dissection') (p. 266 and Figure 8.40). However, usually the patients with ACS due to coronary atherothrombosis present, in case of critical LMT involvement, previous important and predominant subendocardial ischaemia with evident collateral circulation, and, consequently, an ST-segment depression is recorded (NSTE-ACS) (see 'Diagnostic criteria: morphology and voltage' (p. 111). Nevertheless, in rare cases of critical occlusion of LMT or equivalent due to coronary atherothrombosis, an STE-ACS may be seen if the patient does not present previous important subendocardial ischaemia. Figure 4.44 shows a case of 'active' ischaemia due to multiple-vessel-disease involvement (critical LMT + LCX + proximal LAD) (see footnote and section

Figure 4.43 The algorithm to locate the zone of LAD occlusion in case of ACS with predominant ST-segment elevation in precordial leads. In the lower right side is presented an example to calculate the formula: sum of ST-segment deviations in VR, V1 and V6 (remember that – (–2 mm) = +2 mm) and in the lower left side the sensitivity, specificity and positive and negative predictive value of all the criteria.

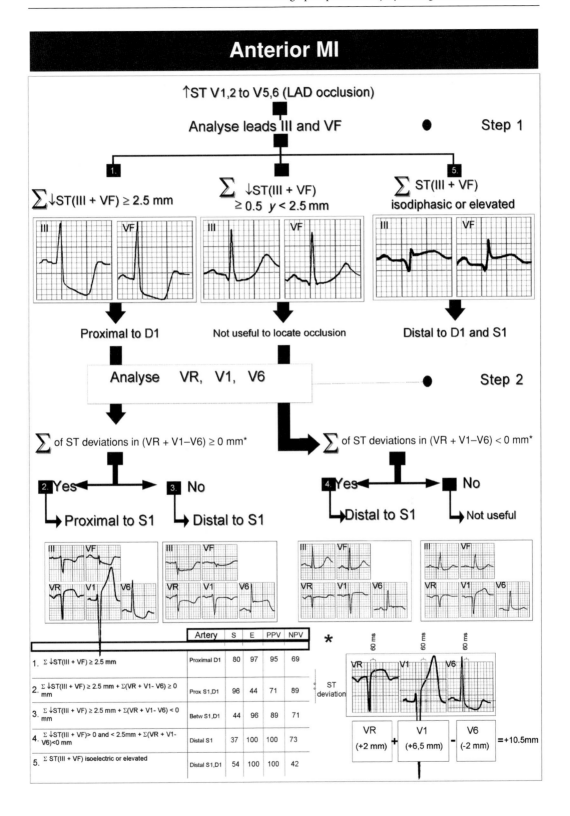

'ST-segment changes in patients with active ischaemia due to multivessel disease') (p. 105). We would like to emphasise that cases of LMT critical occlusion (or equivalent) with ST-segment elevation are infrequently seen especially because they present a highest risk of cardiogenic shock, ventricular fibrillation and sudden death before arriving at emergency services.

(b) **When the ST segment is isoelectric (between <0.5 mm ↑ and <0.5mm ↓ of ST segment) or shows elevation in II, III and VF,** the occlusion is distal to D1. Then, leads VR, V1 and/or V6 should be assessed to know whether the occlusion is **proximal or distal to S1.** We use the formula Σ ST**deviations in VR + V1 − V$_6$** (Fig. 4.43). If the sum is <0 (**which occurs most frequently),the occlusion is also distal to S1** (Figure 4.23). When the formula is ≥0, **the S1 takes off after the D1 branch and the occlusion is distal to D1 but proximal to S1** (Figure 4.25). The comparison of ST-segment elevation in II and III also helps to differentiate both locations. When the occlusion is distal to D1 and S1, ST-segment elevation in II > III, because the injury vector is directed to the apex (see Figure 4.22). On the contrary, if the occlusion is distal to D1, but proximal to S1, the injury vector will point downwards and rightwards, because the most important area at risk is the lower anteroseptal and therefore the ST-segment elevation in III > II (see Figure 4.25).

(c) **When the ST segment is slightly depressed** (<2.5 mm in III + VF), it is harder to classify with respect to D1, but when the sum of ST-segment **deviations in VR + V1 − V6** ≤ 0, the occlusion is probably distal to S1 and D1 (Figure 4.43).

Additionally, when a typical **right bundle branch block** morphology is seen in the course of an STE-ACS, this greatly supports a high septal ischaemia (occlusion above the S1 branch), causing this bundle branch, since first septal (S1) perfuses the right bundle branch (Figure 4.66). This sign is quite specific, but not very sensitive (Engelen et al., 1999).

2. Most striking ST-segment elevation recorded in II, III and VF (Figure 4.45): ST-segment depression may be seen in V1–V3 as a mirror pattern of inferolateral involvement, although it is usually not present when the occlusion of RCA is proximal to RV marginal branches (see below). **This corresponds to an RCA or LCX occlusion** (Birnbaum et al., 1994; Fiol et al., 2004b; Herz et al., 1997; Kosuge et al., 1998; Lew et al., 1986; Saw et al., 2001; Tamura et al., 1995a, b).

In these cases it may be useful to assess the ST/T in V4R to know whether the occlusion is located in the proximal or distal RCA or in the LCX (Figure 4.32) (Wellens, 1999). Since V4R is sometimes not recorded and because abnormalities occurring in this lead are often quite transient, **we use a sequential approach based on the ST-segment changes seen in the 12-lead surface to know weather the RCA or the LCX is the culprit** artery (Fiol et al., 2004b) (Figure 4.45).

Step 1: assess the ST segment in lead I. In the case of depression, the occlusion is located in the RCA, and in the case of elevation, it is located in the circumflex artery (LCX). **When the ST segment is isoelectric, one should proceed to Step 2.**

Step 2: check how is the ST segment in II, III and VF. When the ST-segment elevation in II ≥ III, the occlusion is located in the LCX. **When the ST-segment elevation is III > II, one should proceed to Step 3.**

Step 3: The following relation should be assessed: $(\Sigma \downarrow ST\ in\ V1\text{–}V3)/(\Sigma \uparrow ST\ in\ II, III, VF)$. When the ratio is greater than 1, the culprit artery is the LCX; when it is equal to or lower than 1, the culprit artery is the RCA.

With this sequential approach one may distinguish whether the RCA or the LCX is the culprit artery in over 95% of all cases.

Figure 4.44 (A) The ECG at basal state in a patient with STE-ACS. (B) The ECG during anginal pain. This is a case of 'active' ischaemia due to critical multiple-vessel occlusion. At a first glance looks like LAD occlusion proximal to the D1 and probably not to S1 (ST-segment depression in V1 and slightly elevated in V6). However, the presence of ST-segment elevation in VR arise the suspicion that either was an atypical case of LAD occlusion proximal to S1 and D1 or the global ECG was explained by multiple critical vessel occlusion as was the case (LMT + LAD + CX). The ischaemia due to LCx involvement may explain the ST depression in V$_1$.

(A)

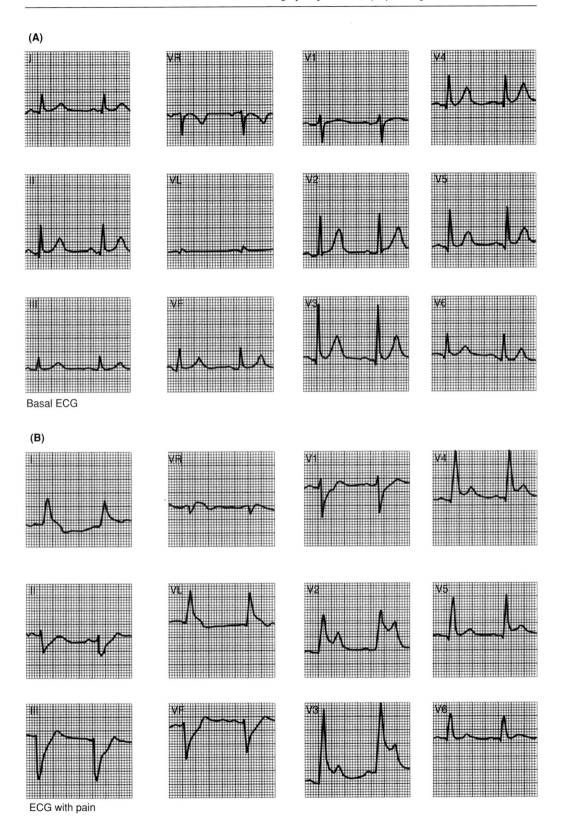

Basal ECG

(B)

ECG with pain

There are many other criteria or combinations of criteria that have been used to differentiate RCA from LCX occlusion. The association of ST-segment elevation in III > II + ST-segment depression in VL has good specificity and positive predictive value for the diagnosis of RCA occlusion (Kabakci, 2001).

Once the RCA has been accurately determined to be the culprit artery, **it is important to know whether the occlusion is proximal or distal** (Figure 4.46). For that matter, **lead V1** is important and, to a lesser degree, leads **I** and **VL**. Generally, an ST-segment isoelectric or elevated is seen in V1 in case of proximal occlusion (Figure 4.46A) and ST-segment depression in V1–V3 in distal occlusion (Fiol et al., 2004a) (Figure 4.46B). This change may persist up to V3–V4, but the ST-segment elevation is V1 > V3–V4. In the distal LAD occlusion, ST-segment elevation may also be seen in the precordial and inferior leads (Figure 4.23). However, in this case (a) the ST-segment elevation in the precordial leads is higher than that in the inferior leads; and (b) the ST-segment elevation is V3–V4 > V1 (Sadanandan, 2003). Furthermore, generally in the RCA proximal occlusion, there is ST-segment depression in lead I and VL, and in case of distal LAD, there is usually not clear ST-segment depression in the same leads (Figures 4.32, 4.46A and 4.23, and Table 4.2).
3. Most striking ST-segment elevation in the lateral wall leads, I, VL and V5–V6: In this case the STE-ACS may be due to **diagonal occlusion** (or LAD incomplete occlusion, involving the diagonal branches), or the **first-second OM (compare Figures 4.27 and 4.40) or,** occasionally, **the ramus intermedius branch occlusion**.

In the acute phase, the diagnosis of a **first diagonal branch** occlusion is favoured by the **presence of a** more significant ST-segment elevation in I and VL and often some precordial leads than in the inferior leads (in which ST-segment depression is usually seen). Instead, in an OM occlusion, a slight ST-segment elevation may be seen in both groups of leads, since the injury vector is not so upwardly directed and even may be downwardly directed, in which the ST-segment elevation may be seen only in inferior leads.

In case of first diagonal branch occlusion, evident ST-segment elevation is often seen in precordial leads (from V2–V3 to V4). This is explained by the direction of the injury vector, which points somewhat anteriorly. On the contrary, this does not occur when the OM branch is occluded. In this case a slight ST-segment depression or just minimal ECG changes are seen, since the OM occlusion generates an injury vector that is directed somewhat posteriorly. In a few occasions of first diagonal occlusion, perhaps due to a rotation of the heart, or the association of LCX or RCA occlusion, we have seen mild ST-segment depression in V2–V3.

On certain occasions STE-ACS due to marginal branch or diagonal branch occlusions may cause small ECG changes or even present normal ECG.

In the chronic phase, the mid-anterior infarction due to a **first diagonal** occlusion (Figures 5.9A(4), 5.21 and 5.22) may cause a QS morphology in VL, or at least 'qr', and even qr wave in lead I. However, no Q wave is seen in V5–V6. On the contrary, in the infarction secondary to the OM **branch** occlusion, a qr morphology may be seen in V5–V6 and also in I and VL, or merely a low-voltage R wave, with or without RS in V1, but in general no QS morphology in VL (Figures 5.9B(1), 5.23 and 5.24). However, in both situations, the ECG may be normal in the chronic phase.

Sometimes a lateral involvement is seen in some STE-ACS of anteroseptal and inferolateral zone. In the first case, when the occlusion is proximal to D1, but distal to S1 (Figure 4.20), the ST-segment elevation is present in I and aVL (aVL > I) but usually not in V6 (Figure 4.21). In the second case (involvement of the inferolateral zone), ST-segment elevation in V5 and V6 is seen especially when there is a proximal occlusion of dominant RCA (Figure 4.36). When the RCA is quite dominant, the ST-segment elevation in V5–V6 is usually ≥2 mm (Nikus et al., 2004), but in this case usually there is ST-segment depression in leads I and especially in VL (Figure 4.36). On the contrary, in case of LCX occlusion, the ST-segment

---

Figure 4.45 The algorithm to identify which is the occluded artery (RCA vs LCX) in case of ACS with predominant ST-segment elevation in inferior leads and to locate in case of RCA occlusion if it is proximal or distal. See the sensitivity, specificity and positive and negative predictive value of all the criteria.

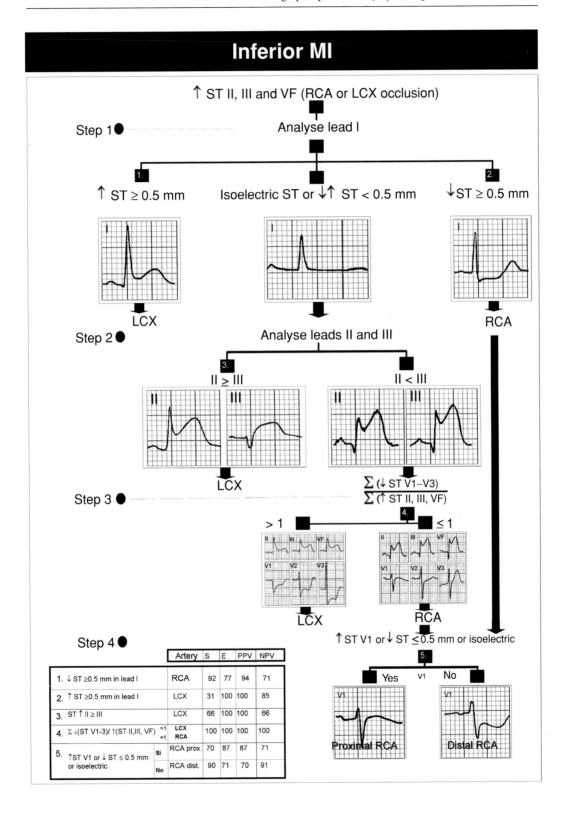

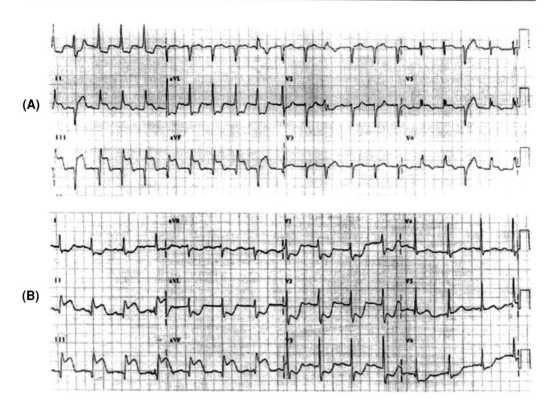

Figure 4.46 (A) The ECG in STE-ACS due to proximal RCA occlusion. ST-segment depression in I and VL (VL > I), as well as ST III > II points to RCA occlusion, while the absence of ST-segment depression in V1 is an accurate criterion of right ventricular involvement (proximal occlusion), since in this case the injury vector points forwards and rightwards. As the RCA is dominant, there is also an ST-segment elevation in V5–V6 (local injury vector – Figure 4.35).

(B) The ECG in STE-ACS due to distal RCA occlusion. In this case, the ST segment in the lateral and inferior leads shows similar behavior than in A (proximal RCA occlusion), but ST-segment depression in V1–V3 indicates distal occlusion, since the injury vector points backwards (towards the inferolateral wall). As the RCA is not very dominant in V6, there is not ST-segment elevation.

elevation is often seen in the majority of lateral leads (I, VL and V5–V6) (Figure 4.38).

4. Atypical ECG patterns seen in STE-ACS (see Table 8.1 and Figure 8.3): The atypical ECG patterns seen in cases of NSTE-ACS are also commented in Part II (see 'Typical and atypical patterns of STE-ACS and NSTE-ACS', p. 210).

(a) In some cases of LCX occlusion, the most striking ECG changes are ST-segment depression in V1–V3 as a mirror image of the posterior leads (STE equivalent). The ST-segment depression is more evident than ST-segment elevation in inferior lateral leads (Figures 4.47 and 8.3C) (p. 97 and 213). Probably, this occurs in cases of occlusion of LCX involving a portion of inferior part of the lateral wall (segments 5 and 11), but especially the in-

ferobasal and mid-inferior segments (4 and 10) of the inferior wall. In these cases if great part of the inferior wall bends upwards, the projection of the injury vector of this area is seen better in the HP than in FP, and more in V3 than in V1 if the involvement of segments 4 and 10 is the most important and points more to V3 than V1. In case of injury, the repercussions of the changes in V3 expressed as ST-segment depression are more evident than the changes of R wave in V3 in case of infarction, because also in normal conditions in V3 there is already an RS pattern and, on the contrary, is never recorded in normal ST-segment depression in right precordial leads. Under these circumstances, an erroneous diagnosis of NSTE-ACS may be established especially because the ST-segment elevation in

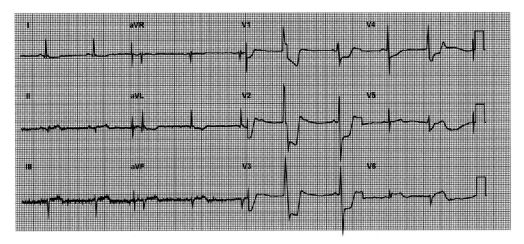

Figure 4.47 Patient with ACS. The most important ECG changes are a ST-segment depression in V1–V3. In spite of that, the presence of an even mild-ST-segment elevation in II, III, VF and V5–V6 assures that this case is an STE-ACS. The ST-segment depression observed in V1–V3 is even more striking in the ventricular premature beats (first QRS in V1–V3).

II, III, VF and V6 is sometimes very scarce. However, in fact the ST-segment depression in V1–V3 is a mirror pattern of the ST-segment elevation in the opposite leads. Check if a mild ST-segment elevation, usually present in II, III, VF and V5–V6, is useful in assuring that, in spite of the larger ST-segment depression from V1 to V3, the diagnosis is consistent with STE-ACS and not with NST-ACS. When the ST-segment depression is seen mainly from V1 to V2–V3, an ST-segment elevation ≥1 mm may be found in the posterior leads.

(b) In an early phase of STE-ACS due to proximal occlusion of LAD, a pseudonormal ECG pattern expressed by a tall and peaked T wave may be seen. This is usually a transient pattern that may be followed by a clear ST-segment elevation (see Figure 8.3A).

(c) In some occasions of LAD occlusion, a negative and deep T wave in precordial leads (V1–V4–V5) may be seen in some moment of the evolution. This corresponds to a pattern seen in cases of LAD proximal occlusion that much probably has reperfused at least partially spontaneously or if remains occluded, present very important collateral circulation that prevents the infarction. However, sometimes if the patient is not treated promptly, it may develop an STE-ACS and impending MI (de Zwan, Bär and Wellens, 1982) (Figure 8.3B). The presence of negative T wave represents that the affected area is still perfused and not completely ischaemic, as happens in the case of ST-segment elevation. Therefore, in this case, coronary angiography has to be performed as soon as possible, but in the absence of angina not as an emergency. However, in case if persistent ST-segment elevation appears, primary PCI if possible or fibrinolysis is mandatory.

On other occasion (see p. 228 and 270), this ECG pattern is seen in cases of STE-ACS due to proximal LAD occlusion, which have been reperfused by treatment (fibrinolysis or PCI), and the ST-segment elevation ECG pattern changes to a negative and often very deep T wave in V1–V4. This is a clear sign of reperfusion after fibrinolytic treatment or PCI and evidence of an opened artery. However, we may not be completely sure that another reocclusion will not appear. As a matter of fact sometimes coinciding with angina due to thrombosis intrastent, the ECG first pseudonormalises and finally an ST-segment elevation may appear.

ST-segment changes in patients with 'active' ischaemia due to multivessel disease

All the cases of STE-ACS that have been discussed are due to ischaemia generated by occlusion in one

---

Usefulness of the ECG in ACS with ST-segment elevation and in the Q-wave infarction

ACS with ST-segment elevation STE-ACS

It is possible to know, generally with accuracy, which the involved artery is and the site of occlusion. This is of critical importance in knowing the area at risk and for risk stratification.

↓

This is achieved by

1. analysing the ST-segment deviations in the different leads (Table 4.1 and 'Correlation between the ECG changes, the occlusion site and the area at risk'). (p. 222)

2. quantifying the burden of ischaemia (see 'Quantification of the burden of ischaemia by the summation of ST-segment deviations') (p. 224)

3. defining the grade (intensity) of ischaemia (see 'To define the grade (intensity) of ischaemia through the ST/T morphology') (p. 224)

Q-wave infarction

The location of the infarcted area may be identified with accuracy.

↓

This is obtained by analysing in which leads Q wave of necrosis or R equivalents are recorded (Figure 5.9) (ECG–CMR correlation).

---

culprit vessel, though stenosis may be present in more than one vessel.

Multiple unstable plaques may be present in more than one culprit artery in patients with ACS. Recently, it has been demonstrated that this may be detected in a few cases (3%) by the presence of a new ST-segment elevation in other area. **The electrocardiographic changes that could suggest that the ischaemia in different cardiac areas is due to significant lesions in two or more vessels are not well known.** However the following clues allow us to suppose that the electrocardiographic patterns may be explained by critical involvement of two or more vessels.

1. In a patient with STE-ACS with **ST-segment elevation in II, III and VF, the presence of ST-segment depression in precordial leads beyond V2–V3 with maximal changes in V4–V5** represents a group of highest risk (Birnbaum and Atar, 2006). This can be explained by occlusion of the RCA, plus a significant obstruction in the LAD.

2. The presence of **ST-segment elevation in the right precordial leads (V1–V3) and ST-segment depression in the left-sided leads (aVL, I and V4–V6)** suggests multivessel involvement (Kurum et al., 2002). In the STE-ACS due to the LAD occlusion proximal to D1 and S1 (single-vessel disease), an ST-segment elevation may also be recorded from V1 to V4, and ST-segment depression in V5–V6. However, in case of occlusion proximal to D1 and S1, the ST-segment depression is not usually evident in lead I and is not present in aVL (see Figures 4.18 and 4.19).

3. It has been shown that in an STE-ACS due to distal to D1 and S1, occlusion of long LAD generates the **ST-segment elevation in precordial leads and in II, III and VF.** However, this morphology may also be explained by an occlusion in LAD in presence of a total RCA occlusion with collateral vessels from the LAD to the RCA, even in the absence of a considerably long LAD. There is not any ECG criterion that may help us to differentiate these two cases, because in both situations the ST-segment elevation in precordial leads is more important than in inferior leads.

4. The presence of **slight ST-segment depression in V2–V4 in STE-ACS due to D1 occlusion (ST-segment elevation in I, aVL and V5–V6, and ST-segment depression in II, III and VF)** suggests the presence of multivessel disease, especially D1 + LCX or RCA.

5. When in a patient with STE-ACS **in precordial leads there are some criteria that do not fit well with the presumed place of occlusion, the presence of ischaemia due to critical multivessel disease may be suspected** (see Figure 4.44). It looks like a LAD occlusion proximal to D1 but was not clear if the occlusion was also proximal to S1 (ST-segment elevation in VR and ST-segment depression in V1). The case corresponds to a critical

STE-ACS: ST-segment elevation in the inferolateral leads

ECG criteria (ST-segment elevation and depression) supporting an occlusion of the RCA, LCX, D1 and OM

1. **Occlusion of the RCA**
   a. There is usually an ST-segment depression in I and VL; in general VL > I.
   b. The ST-segment elevation in III is usually higher than that in II.
   c. The ST-segment depression in the right precordial leads is usually lesser than the ST-segment elevation in the inferior leads. This is especially true when the occlusion is proximal to the RV branches, in which the ST segment in V1 is usually isoelectric or elevated.
   d. When the RCA is quite dominant, an ST-segment elevation is seen in V5 and V6, but not in I and aVL. An ST-segment elevation ≥2 mm in these leads indicates that the RCA is very dominant.

2. **Occlusion of the LCX proximal to first OM branch**
   a. There is usually an ST-segment elevation in I and VL.
   b. The ST-segment elevation in II is usually equal to or higher than that in III.
   c. The ST-segment elevation in II, III and VF is usually lesser than the ST-segment depression in the right precordial leads. Sometimes, this is quite apparent.
   d. When the LCX is quite dominant, it may present the above-mentioned criteria but in some cases there is ST-segment depression in VL, but very rarely in I.

3. **Occlusion of the OM**
   a. There is usually ST-segment elevation in the so-called lateral leads, I and VL and V5–V6, and also inferior leads; usually, II > III.
   b. Sometimes, this change is present only in the inferior leads, especially II and VF.
   c. There is often a slight ST-segment depression in V1–V3.

4. **Occlusion of the D1**
   a. An ST-segment elevation may be seen in the so-called lateral wall leads, especially in I and VL. In fact, these leads face the anterior and often the mid-low lateral wall, but not the high-lateral wall. Since the injury vector is directed more upwards and, generally, anteriorly with regards to what occurs in an OM occlusion, it is usually recorded in the inferior leads in an ST-segment depression.
   b. ST-segment elevation may be seen in the precordial leads, sometimes from V2–V3 and occasionally with evident elevation. In turn, the ST segment in V2–V3 is usually isoelectric or depressed in the OM occlusion (compare Figures 4.27 and 4.40). Rarely, in case of D1 occlusion, slight ST-segment depression may be seen in precordial leads, especially in case of associated LCX or RCA occlusion (Figure 4.28).

occlusion of both LAD proximal to S1 + D1 and LCX plus 70% occlusion of LMT. The involvement of proximal LAD + LCX explains the ST-segment depression in V1 in spite of ST-segment elevation in VR (see Figure 4.44 and p. 98). In our opinion, when there is some discrepancy in the ECG findings, ischaemia due to multivessel occlusion has to be suspected.

6. The recurrence of ST-segment elevation in a different territory after fibrinolytic therapy is a manifestation of multiple unstable coronary plaques (Edmond et al., 2006).

The importance to recognise the culprit artery before performing PCI in case of ACS in critical multivessel disease will be emphasised in the second part of this book (see 'The dynamic changes of ST segment from the prehospital phase to the catheterisation laboratory'). (p. 226).

ST-segment elevation in other clinical settings (Figures 4.48–1.114)

In Table 4.3 the most frequent causes of ST-segment elevation, aside from IHD (typical and atypical ACS), are shown. At the time of making the differential diagnosis in clinical practice, out of all these different entities the possibility of a pericarditis or an early phase acute myopericarditis (Figures 4.48 and 4.49) should be kept in mind. These also cause chest pain that may complicate the diagnosis.

Table 4.3 Most frequent causes of ST-segment elevation, aside from ischaemic heart disease.

1. **Normal variants**: Chest abnormalities (Figures 4.13 B(6) and, 4.52C), early repolarization (Figures 4.50, 7.3 and 7.4) and vagal overdrive. In vagal overdrive, ST-segment elevation is mild and generally presents early repolarization pattern. T wave is tall and asymmetric.
2. **Sportsmen**: Sometimes an ST-segment elevation exists which may mimic an acute coronary syndrome with or without negative T wave, which may be prominent (Figures 4.51 and 3.33). No coronary involvement has been found, but this pattern has been observed in sportsmen who die suddenly. Therefore, its presence implies the need to rule out hypertrophic cardiomyopathy.
3. **Alteration secondary to repolarization changes** (LBBB, LVH, WPW and pacemakers)
4. **Acute pericarditis** in its early stage and **myopericarditis** (Figures 4.48 and 4.49)
5. **Pulmonary embolism** (Figure 4.54): frequently accompanied by RBBB
6. **Hyperkalaemia**: The presence of a tall and peaked T wave is more evident than the accompanying slight ST-segment elevation. Sometimes ST elevation may be evident, especially in right precordial leads (Figure 4.55).
7. **Hypothermia** (Figure 4.56)
8. **Brugada's syndrome**: May present typical ST-elevation pattern (concave in respect to the isoelectric line) or atypical ST-elevation pattern (convex in respect to the isoelectric line) (Figure 4.52; Wilde, et al. 2002).
9. **Arrhythmogenic right ventricular dysplasia** (Figure 4.53)
10. **Metabolic anomalies (diabetes)**
11. **Pheochromocytoma**
12. **Dissecting aortic aneurysm** (Figure 7.4) (mirror pattern of LVH)
13. **Neuromuscular and cerebrovascular diseases**
14. **Pneumothorax**: Especially left sided. An important ST elevation can be exceptionally observed, probably in relation to coronary spasm triggered by pneumothorax.
15. **Toxicity secondary to cocaine abuse, drug abuse, etc.**

We should remember that myocardial involvement is not always diffuse in acute pericarditis or my-opericarditis and that the ST-segment elevation in pericarditis is not very important but can be concave with respect to the isoelectric line and can certainly mimic an ACS, especially if there is an associated myocarditis, in which there is very often a moderate increase of cardiac enzymes. The ECG and clinical evolution of the patient is quite important in establishing the correct diagnosis (Figures 4.48 and 4.49) (Guizton and Lacks, 1982). Typically, pericarditis frequently presents PR-interval deviations (elevation in VR and depression in II) due to atrial injury (Guizton and Lacks, 1982). The presence of precordial pain related with deep inspiration favours pericarditis. Also, the typical evolution of ECG in four phases (Figure 4.48A) supports this diagnosis. However very often the ECG in pericarditis is atypical and may even present dynamic changes of T wave before the ST-segment elevation.

The ST may be mildly elevated in V1–V2 as a normal variant presenting ascending slope of the T wave, a little convex with respect to isoelectric line (Figure 3.1B). Also, the ST-segment elevation in people with vagal overdrive or in cases of early repolarisation is usually mild (1–3 mm) and convex with respect to the isoelectric line and is often observed in many leads, especially in HP (see Figure 4.50). Characteristically, the ST-segment elevation in early repolarisation normalises during the exercise test, which is important in cases of doubt (Figure 7.3). Other different repolarisation abnormalities have also been described outside IHD, including the ST-segment elevation seen in sportsmen, which although usually has no clinical significance; sometimes it has a striking morphology. In these cases it is mandatory to rule out hypertrophic cardiomyopathy and IHD (Figure 4.51).

Brugada's syndrome (Figure 4.52) should be borne in mind due to its potential harmfulness. The ST-segment elevation in the right precordial leads is the key sign in the ECG of patients with Brugada's syndrome, which represents a risk marker for malignant arrhythmias (Wilde et al., 2002). The most typical electrocardiographic patterns are seen in Figure 4.52A. Furthermore, atypical Brugada's syndrome (Figure 4.52B) should be distinguished from the

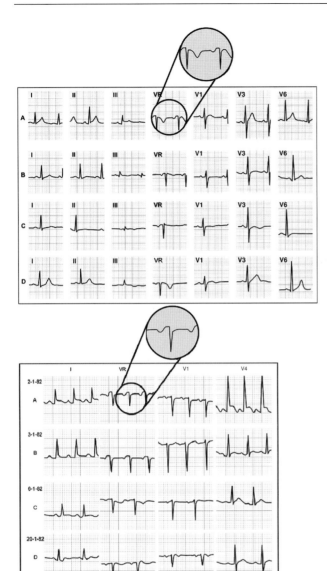

Figure 4.48 Above: Case of acute idiopathic pericarditis with the four electrocardiographic patterns that may be present: (A) The ST-segment elevation with the PR deviations (elevation or depression) in some leads. See especially the PR interval elevation in VR and a 'mirror' image in II. (B, C) Flattening of the T wave. (D) Normalisation of the ECG. Below: Other example of pericarditis with associated myocarditis. In the first phase can be seen in some leads ST-segment elevation, concave with respect to the isoelectric line. Lead VR also shows a clear elevation of the PR interval.

ST-segment elevation seen in athletes and chest abnormalities. The ST-segment elevation morphology in Brugada's syndrome is usually seen only up to V3, and it may reach up to V4–V5 in athletes. Also, usually the r' wave in V1 in athletes and pectus excavatum (Figure 4.52C, D) is tiny and narrow compared with the atypical pattern of Brugada's syndrome (Figure 4.52B). In case of ECG pattern type B it is recommended to rule out Brugada's syndrome (good history taking, to check changes of morphology after ajmaline test, etc.).

In arrhythmogenic right-ventricular dysplasia (Figure 4.53), an atypical pattern of RBBB in V1 with often some ST-segment elevation, especially in right precordial leads, may be seen.

Two other entities, which are important due to their very poor prognosis, may cause ST-segment elevation: pulmonary embolism (Figure 4.54) and dissecting aortic aneurysm (Figure 7.4). An example of ST-segment elevation in massive pulmonary embolism is shown in Figure 4.54, which coincides with the development of

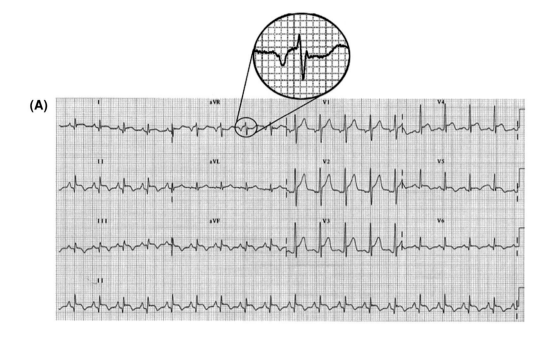

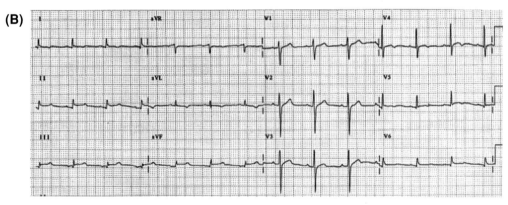

Figure 4.49 (A) A 39-year-old patient with long-standing precordial pain without ischaemic characteristics. There is an ST-segment elevation in many leads and in someone with final negative T wave but without Q waves and with PR elevation in VR with depression in II. The clinical history, ECG and the follow-up (B) with an ECG that shows a typical evolution of pericarditis confirms this diagnosis. In this case was small elevation of troponin I that may be seen frequently in cases of pericarditis.

an RBBB pattern due to the sudden dilation of the RV.

Figures 4.55 and 4.56 are examples of hyperkalaemia and hypothermia that may also present ST-segment elevation in some leads. An ST-segment elevation may also be seen in other situations (Table 4.3), such as certain ionic or metabolic disorders, pneumothorax, etc., and, obviously, in secondary repolarisation abnormalities, such as mirror patterns (e.g. in V1–V2 in LVE or in LBBB).

Electrocardiographic pattern of subendocardial injury in patients with narrow QRS: diagnosis and differential diagnosis

The ECG pattern of subendocardial injury (ST-segment depression) is found in different clinical settings of IHD (Figures 4.57–4.64), but may also be observed in other situations (Figure 4.65). We will now discuss the diagnostic

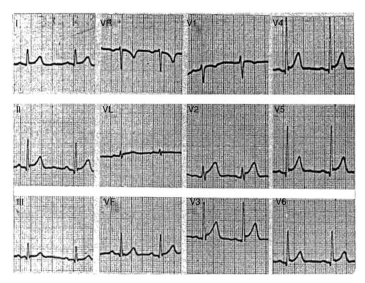

Figure 4.50 ECG of a young 40-year-old man. Typical example of early repolarisation (ST-segment elevation particularly evident in V2–V5 and in some leads of FP).

and location criteria of this pattern, and later on in Chapter 2 we will comment about the specific characteristics of the ECG pattern in different clinical settings of IHD, especially in relation with prognosis.

ST-segment depression in IHD

Diagnostic criteria: morphology and voltage (Figures 4.57–4.64)

There are electrocardiographic criteria based on ST-segment abnormalities (Table 4.4 and Figure 4.57) indicative of a positive exercise stress test in patients with suspicion of IHD or after MI evaluation. Some variables could also cause false-positive and false-negative results (Table 4.5). Characteristically, the ST-segment depression is observed in leads with dominant R wave, especially in V4–V6, I and VL, or even in inferior leads but is not seen as a most evident change only in V1–V3. Recently, it has been reported (Polizos and Ellestad 2006) that 1-mm upsloping ST-segment depression at 70 milliseconds past the J point has a sensitivity and specificity of 82 and 90%, respectively, compared with SPECT image. If we use only as abnormal criteria the horizontal and downsloping ST segment, the sensitivity and specificity compared

with SPECT are lower (65 and 88%). In the absence of clinical signs, false-positive results are frequently found, sometimes with evident ST-segment depression and/or negative T waves secondary to hyperventilation or other causes (Figure 4.58; see Plate 3). Furthermore, hyperventilation can cause repolarisation abnormalities in the form off lattened or negative T waves or even a generally mild ST-segment depression. These changes can be misleading, especially if they appear during an exercise test. The development of repolarisation abnormalities in relation with a provoked hyperventilation, prior to the exercise stress test, aids in the definitive diagnosis.

Small ST-segment depressions in an isolated ECG must be assessed with caution. But in the presence of recent chest pain or in the course of an ACS, ST-segment depressions of 0.5–1.0 mm that appear in sequential ECGs in two or more consecutive leads*can be considered diagnostic in themselves (Holper et al., 2001). However for other authors (McConahay, McCallister and Smith,

---

*In the horizontal plane, there is no problem – V1–V6 are consecutive leads – but in frontal plane, the consecutive leads are the following: VL, I, –VR, II, VF and III (Wagner and Pahlm, 2006).

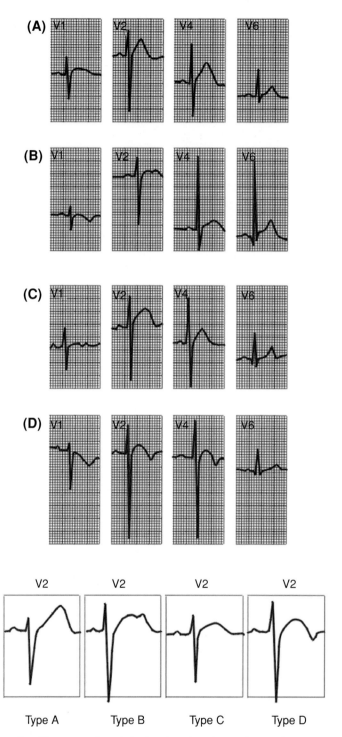

Figure 4.51 Above: Examples of four types of repolarisation alterations that can be seen in sportsmen without heart disease (Plas, 1976). Below: Drawings of more typical changes in V2.

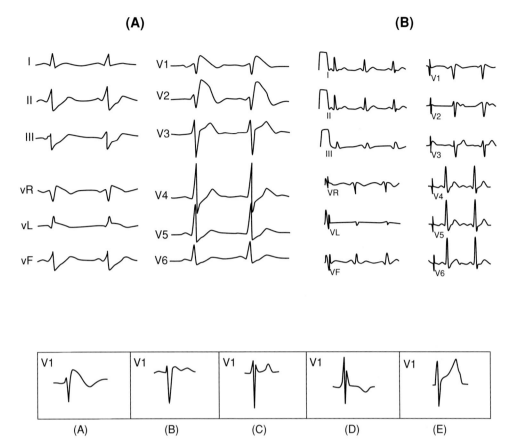

Figure 4.52 Above: Example of the ST-segment elevation in Brugada's syndrome. Typical (A) and atypical (B) patterns. Below: V1. (A, B) Typical and atypical patterns of Brugada's syndrome. (C) The ECG pattern seen in pectus excavatus (see Figure 3.1G). Observe the narrow r' compared to r' of (B) and similar to r' of (D). (D) ECG pattern seen in some athletes probably a marker of mild-RV enlargement. (E) Normal variant.

1971), in order to increase the specificity, an ST-segment depression >1 mm is more convenient (p. 234). It is important to demonstrate that these findings represent new changes, as, frequently, ST segment with mild depression is found in chronic coronary patients.

The morphology of ST-segment depression is more difficult to assess in the presence of a wide QRS complex or LVE. In this situation mixed repolarisation changes can be observed (alterations secondary to LVH or LBBB and primary alterations due to ischaemia) (see 'ECG pattern of injury in patients with ventricular hypotrophy and/or wide QRS') (p. 120).

Location criteria: from the ECG to the occluded artery (Tables 8.1 and 8.2)

The electrocardiographic pattern of subendocardial injury in patients with ACSs is recorded in different leads, depending on the coronary artery involved and the location of the injured area. When the ischaemia is due to left main trunk (LMT) subocclusion or equivalent, or 3 proximal vessel diseases, the involvement of the left ventricle is **circumferential.** In case of single vessel disease or when in presence of multivessel disease, the "active ischaemia" is due to a culprit artery or two distal occlusions the involvement is considered **regional** (Sclarovsky 1989). The correlation between these

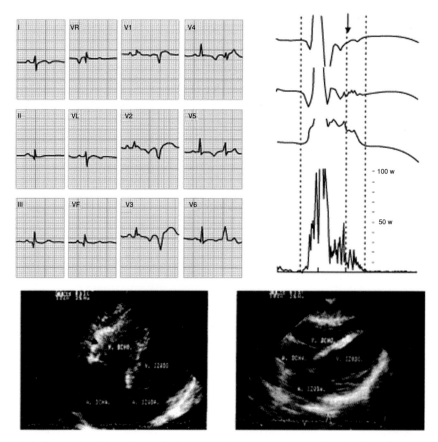

Figure 4.53 Arrhythmogenic right ventricular dysplasia (ARVD). Note the image of atypical right bundle branch block, negative T wave in the V1-V4 leads, and premature ventricular complexes of the right ventricle. QRS duration is much longer in V1-2 than in V6. On the right very positive late potentials are seen in the signal averaging ECG. Below: typical echocardiography image of right ventricle dyskinesia (see arrow) in a patient with ARVD.

two types of involvement and the ECG is not so exact as in cases of transmural injury (STE-ACS), especially the cases of regional involvement. However, there are some morphologies that provide useful information. Following, these will be commented on. In the second part of this book the clinical and prognostic aspects of these patterns will be discussed in detail (see p. 233).

ST-segment depression

(a) Circumferential involvement: A new ST-segment depression is seen in many leads (≥7) with or without dominant R wave, and in some leads (V3–V5) the ST-segment depression may be very significant (≥5 mm). A mirror pattern is seen in VR and sometimes in V1 (Table 8.1, and Figures

4.59–4.61). These cases correspond to LMT incomplete occlusion or three-vessel disease (Yamaji et al., 2001; Kosuge et al., 2005; Sclarovsky, 2001; Nikus, Eskola and Sclarovsky, 2006). Usually, cases with negative T wave in V4–V6 correspond to LMT incomplete occlusion (Figure 4.59). Cases with three-vessel disease more frequently present terminal positive T wave in V3–V5 and, often, a smaller depression of ST (Figure 4.60). According to Kosuge et al. (2005) in patients with NSTE-ACS, the presence of ST-segment elevation in aVR usually ≥1 mm is the best predictor of LMT/three-vessel disease.

Figure 4.9 shows how in case of LMT incomplete occlusion the circumferential diffuse subendocardial injury explains the ST-segment changes. However, we have to remind that rarely cases of critical

ACS: diagnostic criteria according to the ST-segment depression in patients with a narrow QRS complex (measured at 60 ms from the J point)

- Flattened or downsloping ST-segment depression at least ≥0.5 mm in at least two consecutive leads.

- Changes should be of new onset or dynamic.

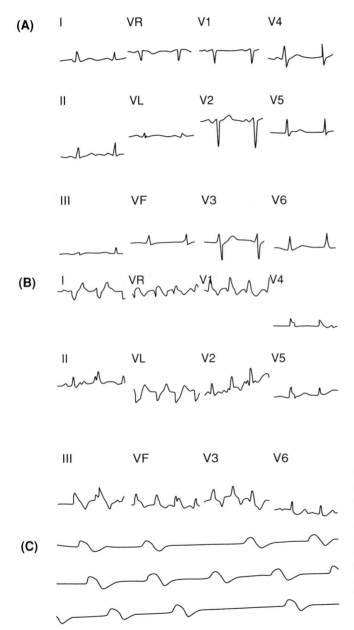

Figure 4.54 (A) Preoperative ECG of a 58-year-old patient without heart disease. (B) In a postoperative period the patient suffered from massive pulmonary embolism with the ECG showing an ÂQRS pointing sharply to the right, complete right bundle branch block with the ST-segment elevation in some leads and sinus tachycardia. The P wave is visible in the majority of leads with occasional premature beats. (C) Patient died within minutes: the ECG in agonic rhythm.

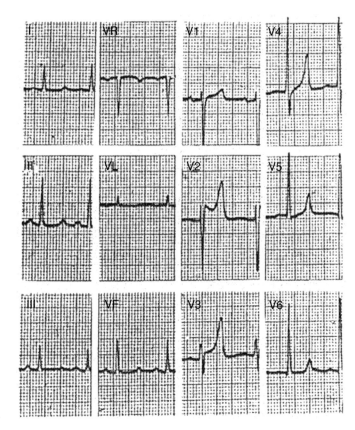

Figure 4.55 A 20-year-old patient with chronic renal failure submitted to periodical haemodialysis during last years, presenting with significant hypertension (230/130). The potassium level is elevated (6.4 mEq/L). Observe a tall and peaked T wave, as well as the ST-segment elevation in V2–V3. A relatively long QT interval is due to the ST-segment lengthening produced by coexisting hypocalcaemia (see V6 and I).

or even total LMT occlusion, as happens in coronary dissection, and some rare cases of LMT critical occlusion due to atherothrombosis without important previous subendocardial ischaemia and no collateral circulation may present an ACS with STE-ACS (Figure 4.44). These patients are rarely seen because they usually present catastrophic haemodynamic impairment and/or sudden death due to ventricular fibrillation (see p. 234).

(b) Regional involvement: The cases with regional involvement present the greatest difficulties to locate through the correlation with ECG patterns the place of occluded artery. Although with limitations we may distinguish two types of patterns:

–**New ST-segment depression not very striking (<2–3 mm) and generally seen in fewer than six leads** more frequently in lateral than in inferior leads (Table 8.1B, and Figures 4.62–4.64): This

---

Patients with an ACS due to proximal LAD involvement may present the following:

(a) **A clear STE-ACS with ST-segment elevation in precordials and ST-segment depression in inferior leads** (see Table 4.1).

(b) **Atypical pattern of STE-ACS: deep negative T wave from V1 to V5–V6** (Figures 3.21 and 8.3).

(c) **NSTE-ACS: a flat or slightly negative T wave in V1–V3 and also a negative U wave may be seen** (Figure 8.23).

(d) **NSTE-ACS: an ST-segment depression especially seen in precordial leads usually more evident in V2–V3 to V4–V5** with T wave with a final positive deflection (Nikus, Eskola and Virtanen, 2004).

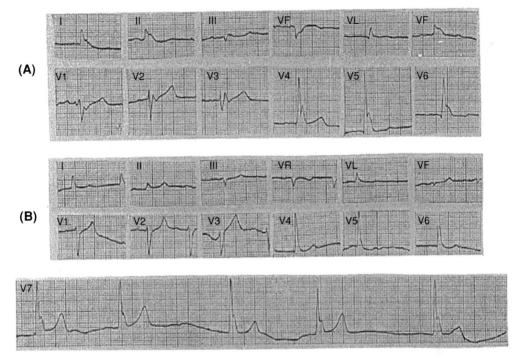

Figure 4.56 (A) A 76-year-old patient with hypothermia and the ECG typically seen in this condition. Note the J, or Osborne wave, typical of hypothermia at the end of the QRS complex and/or the ST-segment elevation; sinus bradychardia; long QT interval and an irregular baseline (lower strip). (B) When the problem was resolved after warming, the J wave disappeared completely (long recording of V4 during hypothermia).

Table 4.4 Electrocardiographic criteria of the positive exercise test.

- Horizontal or downsloping ST depression ≥ 0.5 mm in at least two consecutive leads usually with RS or R morphology (see p. 111; Gibbons, et al. 2002, Ellestad, 2004, Aros, et al. 2000). The criteria is more specific if the ST depression is ≥ 1 mm
- ST segment elevation ≥ 1 mm

Also suggestive are

- Horizontal or downsloping ST depression ≥ 1 mm in at least two consecutive leads beyond 70 ms (SE ≅ 65% and SP ≅ 90%)
- Upsloping ST-segment depression ≥ 1 mm beyond 70 ms from the J point. Using also this criterion, the SE increases (≅ 90%)
- Inverted U wave
- Appearance of serious ventricular arrhythmias at not important exercise level (<70% of the predicted maximum heart rate)

Table 4.5 The most frequent false-positive and false-negative results of exercise test.

False-positive results

- Drugs: digitalis, diuretics, antidepressant, sedative drugs, oestrogens, etc.
- Heart diseases: cardiomyopathy, valvular heart disease, pericarditis, hypertension, ECG alterations (left bundle branch block, WPW, repolarisation alterations, etc).
- Miscellaneous: thoracic abnormalities (pectus excavatum), female sex, hyperventilation, glucose intake and ionic disorders etc.

False-negative results

- Drugs: beta-blocking, antianginal agents
- Inadequate exercise: early termination of the exercise test and inadequate physical training level
- Technical problems

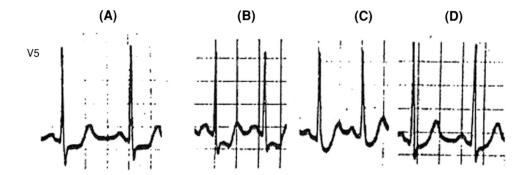

V5

(A)   (B)   (C)   (D)

Figure 4.57 Different types of subendocardial injury patterns that appeared in the course of an exercise test: (A) Horizontal displacement of the ST segment, (B) descendant displacement, (C) concave displacement and (D) ST-segment depression from J point with ascendant morphology and with rapid upsloping. This usually is seen in normal cases (Figure 4.2). The coronary angiography was abnormal in (A), (B) and (C), and normal in (D). These changes are especially visible in leads with dominant R wave especially V3–V4 to V5–V6, I and VL, and/or inferior leads present dominant R wave.

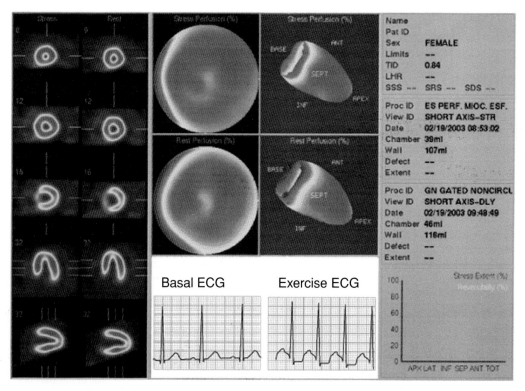

Figure 4.58 Patient with atypical precordial pain and a clearly positive exercise test (marked ST-segment depression) without pain during the test. The SPECT test was normal (see homogeneous uptake in red), as well as coronary angiography. It is a clear example of a false-positive exercise test. This figure can be seen in color, Plate 3.

ST-segment depression may appear during an exercise test (Figures 4.62–4.64) or occurs in a dynamic way during an ACS (Figure 4.63). The cases with worst prognosis present ST-segment depression in V4–V6 and some leads of FP and the T wave is negative in V4–V6 (Birnbaum and Atar 2000) (Figure 4.63) (see p. 237). In spite that sometimes the ECG changes are small, the patient may present severe coronary atherosclerosis (Figure 4.62).

–New ST-segment depression usually not very striking and most evident in precordial leads with and without dominant R wave (from V2–V3 to V4–V5): It is accompanied by a positive T wave in V3–V5. In this case the culprit artery is in general proximal LAD occlusion (Table 8.1B; Nikus, Eskola and Virtanen, 2004). Characteristically, as happens in exercise testing, the ST-segment depression is not usually present as the most evident changes in leads with rS morphology (V1–V2).

Very often patients with or without IHD usually present mild ST-segment depression, related or not with the presence of LVH (hypertension or other diseases) or of an unknown cause. This ECG pattern has to be considered as a risk factor for future events but only if there is an increase in the ST-segment depression with exercise or pain, can it be considered as a suggestive of 'active' ischaemia. (fig 4.68B)

ST-segment depression in other clinical settings (Figure 4.65)

In Figure 4.65 the most frequent causes of ST-segment depression, aside from IHD, are shown. The most striking changes are those secondary to the digitalis effect (Figure 4.65A), ionic abnormalities (Figure 4.65B) and those seen in different heart diseases, such as mitral valve prolapse (Figure 4.65C). During and following a paroxysmal tachycardia, ST-segment/T-wave abnormalities may be seen with non-demonstrable ischaemia. The negative T wave is sometimes more striking than the ST-segment depression (Figure 3.36).

Frequently, the ST-segment depression and/or the negative T wave in the course of a paroxysmal tachycardia are mild, but diffuse and often quickly reversible when the crisis ceases. The paroxysmal tachycardia is sometimes accompanied by chest

(A)

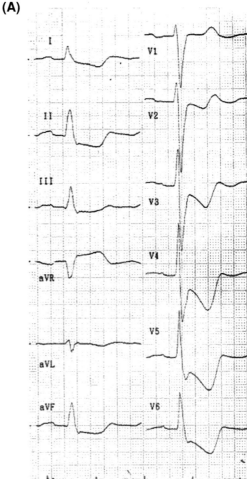

(B)

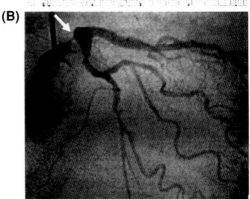

Figure 4.59 (A) The ECG of a patient with ACS and the ECG typical of tight but incomplete occlusion of the left main coronary artery (see coronary angiography) (B) in the presence at basal state of important and circumferential subendocardial ischaemia. There is ST-segment depression in more than eight leads and clear ST-segment elevation in VR. Note that the maximum depression occurs in V3–V4 without final positive T wave in V4–V5.

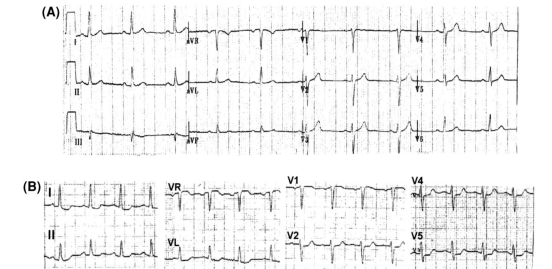

Figure 4.60 (A) Normal control 'ECG of a patient with chronic ischaemic heart disease'. (B) During an NSTE-ACS diffuse and mild-ST-segment depression in many leads, especially seen in I, V5 and V6 with small ST-segment elevation seen in III, VR and V1. The coronary angiography shows three-vessel disease with severe proximal obstruction in LAD + LCX.

pain of doubtful significance. When the pain is suggestive of angina, especially in a patient with risk factors, it is advisable to perform a coronary angiography, which is generally negative.

The occurrence of false-positive cases of ST-segment depression during an exercise stress test has already been addressed. These are due to different causes (hyperventilation, drugs, etc.) or are of unknown origin (Table 4.5 and Figure 4.58). In some circumstances (neurocirculatory asthenia, hyperventilation, etc.), their origin is unknown or difficult to explain.

ST-segment depression, mild and generally with non-descending slope, can be observed in the absence of evident heart disease, especially in women and the elderly. They are sometimes hypertension related, especially when there is concurrent LVE. It is especially important to check the appearance of these ST-segment depressions during exercise or if changes in clinical situations are suggestive of an ACS.

Diagnosis of the electrocardiographic pattern of injury in patients with LVH and/or wide QRS complex (Figures 4.66–4.68)

In cases of LVH with strain pattern and/or wide QRS complex, the electrocardiographic diagnosis of injury pattern is frequently more difficult, especially in the presence of an LBBB or pacemaker. However, in some ACS, especially those secondary to the total proximal occlusion of an epicardial coronary artery, ST-segment elevation are well seen in the presence of complete RBBB (Figure 4.66), and also in the course of ACS the presence of complete LBBB or pacemaker allows us to visualise usually very well the ST-segment elevation (Figures 4.67 and 4.68A).

Sgarbossa et al. (1996b; 2001) have reported that in cases compatible with acute MI, **a diagnosis of evolving infarction associated with a complete LBBB is supported by the following criteria** (Figure 4.67):

(A)

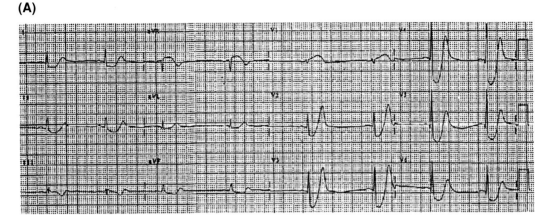

(B)

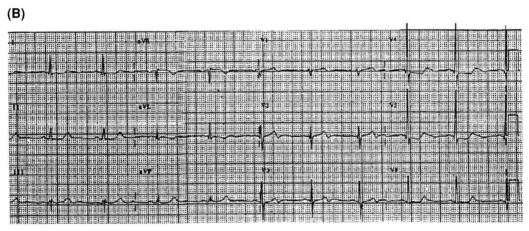

Figure 4.61 (A) The ECG of a patient with an NSTE-ACS that presents during angina a huge ST-segment depression in many leads more prominent in precordial leads V3–V5 with positive T wave and with ST-segment elevation in VR and V1. (B) ECG at rest with signs of mild subendocardial injury.

1 ↑ ST > 1 mm concordant with the QRS complex
2 ↓ ST > 1 mm concordant with the QRS complex
3 ↑ ST > 5 mm non-concordant with the QRS complex (e.g. in V1–V2)

This last criterion is of less value when the QRS complex has an increased voltage (Madias, Sinha and Ashtiani, 2001).

These criteria have been studied by other authors (Kontos et al., 2001), who have confirmed that they are highly specific (100%), especially in the presence of concordant ST-segment elevation or depression, though they are not very sensitive (10–20%).

Recently, it has been reported (Wong et al., 2005, 2006a, b) that patients with RBBB or LBBB have different prognoses, depending on the ST-segment morphology and QRS duration (p. 248).

Similar criteria are also useful for the diagnosis of infarction in the presence of a pacemaker (Sgarbossa et al., 1996a).

Occasionally, the presence of an intermittent RBBB (Figure 4.66) or LBBB (Figure 4.67) allows for the visualisation of the underlying repolarisation abnormality, such as ST-segment deviation (Figures 4.66 and 4.67) or a negative T wave (Figures 3.34 and 3.41). Therefore, the evidence that

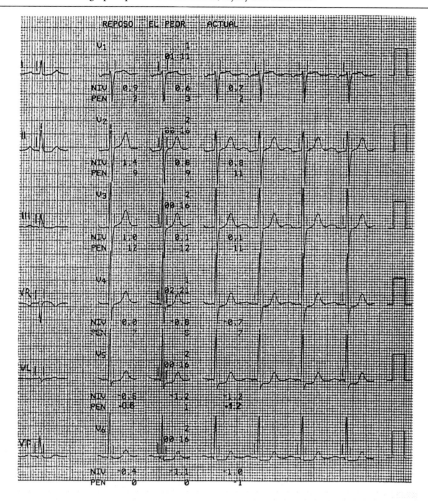

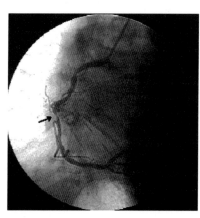
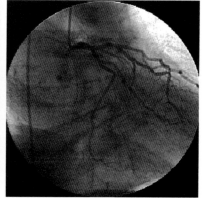

Figure 4.62   Above: (Left) A 65-year-old man with typical in-crescendo angina, and practically normal ECG at rest. Only in some leads there is an ST-segment depression but not higher than 0.5 mm. (Right) During exercise test appears anginal pain and an evident, but not huge, increase in the ST-segment depression (greater than 0.5 mm), in spite that the patient presents not very striking ECG changes. Below: The coronary angiography shows in proximal three-vessel disease. The patient was submitted to a triple bypass.

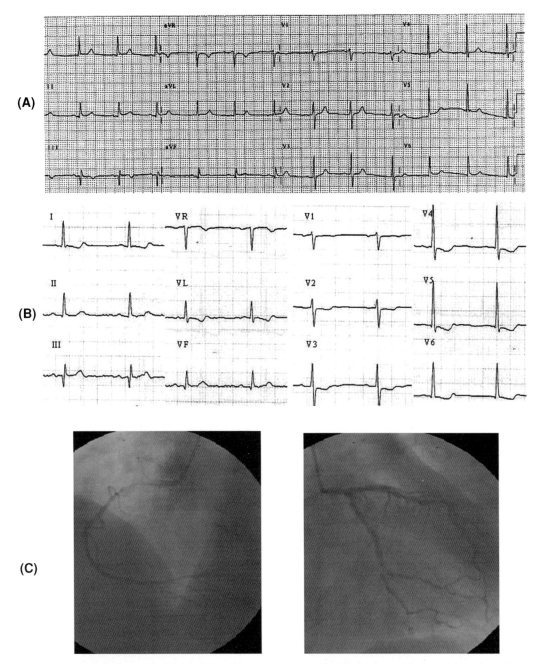

Figure 4.63 (A) ECG without pain. (B) ECG during pain in the course of NSTE-ACS. The ECG shows ST-segment depression not very prominent (<3 mm) in V4–V6 and I and VL with negative T wave in V4 and V5. No clear mirror image can be seen. (C) Coronary angiography shows a three-vessel disease.

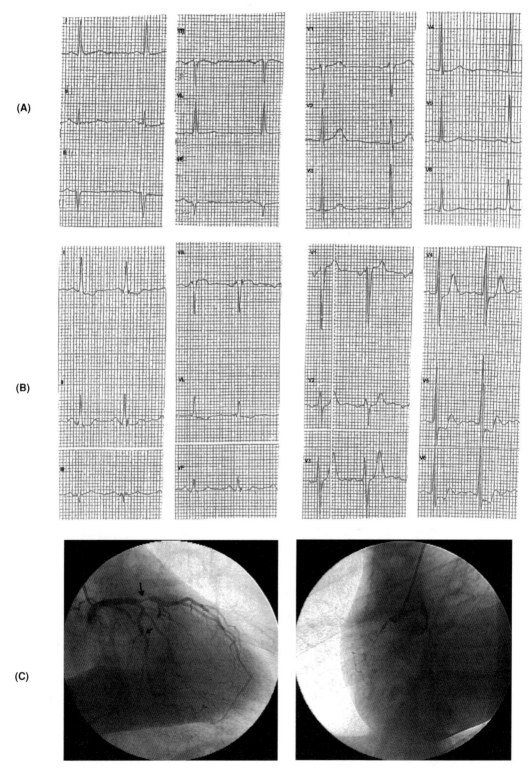

Figure 4.64 (A) Patient with precordial pain at exercise and a rest ECG that presents slightly flattened T wave in lateral leads. (B) The exercise test shows a clear ST-segment depression with the presence of the same pain. (C) The coronary angiography shows obstructive lesions in the three main vessels (complete occlusion in RCA).

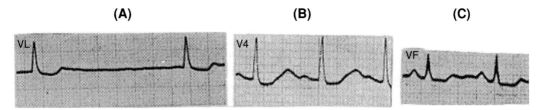

Figure 4.65 Non-ischaemic ST-segment depression.
(A) ST-segment depression secondary to digitalis effect: note the typical digitalis 'scooped' pattern with a short QT interval in a patient with slow atrial fibrillation.
(B) Example of hypokalaemia in a patient with congestive heart failure who was receiving high doses of furosemide. What seems to be a long QT interval is probably a QU interval (T+positive U waves). (C) Case of mitral valve prolapse with ST-segment depression in inferior leads.

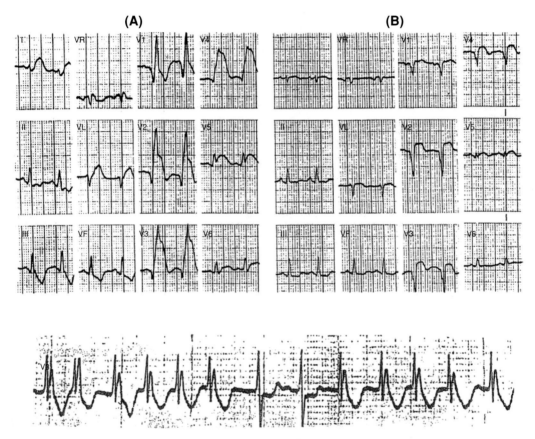

Figure 4.66 Above: (A) Acute phase of evolving Q-wave myocardial infarction of anteroseptal zone. There is a huge ST-segment elevation, especially in I, VL and from V2 to V5, QRS >0.12 s and morphology of complete RBBB that was not present in previous ECG. (B) Twenty-four hours later RBBB have disappeared and subacute anterior extensive infarction becomes evident. There is ST-segment elevation from V1 to V4. The transient presence of new complete RBBB (RBB is perfused by S1) suggests that the occlusion of LAD is proximal to S1 and D1. Below: The ECG of a patient that presents rapid atrial fibrillation and RBBB. In the seventh and eighth complexes can be seen the disappearance of tachycardia-dependent RBBB, and then the morphology of subendocardial injury pattern appears. The complexes with RBBB present also a typical mixed pattern (see Figure 3.27).

(A)   **(B)**   **(C)**

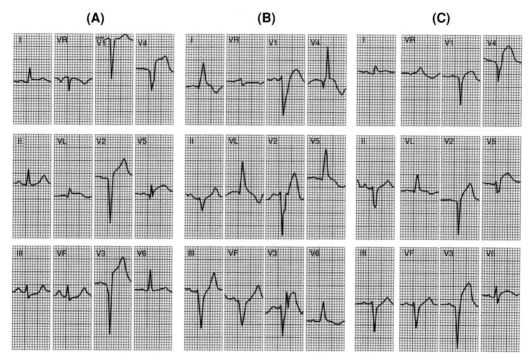

Figure 4.67 (A) Acute MI of anteroseptal zone due to occlusion of LAD proximal to D1 (ST-segment depression in III and VF) but distal to S1 (non-ST-segment elevation in VR and V1 and non-ST-segment depression in V6). (B) After some hours complete LBBB appears (see q in I, VL and V4 and polyphasic morphology in V3) (see the Sgarbossa criteria, concordant ST-segment elevation, in I, VL, V4–V6). (C) The complete LBBB disappears but superoanterior hemiblock remains with the clear evidence of apical-anterior MI (QS from V1 to V4 without 'q' in VL and I) (see Figure 5.9A(2)).

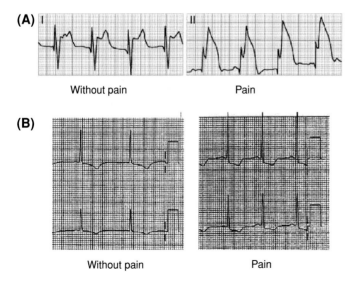

Figure 4.68 (A) Patient with pacemaker and acute STE-ACS. During an angina pain crisis of Prinzmetal type, a marked transient ST-segment elevation is seen. (B) 62-year-old patient with hypertension that presents an NSTE-ACS. Left: Without pain, there is a mixed pattern of LVH with strain+negative T wave. Right: During pain, a clear ST-segment depression appears.

there is somewhat different repolarisation pattern, with a generally more symmetric and deeper T wave, in the presence of a bundle branch block, is very much in favour of mixed origin of the ECG pattern (Figures 3.40, 3.41 and 4.66).

In cases of LVH with strain pattern, often also some type of mixed patterns may be seen (Figure 3.27). The diagnosis, however, may usually be performed if sequential changes appear (increase in ST-segment depression already present) (Figure 4.68B).

CHAPTER 5

Electrocardiographic pattern of necrosis: abnormal Q wave

Limits of the normal Q wave

How the width and height of the Q wave and other ECG parameters are measured is shown in Figure 5.1. Normal Q waves in different leads show the following characteristics:

Leads I and II: In the presence of a qR morphology, the 'q' wave is usually narrow (less than 0.04 s) and not very deep (less than 2 mm), though it can measure up to 3 or 4 mm, on occasion. In general, it never measures more than 25% of the following R wave. The R wave is usually more than 5–7 mm. It is not a normal qrS morphology in these leads.

Lead III: The 'q' wave, if present, is narrow (less than 0.04 s), not very deep, and is generally followed by a low-voltage 'r' wave (qrs or qrsr' complex). In horizontal hearts it may be seen in normal cases, a relatively deep 'Q' wave, with a Q/R ratio ≥1, which usually disappears during deep respiration or in standing position.

VR lead: QS or Qr morphologies are frequently found, the Q wave sometimes being ≥0.04 seconds. In the presence of 'rS' morphology, the normal 'r' wave must be narrow and not tall; when it measures 1 mm or higher, though it may be normal, it is mandatory to rule out the presence of heart disease. In patients with MI the presence of r > 1mm suggests low-lateral involvement.

VL lead: The 'q'-wave duration is normally shorter than 0.04 seconds and its depth is less than 2 mm. Occasionally, in normal individuals, 'q' wave measures more than 25% of the following 'R' wave. However it is not a normal qrs morphology. In some vertical hearts with no underlying cardiac disease, a narrow 'QS' morphology without notches and/or slurrings may be seen in VL. This pattern must be considered to be the expression of left intracavitary morphology. In these cases, P and T waves are usually flat or negative as well. It is not normal for an R wave to be of lower voltage than the Q wave.

Lead VF: The 'q'-wave duration is normally shorter than 0.04 seconds and not deeper than 2 mm or, at the most, 3 mm. Generally, it never has a voltage higher than 25% of the following 'R' wave. Nevertheless, when the following 'R' wave is of low voltage, the Q/R ratio lacks diagnostic value. 'Q' waves usually with QR morphology may be seen in some normal individuals and usually disappear in the sitting or standing position or with deep inspiration. A QS complex which turns into an rS complex with deep inspiration has been shown to be usually normal, although exceptions may occur. In turn, the QS complex turning into a Qr complex during deep respiration is probably abnormal.

Precordial leads: Normally, a 'q' wave is seen in V5–V6. In a heart with levorotation, a 'q' wave may be seen as from V3, but only in complexes with qRs morphology, while 'q' waves are not usually seen in any precordial lead in dextrorotated heart. Q waves are never present in V1 or V2. The 'q'-wave duration in the precordial leads is usually shorter than 0.04 seconds and of less than 2 mm in depth, or it does not exceed 15% of the following R wave. It is not normal a qrs morphology in V6 with r < 6–7 mm. Normal 'q' waves that are recorded in the intermediate precordial leads become deeper towards the left precordial leads and are followed by a tall R wave. The R wave in the left precordial leads is usually higher than 5–6 mm. Normal 'q' waves should exhibit no significant slurring in any lead.

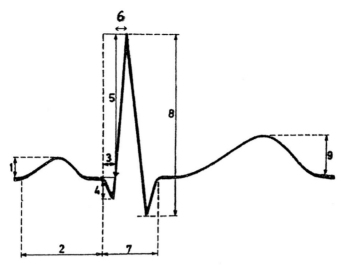

Figure 5.1 Measurement of ECG parameters: (1) voltage of the P wave: vertical interval from the superior border of the baseline to the peak of P wave; (2) PR interval: from the onset of P wave to the onset of QRS; (3) Q-wave duration: from the point where the superior border of PR starts to descend up to the left border of the ascending arm of R wave; (4) Q-wave voltage: from the inferior border of PR to the peak of Q wave; (5) voltage of R wave: vertical distance from the superior border of PR to the peak of R wave; (6) intrinsic deflection: horizontal distance between the onset of QRS and R peak; (7) QRS duration: horizontal distance from the beginning of the descent of the superior border of PR to the end of the ascendant arm of S wave or descendent arm of R wave; (8) QRS voltage: vertical distance from the most negative to the most positive peak of QRS complex; (9) voltage of T wave: vertical distance between the superior border of the baseline and the peak of T wave.

Changes of QRS due to MI: abnormal Q wave of necrosis and fractioned QRS

In presence of infarction, a **significant diastolic depolarisation** exists in the infarcted area. Thus, **such an area is non-excitable and does not generate a TAP (Figure 2.1(4))**. When diastolic depolarisation is not only significant but also extensive, affecting the entire or a large area of the ventricular wall, the ECG usually records an abnormal Q wave (**Q wave of necrosis**). **The Q wave of necrosis** is generated asa consequence of the change induced by infarction in areas of LV that depolarises the first 40–50 milliseconds (see p. 131 'Theories to explain the Q wave of necrosis', and Figures 5.2 and 5.3).

Anomalies in the mid-late part of QRS (as slurrings, rsr' or very low voltage QRS in left precordial leads) may occur, either isolated or with Q wave, as a consequence of necrosis of areas of late depolarisation (Horan and Flowers, 1972; Horan, Flowers and Johnson, 1971). Recently, it has been reported (Das et al., 2006) that in coronary patients the presence of these anomalies known as **fractioned QRS** has more accuracy to diagnose necrosis than the existence of Q wave (Figures 9.3 and 9.4). However, it is important to remind that these morphologies may sometimes be seen in normal individuals. In Chapter 2 we will comment on more aspects of these changes when we discuss the MI of areas of late depolarisation (see 'Infarction of the basal parts of left ventricle') (p. 291).

Measurement and assessment of Q and R waves can be done according to the Minnesota code (Blackburn et al., 1960) (Figure 5.1). To define a wave as having QS morphology, one should have on mind the following aspects: (a) the presence of an R wave (R > 0.25 mm) in any of the complexes of a given lead cancels the possibility of QS existence; (b) positive deflection (R > 1 mm) that follows any negative deflection is classified as R wave and cancels QS definition if existing in the majority of complexes in a given lead. Finally, one should not confound an rsR' pattern with an ST-segment elevation. Sometimes in Brugada's syndrome there is ST-segment elevation in V1 but not terminal R, although it has been considered that the morphology was of RBBB.

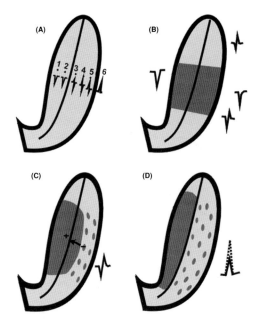

Figure 5.2 (A) Normal ventricular depolarisation does not generate measurable potentials in the subendocardium (1 and 2) because it is quite rapid, as this area is rich in Purkinje fibres. Starting at the limit with the subendocardium (3), morphologies with an increasingly tall R wave (rS, RS and Rs) are being generated, until reaching an R-wave morphology in the epicardial recording (6). Consequently, when an experimental necrosis is produced, it generates only a Q wave when it reaches the subepicardium, because then measurable necrosis vectors are generated. These vectors will become larger, as they are moving away from a necrotic area that also becomes larger. This generates qR morphologies in (3), QR in (4) and (5), until attaining a QS complex when the necrosis is transmural. Likewise, in clinical practice, a transmural infarction gives rise to a QS complex (B), and an infarction that involves the subendocardium and part of the subepicardium, not being necessarily transmural (C), generates QR morphology. Finally, an infarction that involves the subendocardium and part of the subepicardium, but in patches, sparing areas of subepicardium close to the subendocardium, allows for the development of normal depolarisation vectors from the onset, but smaller which will be recorded as an R wave, although with a lower voltage (D).

The presence of Q wave does not invariably imply that the tissue is irreversibly injured – i.e. dead – because in some cases when the ischaemia resolves, such as in coronary spasm, the Q wave may be of a transient nature (Table 5.5, p. 175).

On the other hand, we have to remind that Q wave of infarction may be seen in absence of infarction (**Q wave without infarction**) (see 'Differential di-

agnosis of the infarction Q wave' p. 168) or that MI may exist without Q waves (**infarction without Q wave**) (see 'Myocardial infarction without Q wave or equivalent' p. 289).

Further ahead (see 'Diagnosis of Q-wave MI in the presence of abnormal intraventricular conduction'), (p. 170) the characteristics of an abnormal Q wave in the presence of abnormal intraventricular conduction will be dealt with.

Electrophysiological mechanism of Q wave of necrosis

Ventricular activation and morphology of the normal QRS complex and of the MI with and without Q wave (Q-wave MI vs non-Q wave MI)

Since almost 50 years (Cabrera, 1958), it has been considered that subendocardium depolarisation was silent from an electrical point of view, because, as it is an area rich in Purkinje fibres, the electrical stimulus is distributed with such a velocity through this network that the time it takes does not allow for the creation of wavefronts with measurable potentials (Figure 5.2A). Consequently, a QS morphology is recorded in the subendocardium, as well as in the left-ventricular cavity (Figure 5.2A(1–2)). Only when the stimulus reaches the subepicardium, wavefronts begin to be generated, with the positive electrical charges directed towards the epicardium, thereby producing the R wave of the ventriculogram (Figure 5.2A(3–6)).

It can thus be understood why exclusively subendocardium experimental infarction does not generate changes in the QRS complex and, therefore, does not give rise to the development of Q waves. If part of the subepicardium is affected, a **QR morphology** is recorded (Figure 5.2C), as vector of infarctions that move away from the area are generated. Thus, increasingly deep Q waves can be observed as the involved subepicardium area increases. When the infarction is entirely transmural and homogeneous, a **QS complex is recorded** (Figure 5.2B). When the infarction spares the subepicardium area that is in contact with the subendocardium, the activation fronts are generated and give rise to an R wave, although the voltage of the R wave decreases in accordance with the patched ventricular subepicardium areas involved (**non-Q-wave infarction**) (Figure 5.2D). Thus, it is logical that in the clinical

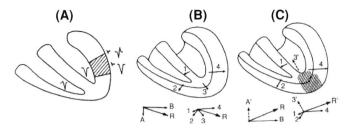

Figure 5.3 (A) Under normal conditions, the overall QRS vector (R) is made up of the sum of the different ventricular vectors (1 + 2 + 3 + 4). (B) When a necrotic (infarcted) area exists, the vector of infarction has the same magnitude as the previous vector, but has an opposite direction (3'). This change of direction of the initial depolarisation electrical forces of a portion of the heart, the necrotic (infarcted) area, also implies the change of the overall vector direction (R'). (C) The development of a necrosis Q wave when a transmural infarction with homogeneous involvement of the left ventricle exists may be explained because the necrotic tissue, which is non-activable, acts as an electrical window and allows for the recording of the left ventricular intracavitary QRS (which is a QS complex) from outside. The QS complex in left ventricle is explained because the normal activation vectors, 1, 2 and 3, are moving away from that cavity.

setting transmural infarctions with homogeneous involvement of all wall generates a QS or QR morphology in most cases, according to the place from which they are recorded (Figure 5.2B, C) or similar 'mirror' pattern morphologies (R wave in V1–V2 in some cases of the lateral infarction).

As we have previously affirmed, predominantly subendocardium infarctions can generate an infarction Q wave if they affect subepicardium areas of the ventricular wall that are in contact with the subendocardium, even though the wall is not homogeneously or necessarily transmurally affected. This occurs because in these situations a vector of infarction can arise (Q wave) (Figure 5.2C). Only when the stimulus reaches normal areas will an R wave be generated (QR complex).

Currently, the CMR images with gadolinium injection have demonstrated in very elegant manner (Mahrholdt et al., 2005a, b) how, after coronary occlusion, a wavefront of infarction starts in the subendocardium and evolves to a transmural infarction. With this technique it has been defined that there are infarctions predominantly in the subendocardium or transmural but never subepicardial (Figures 1.5 and 8.6) (see p. 216).

Theories to explain the Q wave of necrosis

The explanation of the Q wave of necrosis can be made on the basis of **the theory of the electrical window of Wilson or on the formation of a vector of infarction.** According to the **first theory**, the transmural and homogeneous infarcted area acts as an electrical window. Consequently, the electrode that faces that area records the negativity of the intracavitary QRS complex (Q wave of necrosis). It should be reminded that a QS morphology is recorded within the left-ventricular cavity, since all the vectors are directed away from this cavity (Figure 5.3A). Thus, when compromise of the wall is important, even when we now know that it is not always transmural and homogeneous, a pathologic Q wave (QS complex) or QR complex in the bordering zones is recorded (Figure 5.3A).

According to the **vector of infarction theory**, the infarction Q wave is of the same magnitude but in opposite direction to the one normally generated by the infarcted area (Figure 5.3B, C). **The vector of infarction, thus, moves away from the infarcted area** (see Figs. 5.3–5.5). For this reason, the beginning of ventricular depolarisation changes its

In summary, according to what has been discussed, it is understood that in the presence of an infarction that may affect extensive areas of the entire wall, but with predominant subendocardial compromise, one can find pathological Q waves on some occasions (Figure 5.2C) yet not on others (Figure 5.2D).

CE-CMR correlations have confirmed this concept (see p. 10 and 140). More information referring to non-Q-wave infarctions is dealt with in the second part of this book (see 'MI without Q wave or equivalent') (p. 289).

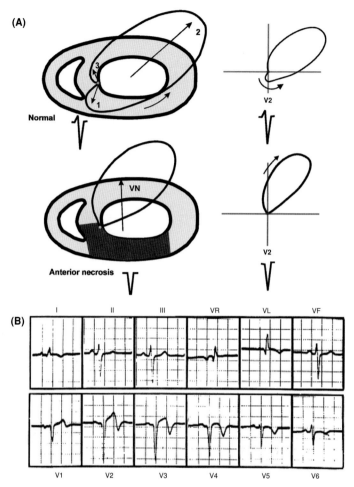

Figure 5.4 (A) Observe the comparison between the normal activation and the activation in case of an extensive anterior infarction. The vector of infarction is directed backwards and through the correlation loop–hemifield explains the appearance of the Q wave in anterior leads. (B) Example of MI of anteroseptal zone.

direction when the infarcted area corresponds to an area that depolarises within the first 40 milliseconds of ventricular activation, which is what occurs with most of the LV, with the exception of the basal areas. Thus it is clear that the basal areas of the heart do not generate Q wave. Therefore, the old concept that R wave in V1 is a mirror image of Q wave recorded in the back leads may not be any more accepted as generated in the basal part of inferoposterior wall of the heart (segment 4). Very recently (Bayés de Luna, 2006a), the correlation with cardiovascular magnetic resonance has demonstrated that the pattern RS in V1 is due to lateral MI (specially segments 11 and sometimes 12 and not to infarction of inferobasal segment 4 – old posterior wall) (see p. 139).

Diagnostic criteria of Q-wave MI and its location in different walls of the LV, in patients with normal intraventricular conduction

Introduction

In Figures 5.4 and 5.5 the changes that, as a consequence of the presence of the vector of infarction, are generated in the ventricular depolarisation loops in the presence of two prototype infarctions (anteroseptal and inferolateral areas, respectively) are represented. Said changes explain the presence of Q waves in the different leads by means of the loop–hemifield correlation. Some of the ECG morphologies and the QRS loops correlations in the seven types of infarctions, according to the classification

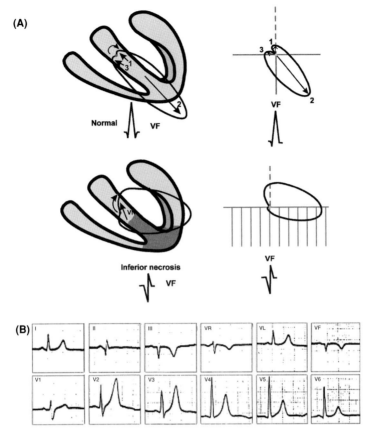

Figure 5.5 (A) See the comparison between normal activation and activation in case of inferolateral infarction. The vector of infarction is directed upwards and a loop–hemifield correlation explains the appearance of a Q wave in inferior leads. (B) Example of MI of inferolateral zone.

used in this book, are shown in Figure 5.6. In this figure the morphology of the loops is in agreement with the changes in direction of the ventricular activation forces, related with the vector of infarction. In the majority of QRS loops, the minimum number of milliseconds has been drawn in the initial part of the activation that must be affected to generate an infarction Q wave or R wave in V1. Naturally, this number varies according to the ventricular activation sequence, being lower, e.g. in the septal infarction (Figure 5.6A-1), than that in the lateral infarction (classically considered posterior infarction – see p. 138) (Figure 5.6B-1).

The leads that face the vector of infarction tail record morphologies with the Q wave of necrosis (QS or QR complexes). **Throughout this book we will use this concept – vector of infarction and changes that it generates in the morphology of the QRS loop and its projection in its respective** hemifields – **to explain the different electrocardiographic patterns that are observed in infarctions located in different areas of the heart** with important and often transmural involvement (**Q-wave infarction**).

ECG criteria of Q wave (or equivalent) MI

Since the early beginning of the ECG, criteria have been sought that would allow for the diagnosis of MI. They consist in the presence of the **necrosis Q wave** or equivalents, especially the presence of RS morphology in V1 as a mirror image of Q wave recorded in the back leads. The presence of Q wave or RS in V1 as a mirror image is consequence of the changes in the first 40–50 milliseconds induced by necrosis (vector of infaction).

Recently, it has been demonstrated by CMR (Moon et al., 2004) that the presence of Q wave is not indicative of transmural MI (p. 275). However,

ECG pattern	(A)	(B)	(C)
A **Anteroseptal zone**			
A - 1 ① Septal — Q in V1–V2			
A - 2 ② Apical anterior — Q in V1–V2 to V4–V6			
A - 3 ③ Extensive anterior — Q in V1–V2 to V4–V6 and/or I and VL			
A - 4 ④ Mid-anterior — QS (or qr) in VL and even in I sometimes 'q' in V2–V3			
B **Inferolateral zone**			
B - 1 ⑤ Lateral — RS (Rs) in V1 and/or 'qr' in V5–V6 and/or 'qr' (qrs) in I and VL			
B - 2 ⑥ Inferior — Q (QS, QR, Qr, qs) wide 'q' in II III, VF			
B - 3 ⑦ Inferolateral — Criteria 5 + 6			The loop is usually more to the right in case of very dominant LCX

Table 5.1 Criteria for Q-wave abnormality according to the classical criteria (Friedman, 1985).

Leads	Width (s)	Depth (mm)	Q/R Ratio (%)
I, II, VF	$\geq 0,04$	≥ 2	>25
V1–V3		Q wave is normally absent in these leads.	
V4–V6	≥ 0.04	≥ 2	15
VL	≥ 0.04	$\geq 2^{\dagger}$	>50
III*	≥ 0.04	≥ 2	>25

* To be considered a Q wave in III abnormal usually is required the presence of abnormal Q in II and/or VF. However the presence of QS pattern is often abnormal. Sometimes Q in lead III may be as much as 6 mm deep normally. Check the decrease or disappearance of Q with deep inspiration.
† QS may be seen in normal hearts in VL, usually in the presence of negative P wave (vertical heart) and in the absence of abnormal 'Q' in I and V6.

it is important to differentiate between MI with and without Q wave, because the former usually encompasses larger area (p. 276). It has already been described that the infarction of late depolarisation zones is responsible for the changes of the middle-late part of QRS (Horan, Flowers and Johnson, 1971) that are expressed by a loss of voltage of R wave especially in V5–V6 and/or rsr' morphology or slurrings in QRS in some leads (**fractioned QRS**) (Das et al., 2006) (see p. 291).

The criteria of Q-wave MI encompass increase of the width and deepness and changes in the Q/R ratio. These criteria were based especially in epidemiological studies (Minnesotta code – Blackburn et al., 1960; Kannel and Abbott, 1984; Kannel, Cupples and Gagnon, 1990) and in **different ECG–VCG correlations (Friedman, 1985). According to this, Q waves were considered abnormal (Table 5.1)** when in leads I, II and VF they were ≥ 0.04 seconds, equal to or greater than 2 mm in depth with a Q/R ratio >0.25. The same consideration is for VL but with Q/R ratio >0.50 in the presence of positive P wave. When the voltage of R is low (5 mm or less), Q/R ratios are not useful for diagnosis. In VL the QS pattern may be seen as a normal variant usually in the presence of negative P and asymmetric negative

T wave and in the absence of abnormal Q wave in I and V6. Regarding Q wave in III, its significance depends on whether Q waves are also present in VF and II. Also is suggestive of MI the presence of $R >$ I mm in VR in the presence of Q in inferior leads. The only presence of Q in lead III especially if is not wide (>40 ms) is usually normal and frequently disappears with deep inspiration (Figure 5.42). These criteria present a high specificity (>90%) but low sensitivity ($\cong$50–60%).

With the aim to increase the sensitivity, different ECG–VCG correlation studies have been performed (Starr et al., 1974, 1976; Warner et al., 1982), considering abnormal a width of Q wave ≥ 0.03 seconds in inferior leads instead of ≥ 0.04 seconds and a Q/R ratio >0.20 instead of >0.25 in the same leads (Rios, 1977). However this was accompanied by a loss of specificity. Later, in year 2000, the consensus document of ESC/ACC (Alpert et al., 2000; Wagner et al., 2000) established a new definition of MI and considered the ECG changes that are seen in stabilised MI (see Table 5.2). However, the criterion given in this table does not include when Q wave in III or RS in V1 are abnormal. Recently, Jensen et al. (2006) in a retrospective study, and using as a gold standard for diagnosis of MI the myocardial perfusing imaging studies, compared the classical criteria (Table 5.1) and the criteria of the ESC/ACC consensus document (Table 5.2). This study shows the comparative sensitivity, specificity and positive and negative predictive value of both criteria. This comparison suggests that the ECG criteria of ESC/ACC consensus are much less specific (60% vs 97%), resulting in an inappropriately high number of false-positive results. Would it be important **to perform a prospective study using CE-CMR as a gold standard and comparing the classical criteria exposed in Table 5.1 with the ECG criteria that have demonstrated to present the highest sensitivity and specificity in our comparative study with CMR** and also with the VCG criteria (see p. IX). (Bayés de Luna, 2006a; Wagner, 2001) (Table 5.3 and Figure 5.9).

We have to understand that there are subtle changes in the first part of QRS that may be useful to diagnose MI (Figure 5.7A) and that, on the other

Figure 5.6 QRS-loops–ECG correlations found in seven different ECG patterns of Q-wave MI according to the classification presented in Figure 5.9. The numbers around the loops represent the minimum number of milliseconds affected by the necrosis that are necessary to generate a 'Q' wave. However, other patterns of QRS loops may also be seen (see some examples in the next figures).

Table 5.2 Electrocardiographic changes in established MI.

1. Any QR wave in leads V1 through V3 ≥ 30 ms
2. Abnormal Q wave in leads I, II, VL, VF or V4 through V6 in any two contiguous leads of at least 1 mm in depth, although criteria for QRS depth require more research
3. Criteria to establish the diagnosis of posterior MI are not clear and require further research

Adapted from Consensus ACC/ESC 2000 (Alpert, et al. 2000; Wagner, et al. 2000, Table 6.2).

(A)

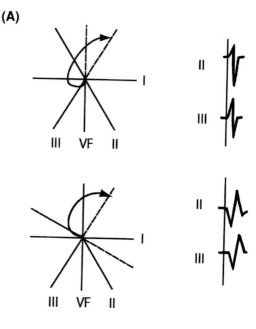

hand, sometimes a cancellation of vectors of necrosis, when the infarction encompasses two walls, explains that the ECG pattern does not reflect the true extension of the infarcted area (Figure 5.7B).

To measure and quantify the mass of the infarcted area, a score system has been developed by Selvester, Wagner and Hindman (1985), although currently CMR is the gold-standard technique for quantification of infarcted mass (see 'Quantification of the infarcted area' p. 285).

(B)

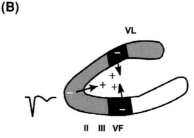

Table 5.3 Characteristics of the 'necrosis Q wave' or its equivalent*.

1. Duration: ≥30 ms in I, II, III[†], VL[‡] and VF, and in V3–V6. Frequently presents slurrings. The presence of a Q wave is normal in VR. In V1–V2, all Q waves are pathologic; usually also in V3, except in case of extreme levorotation (qRs in V3)
2. Q/R ratio: Lead I and II >25%, VL >50% and V6 >25% even in presence of low R wave[†]
3. Depth: above the limit considered normal for each lead, i.e. generally 25% of the R wave (frequent exceptions, especially in VL, III and VF)
4. Present even a small Q wave in leads where it does not normally occur (for e.g. qRs in V1–V3).
5. Q wave with decreasing voltage from V3–V4 to V5–V6,
6. Equivalents of a Q wave: V1: R-wave duration ≥40 ms, and/or R-wave amplitude >3 mm and/or R/S ratio >0.5.

* The changes of mid-late part of QRS (low R wave in lateral leads and fractioned QRS, p. 129) are not included in this list, which mentions only the changes of first part of QRS (Q wave or equivalent).

[†] The presence of isolated Q in lead III usually is non-pathologic. Check changes with inspiration (see Figure 5.42). Usually in III and VF, Q R ratios are not valuable when the voltage of R wave is low (<5 mm).

[‡] QS morphology may be seen in VL in a normal heart in special circumstances (see Table 5.1).

Figure 5.7 (A) Two examples of how the VCG loops may explain some ECG criteria of inferior MI. (1) In case of superoanterior hemiblock (SAH) the presence of 'r' II < III favours associated infarction even in the absence of 'q' wave because sometimes in case of small inferior infarction the area where the depolarisation begins in case of SAH is preserved (see Figure 5.58). (2) Also the VCG explains that Q wave in III starts later than that in II because the first part of the loop fails in the border between positive and negative hemifield of III. (B) Proximal occlusion of a very long LAD whole anterior wall and a part of inferior and lateral wall are involved. In this situation, in some cases the ECG pattern may do not reflect the infarcted area due to the cancellation (more gray areas) of the vector of the middle segment of anterior wall (which explains the Q wave in VL) and the vector of inferior necrosis (which explains the Q wave in inferior leads). In this case only Q waves in some precordial leads may be recorded. The more basal part of anterior wall that is also usually infarcted does not generate Q wave of necrosis due to late depolarisation.

Location of Q-wave MI

The characteristics of Q-wave MI in different leads to locate MI were based on anatomic correlations (Myers et al., 1948a, b; Horan and Flowers, 1972; Horan, Flowers and Johnson, 1971). Some studies performed on haemodynamic (Warner et al., 1982, 1986) and imaging (Bogaty et al., 2002) correlations have also been done. In spite of the differences in terminology it was generally considered that the **MI may be clustered in three groups:** MI of **inferoposterior area** (II, III and VF inferior MI, and RS in V1–V2 as a mirror pattern – posterior MI), **anteroseptal area** (V1–V2 septal and V3–V4 anterior) and **lateral area** (I and VL high-lateral and V5–V6 low-lateral MI) (p. 22).

However, as we have stated previously (see p. 23), there are **several limitations** to this classification **that make it necessary to establish a new classification of the location of MI** based on CMR correlation, which is really the gold standard for the non-invasive detection of the infarcted area. In the following pages we will comment about all the aspects of this new classification.

New classification of the location of Q-wave MI based on the correlation between the Q wave and the infarcted area as assessed by CE-CMR

(Bayés de Luna, Batcharor and Malik, 2006; Bayés de Luna, Fiol and Antman, 2006; Cino et al., 2006).

The most important limitations of classical classification (see p. 23) are:

(a) The basal parts of the heart depolarise after 40–50 milliseconds (Durrer et al., 1970). Therefore, the R wave in V1 (equivalent of Q) cannot correspond to an infarction of the inferobasal segment of the inferior wall (classically posterior wall), as has been considered for decades (Perloff, 1964).

(b) An infarction may not be classified as being of one type or another, depending on the involvement or not of a single precordial lead, especially V3–V5, since the QRS morphology recorded from these leads depends on how electrodes are placed and/or on the patient's body-build.

(c) Additionally, classification based on pathological correlations only allow for the precise location of MI of patients that have died, usually the most extensive, and furthermore the heart is evaluated outside of the thorax, in a situation completely different from a normal assessment of the anatomy of the heart in humans. Other limitations have been exposed previously (p. 23).

Gadolinium-enhanced CMR, on the contrary, allows for a real anatomic view of the heart within the thorax and for the real location of the infarcted area in all types of infarction. These correlations have given to us the following crucial information that can now be summarised as follows:

(a) Often the basal part of inferior (former inferoposterior) wall follows the same direction of the mid-apical parts of the wall (Figure 1.12).

(b) In cases that the basal inferior wall (segment 4) bends upward this has not ECG repercussion, even in rare cases that the most part of inferior wall (segments 4 and 10) are truly posterior as may occur rarely in very lean individuals, because the vector of infarction of this part of inferior wall (former inferoposterior wall) faces V3–V4 and does not change the morphology of V1, as it was thought (Perloff, 1964). On the contrary, the infarction vector of lateral wall faces V1 and may explain the RS morphology in this lead (Figures 1.10 and 1.11).

(c) Sometimes, even when the MI involves the segment 4 (old posterior wall), the infarcted area is non-transmural. This is probably due to double perfusion (RCA + LCX) that often receives this basal part.

These anatomical correlations, together with the electrophysiological evidence that the posterior wall (now named inferobasal segment) depolarise after 40–50 milliseconds, allow us **to conclude the following:**

(a) **The posterior wall either does not exist or, at least, does not have any repercussion on the changes of the first part of QRS (Q wave or equivalent).** Therefore, in accordance with the statement of AHA (Cerqueira, Weissman and Disizian, 2002), it is better to delete the word 'posterior' and to consider that the best names for the four walls of the heart are anterior, septal, lateral and inferior.

(b) **The RS pattern in V1 is explained by lateral MI and not by MI of inferobasal (posterior) wall.**

(c) Consequently, **Figure 5.8 shows the difference between the classic concept of inferior, posterior and inferoposterior MI to explain Q in inferior leads and RS in V1, and the new concept**

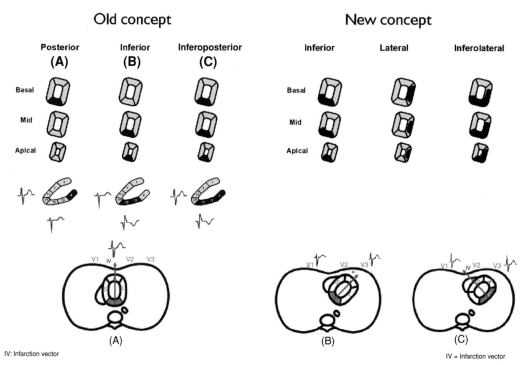

IV: Infarction vector   IV = Infarction vector

Figure 5.8 Above: Left side shows the involved area in case of inferior, posterior and inferoposterior MI with the classical ECG patterns in chronic phase according to the old concept; right side shows that with the new concept exposed in this book the name posterior disappears, the RS pattern in V1 is explained by lateral MI and the MI of the inferobasal segment of inferior wall (classically posterior wall) does not generate Q wave because it is a zone of late depolarisation. Therefore, the MIs of the inferolateral zone are clustered in three groups: inferior (Q in II, III and VF), lateral (RS in V1 and/or abnormal Q in lateral leads) and inferolateral (both patterns). Below: (A) Anatomic position of the heart that explains the old concept (RS in V1 due to involvement of segment 4 (old posterior wall)). (B, C) Anatomic real position according to CMR correlations that explain that lateral MI originates RS in V1 (see Figure 1.12).

of inferior, lateral and inferolateral MI to demonstrate thanks to CMR correlation that the inferobasal (posterior) MI does not originate RS morphology in V1, which is generated by MI of lateral wall (Figures 5.8 and 5.9).

Bearing all this in mind, we study the correlation between the infarcted area in different walls due to occlusion in different locations of three coronary arteries (STE-ACS evolving to Q-wave MI) and leads with infarction Q waves based on two standpoints: (1) **from the CMR to ECG**, and (2) **from the ECG to CMR**.

1. To assess, based on the infarcted areas as defined by CE-CMR, what electrocardiographic patterns best correlate with those areas: from the CMR area of MI to leads with Q wave in the ECG (Figure 5.9). Seven infarcted areas due to first MI have been found to have a good correlation with seven electrocardiographic patterns (Cino et al., 2006). Four of these are located in the anteroseptal zone, while the remaining three in the inferolateral zone, the former being secondary to occlusions in different segments of the LAD and its branches and the latter due to RCA or LCX occlusion

Figure 5.9 Correlations between the different myocardial infarction (MI) types with their infarction area assessed by contrast-enhanced (CE) CMR, ECG pattern, name given to the infarction and the most probable place of coronary artery occlusion. Due to frequent reperfusion treatment usually the coronary angiography performed in the subacute phase does not correspond to the real location of the occlusion that produced the MI. The gray zones seen in bull's-eye view correspond to infarction areas and the arrows to its possible extension.

	Name	Type	ECG pattern	Infarction area (CE-CMR)	Most probable Place of occlusion
Anteroseptal zone	Septal	A1	Q in V1–V2 SE: 100% SP: 97%		LAD
	Apical-anterior	A2	Q in V1–V2 to V3–V6 SE: 85% SP: 98%		LAD
	Extensive anterior	A3	Q in V1–V2 to V4–V6, I and aVL SE: 83% SP: 100%		LAD
	Mid-anterior	A4	Q (qs or qr) in aVl (I) and sometimes in V2–V3 SE: 67% SP: 100%		LAD
Inferolateral zone	Lateral	B1	RS in V1–V2 and/or Q wave in leads I, aVL, V6 and/or diminished R wave in V6 SE: 67% SP: 99%		LCX
	Inferior	B2	Q in II, III, aVF SE: 88% SP: 97%		RCA LCX
	Inferolateral	B3	Q in II, III, Vf (B2) and Q in I, VL, V5–V6 and/or RS in V1 (B1) SE: 73% SP: 98%		RCA LCX

Table 5.4 Proportions of agreement between electrocardiographic patterns and contrast-enhanced cardiovascular magnetic resonance for the different myocardial infarction locations and their 95% confidence interval. (Bayes de Luna 2006a)

Myocardial infarction location		Proportions of Agreement		95% Confidence Interval	
CE-CMR location	*ECG pattern**	*Expected by chance*	*Observed*	*Lower limit*	*Upper limit*
Septal	**A-1**	0.07	0.75	0.35	0.95
Apical- Anterior	**A-2**	0.09	0.7	0.35	0.92
Extensive Anterior	*A-3*	0.04	0.8	0.30	0.99
Mid- Anterior	*A-4*	0.030	1	0.31	1.0
Lateral	**B-1**	0.045	0.8	0.30	0.99
Inferior	**B-2**	0.11	0.81	0.48	0.97
Infero-lateral	**B-3**	0.15	0.8	0.51	0.95
	Composite	0.17	0.88	0.75	0.95

CE-CMR, contrast-enhanced cardiovascular magnetic resonance.
* ECG pattern: **A–1:** Q in V1–V2; **A–2:** Q in V1–V2 to V3–V6; **A-3:** Q in V1–V2 to V4–V6, I and aVL; **A-4:** Q (qs or qr) in aVL (I) and sometimes in V2–V3; **B-1:** RS in V1–V2 and/or Q wave in leads I, aVL, V6 and/or diminished R wave in V6; **B-2:** Q in II, III, aVF; **B-3:** Q in II, III, Vf (B2) and Q in I, VL, V5–V6 and/or RS in V1 (B1) (see Figure 5.9).
From Bayes dc Luna (2006).

(Figure 5.9). The infarcted areas, the coronary arteries potentially responsible for the infarction and the seven electrocardiographic patterns can all be seen in Figure 5.9. The names given to these areas correspond to the part of the LV that is more involved. We have avoided names which represent involvement of more than one wall in order to be more concrete and because semantically a short name sounds much better. However, we know that this does not correspond exactly to the reality. Figure 5.9 shows some of the limitations of these names (i.e. mid-anterior MI also encompasses some part of mid-lateral wall).

To define a Q wave of necrosis we have used the characteristics of Q wave shown in Table 5.3. **According to that, the electrocardiographic criteria of the areas of infarction detected by CE-CMR (septal, apical-anterior, mid-anterior, extensive anterior, lateral, inferior and inferolateral) can be defined with a high specificity and, generally, except for mid-anterior and lateral MI, with relatively good sensitivity.** However, these results have to be confirmed in a larger series. Some of their patterns encompass different morphologies (see Figure 5.9).

2. Once we found that the above-mentioned detected infarcted areas present characteristic ECG patterns, we assess if a post-MI patient with one of the referred electrocardiographic patterns would exhibit an infarct located in the above-mentioned area: from the leads with Q wave in the ECG to CMR areas with MI (Bayés de Luna 2006a). The concordance of such seven patterns with the seven corresponding areas has been shown to be good (>85%), and also the proportion of agreement (Table 5.4) (Bayés de Luna 2006a). Therefore the proper use of these patterns may be very useful to locate the infarction area.

A committee appointed by the International Society of Holter and Non-Invasive ECG (Bayés de Luna 2006b) **has reached an agreement about the names given to the walls of the heart and the different types of Q-wave infarctions that are presented in Figure 5.9.** Following, each of the **seven electrocardiographic patterns will be presented and discussed** (Figure 5.9), focusing on (a) **what is the involved LV** (segments) and, with the expressed limitations, not only what the occluded artery is, but also the most probable site of occlusion causing the infarction; (b) **how the electrocardiographic pattern is generated** based on the changes caused in the QRS loop by the vector of infarction moving away from the infarcted area.

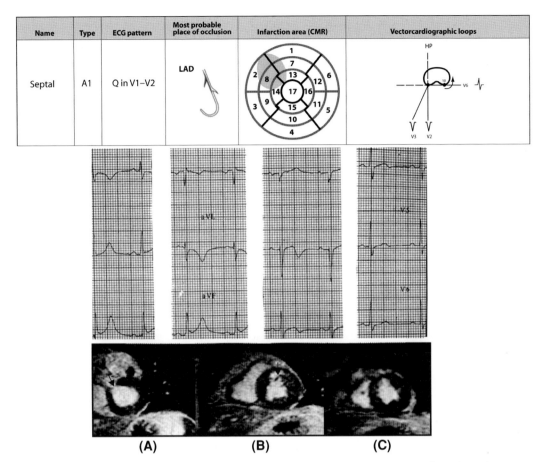

Name	Type	ECG pattern	Most probable place of occlusion	Infarction area (CMR)	Vectorcardiographic loops
Septal	A1	Q in V1–V2	LAD		HP

Figure 5.10 Example of small septal MI (type A1). ECG (Q in V1–V2). Most probable place of occlusion, CE-CMR images and VCG loops (see Figure 5.6). The infarct extension encompasses some anterior and septal segments: 1 and 2 (A), 7 and 8 (B) and 13 and 14 (C) (Figures 1.8 and 5.9).

Types of infarctions in the anteroseptal area: presence of Q waves or their equivalent in the precordial leads and/or I and VL (Figure 5.9A)

A-1. Electrocardiographic pattern type A-1 (Figure 5.9-A1). **Q waves in V1–V2** (Figures 5.10–5.12). This corresponds to **septal infarction.**

(a) When is this pattern observed? Its correlation with the infarcted area and the most probable culprit coronary artery.

It is called septal infarction because it corresponds to infarcted area that involves more or less extensive part of septal wall (especially segments 8, 9 and 14) (Figures 5.10 and 5.11). The mid-inferior segments (especially segments 8 and 9)

must be involved for the Q wave to develop since it is in this area where the first vector has been basically generated. Frequently, a certain extension to the neighbouring segments of the anterior wall exists (1 and 7) (Figures 5.10 and 5.11).

The infarction is generally a consequence of non-complete **LAD occlusion, which has partly or totally involved the septal branches,** but not the diagonal branches, or due to complete distal occlusion of LAD after all the diagonal branches take off. Otherwise, the infarction would be of the A-2 type (apical-anterior). On some rare occasions it may be secondary to the exclusive occlusion of one septal branch (Figure 4.29). This may occur spontaneously or during the course

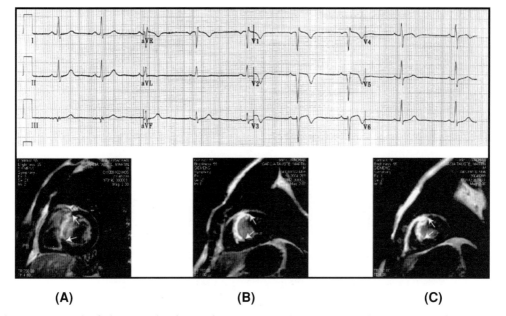

Name	Type	ECG pattern	Most probable place of occlusion	Infarction area (CMR)	Vectorcardiographic loops
Septal	A1	Q in V1–V2	LAD		

(A)   **(B)**   **(C)**

Figure 5.11 Example of a huge septal MI (type A-1) ECG criteria (Q in V1–V2 with rS in V3), most probable place of occlusion (more extended than in Figure 5.10), CE-CMR images and VCG loops. The septal infarction is very extensive encompassing the greatest part of the septal wall less the most inferior, at all levels – basal (A), mid (B) and apical (C). There is small extension towards the anterior wall at mid and apical level (arrows) (Figures 1.8 and 5.9).

of a PCI (Tamura, Kataoka and Mikuriya, 1991), or chemical ablation, in the case of hypertrophic cardiomyopathy.

(b) How does this ECG pattern arise? (Figure 5.12)

Since the high-septal area is depolarised after the first 40 milliseconds, the infarction of this area does not generate vector of infarction that can originate Q waves. In these cases, changes the final portions of the QRS complex may be present. For the typical pattern of this type of infarction to appear, it is required, then, that the infarction involves the middle-low portion of the septum. The other parts may or may not be involved.

The QS pattern in V1–V2 and sometimes in huge septal infarction small r in V3 (rS pattern) (see Figures 5.10 and 5.11) is due to infarction vector that is directed posteriorly and generates changes in the first part of QRS loop, which is also directed posteriorly or, in small infarctions, is very slightly anterior. An example of the ECG–VCG correlation in the acute phase of a septal infarction is shown in Figure 5.12. Therefore, the QRS loop is normal, except for the first few milliseconds, where it is usually not directed anteriorly in the HP (see Figure 5.9A(1) and 5.12).

A-2. Electrocardiographic pattern type A-2 (Figure 5.9-A2): Q wave in V1–V2 to V3–V6

Electrocardiographic pattern of the septal infarction (Figure 5.9A(1))

The ECG patterns of septal infarctions may be a little different, depending on the size of MI:
(a) Small septal MI usually presents QS in V1 and qrS in V2 with a T wave that may be positive or negative in V2–V3.

(b) Large septal MI presents QS in V1–V2 and usually rS in V3 with a negative T wave, but depending on where the V3 electrode is placed, a qrS or rS pattern may or may not be seen in this lead.

(Figures 5.13–5.17). This electrocardiographic pattern corresponds to the so-called **apical-anterior infarction.** Compared to the A-1 pattern, it exhibits a Q wave (QS or qr morphology) beyond lead V2 and usually beyond V3.

(a) When is this pattern observed? Its correlation with the infarcted area and the most probable culprit coronary artery (Figures 5.13–5.16).

It is called **apical-anterior infarction** because it corresponds to infarcted area usually

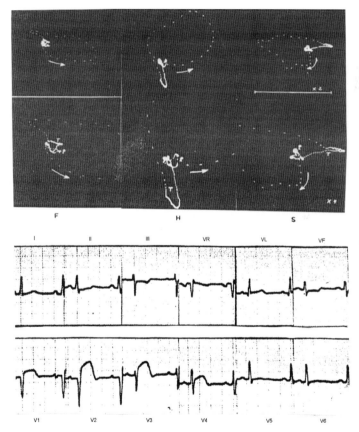

Figure 5.12 ECG–VCG of a patient with evolving Q-wave septal MI. (A) The VCG loops with the beginning of depolarisation directed nearly backwards (see H and S planes). (B) Acute septal MI (ST-segment elevation V1–V4 with Q in V1–V2 and small ST-segment depression in II, III, VF and V6). The presence of mild ST-segment depression in inferior leads do not assure the place of occlusion in relation to D1. However, the ST-segment elevation clearly seen in V1 favours that the occlusion is located proximal to S1 (Σ ST↑ V1 + ST↑ VR + ST↓ V6 > 0) and that the MI involves septal but probably not very much diagonal branches (see Figure 4.43).

Name	Type	ECG pattern	Most probable place of occlusion	Infarction area (CMR)	Vectorcardiographic loops
Apical-anterior	A2	Q in V1–V2 to V3–V6	LAD		

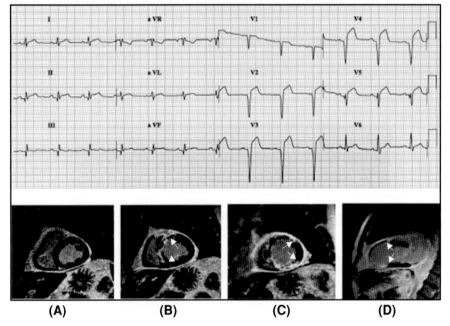

Figure 5.13 Example of apical-anterior MI (type A-2). ECG criteria (Q in precordial leads beyond V2), most probable place of occlusion, CE-CMR images and VCG loops. (A) See the lack of basal involvement. (B) and (C) Transverse transections involving especially in the most apical part, the anterior, septal and inferior wall with small lateral involvement, and in (D) sagittal-like view with important apical-inferior and -anterior involvement.

circumscripted to segments of the apical part of the LV (13, 14, 15, 16 and 17). Sometimes there is more extension to anterior and septal walls, involving at least part of the middle and lower septal area, which generates the first vector but not arriving the infarction to the basal areas of both walls. Generally, the lateral wall is the least involved being the mid segment (segment 12) usually spared. The inferior wall involvement depends on the length of the LAD (the so-called **anteroinferior infarction**).

The typical apical-anterior infarction is a consequence of **LAD occlusion, clearly distal to the D1 and S1**. If there is anteroseptal extension, it is usually due to non-complete **LAD occlusion im-**

mediately below the take-off of the S1 and D1, which involves not only the middle and lower septal branches, but also the diagonal branches below D1. When the LAD is long, an infarction that involves **the apical area, but also a greater part of inferior and septal walls, is generated.** The involvement of the anterior wall, compared to what is observed in a septal infarction, is larger, but the basal anterior wall, usually a part of middle-anterior wall, and the basal and mid-lateral wall are preserved. Should that occur, the LAD occlusion would be proximal to the take-off of the S1 and D1; it would thus be an extensive anterior MI (type A-3 infarction). The inferior wall involvement will be larger when the LAD wraps

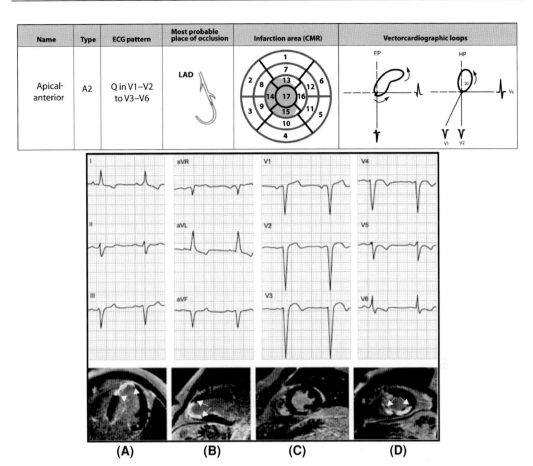

Name	Type	ECG pattern	Most probable place of occlusion	Infarction area (CMR)	Vectorcardiographic loops	
Apical-anterior	A2	Q in V1–V2 to V3–V6	LAD			

Figure 5.14 Other example of apical-anterior MI smaller than the one given in Figure 5.13. In sagittal view (B) it is well seen that the inferior involvement is even larger than the anterior involvement and in mid-transverse (C) and low-transverse (D) transections the MI is seen especially in (D) (septal and inferior involvement). The involvement of the low part of septum is well seen in (A).

the apex. Examples of apical-anterior infarction with more or less anteroseptal extension and with less lateral extension (no involvement of segment 12) with their corresponding correlation with the CMR are shown in Figures 5.13–5.15.

(b) How does the ECG pattern arise? (Figure 5.17)

The typical pattern of apical-anterior MI (QS in V1–V4) with more or less extension up to V6, but not in leads I and VL, is explained by the **infarction vector directing posteriorly, but not rightwards, since not much lateral involvement is present (the 6 and 12 segment are spared). Consequently, the QRS loop is oriented generally posteriorly from the beginning** and, sometimes, with initial forces directed anteriorly, but

which suddenly turn backwards with a clockwise or counter-clockwise rotation; however, due to less involvement of lateral wall, most of the loop is located to the left, which explains why no Q wave (QS or QR) is recorded in leads I and VL (Figures 5.9A(2) and 5.17).

In some infarctions with QS pattern from V1 to V4, the presence of a Q wave is observed in II, III, and VF, with 'qr' or 'QS' pattern. This occurs in typical apical infarctions, but not in case of important anteroseptal extension (Figure 5.16), since in the former, inferior infarction is frequently as important or more than anterior infarction, with the infarction vector of inferior wall and the corresponding loop in the FP, being directed upwards (Figure 5.16A). In

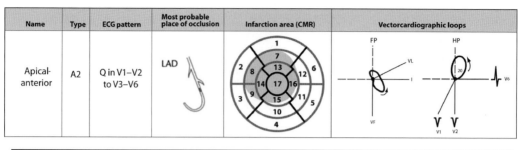

Name	Type	ECG pattern	Most probable place of occlusion	Infarction area (CMR)	Vectorcardiographic loops
Apical-anterior	A2	Q in V1–V2 to V3–V6	LAD		

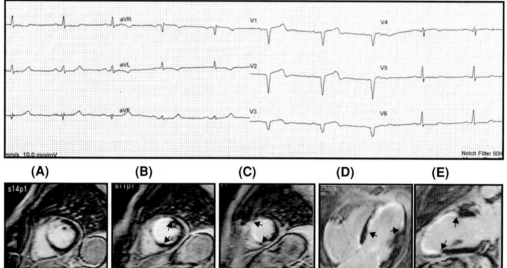

Figure 5.15 The ECG pattern of apical-anterior infarction (type A-2) with important anteroseptal extension as may be seen in this example but preserving the basal area of septum (D) and anterior wall (E). The lateral extension only involves the low part (D). The lack of involvement of segment 12 and lesser involvement of segment 7 are the most important differences between apical-anterior infarction with anteroseptal extension and extensive anterior MI (see Figures 5.15 and 5.18). (A)–(C) CMR image of transverse transection. (D) and (E) the septal and anterior extension.

apical-anterior infarction with anteroseptal extension, in turn the infarction vector of the inferior wall is probably cancelled out by the forces of the infarction vector of the anterior wall, and therefore no Q wave is recorded in II, III and VF (Figure 5.16C). As a matter of fact, if tall R waves are present in inferior leads, the involvement of inferior wall is probably absent (short LAD).

This electrocardiographic pattern (QS in V1 to V4–V6), as has already been mentioned, may be seen in apical-anterior MI with and without evident anteroseptal extension. In case of very distal LAD occlusion the sensitivity of this pattern is lower, since apical infarctions secondary to a very distal LAD occlusion allow for the recording of the first vector (rS in V1–V2), and the Q wave may be seen just in the inferior wall leads; in fact, the ECG may even be normal (Giannuzzi et al., 1989). It should also be reminded that sometimes an rS pattern is seen in V1–V2 in case of apical MI with Q wave in most of the remaining precordial leads, but without a Q wave in leads I and VL. This pattern may be explained by an infarction vector generated in the mid-low-lateral wall facing V1–V3 when the D1 branch is small, and the perfusion of the lateral wall is shared by OM branch and middle or distal diagonal branches.

There are also some rare cases in which **a type A-2 electrocardiographic pattern of apical-anterior MI may be seen in cases of MI due to proximal LAD occlusion.** In these cases

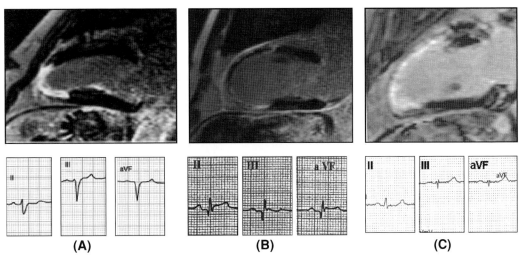

(A)   **(B)**   **(C)**

Figure 5.16 (A, B) Example of apical-anterior infarction with inferior involvement equal to or greater than the anterior. There is Q wave in inferior leads that is not usually seen in cases of apical-anterior MI with anteroseptal involvement greater than the inferior involvement (C).

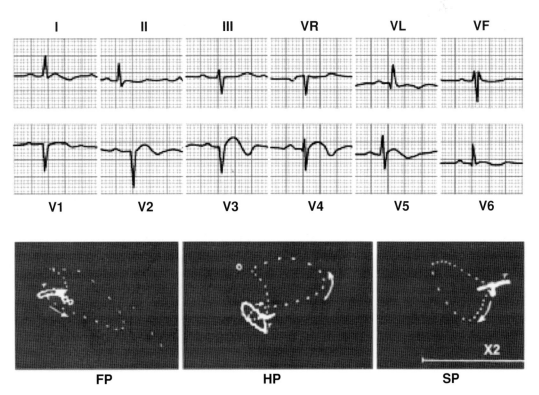

Figure 5.17 ECG and VCG of a patient with apical-anterior MI (Q wave beyond V2). The VCG loop explains the ECG morphology (loop–hemifield correlation).

the LAD is very long and perfuses, in addition to the entire anterior cardiac wall, part of the mid- and low-lateral and septal walls and a large region of the inferior wall. In these situations, which are rare and represent a large infarction, the ECG may be misleading, and a QS pattern may be seen just from V1 to V4–V5, without a Q wave in I and VL, sometimes with a qR pattern in V6. This is probably due to vectors of infarction of inferior and mid-anterior walls being mutually cancelled out, preventing the generation of Q waves in I and VL and in II, III and VF and leading to a **false impression of an apical-anterior infarction** (Takatsu et al., 1988; Takatsu, Osugui and Nagaya, 1986) (see Figure 5.7B).

A-3. Electrocardiographic pattern type A-3 (Figure 5.9-A3): Q waves from V1 to V3–V6, I and/or VL (Figures 5.18 and 5.19). This pattern corresponds to **extensive anterior infarction**. Compared to the A-2 pattern, this one also exhibits a Q wave (QS or QR) in VL and, sometimes, in lead I.

(a) When is this pattern recorded? Its correlation with the infarcted area and the most probable culprit coronary artery.

It is called **extensive anterior infarction** because it corresponds to large areas of not only the anterior and septal walls, but also the low- and

mid-lateral walls (segments 12 and 16), including at least part of the anterior and/or septal basal areas. The lateral basal area is not involved, since it is perfused by the LCX. However, the middle and apical lateral segments are usually involved and it explains the presence of Q in VL and/or I leads. Inferior wall involvement depends on the length of LAD. Thus, the segments more compromised are 7, 8, 13, 17 and 14 and parts of segments 1, 2, 9, 12, 15 and 16 (Figures 5.18 and 5.19).

The pattern of the extensive anterior infarction is usually explained by **proximal LAD occlusion, above the take-off of the S1 and D1 branches**. Naturally, the infarction also extends to the apical area and here the four walls are always involved (except when the LAD is very short). But the difference with the apical-anterior infarction lies in that in the latter; although anteroseptal wall may be involved, the basal portion of LV is spared and the involvement of lateral wall is lesser. The extensive anterior infarction, on the other hand, reaches the mid-lateral wall and the basal areas in some walls, generally the anterior and septal walls, but not lateral wall (Figure 5.18), because as we have already said the basal segments of lateral wall, even the anterior portion, are perfused by the LCX (OM) (see Figure 5.4C).

(b) How is the ECG pattern explained? (Figures 5.18 and 5.19)

Electrocardiographic pattern of apical-anterior infarction (Figure 5.9A(2))

• A Q wave in V1 to V3–V6 may be seen in apical-anterior infarction with or without anteroseptal extension. The presence of a Q wave in II, III and VF supports that inferior infarction being equal to or more important than anterior infarction; is a typical apical infarction.
• A QS pattern from V1–V2 to V3–V6 may be due in some rare cases to the proximal occlusion of a very long LAD and, as a result, the infarction is larger. It is explained by the cancelling out of the inferior and mid-anterior vector of infarctions, which precludes the recording of a Q wave in the inferior and VL leads (Figure 5.7B).
• The smallest apical-anterior infarctions due to very distal LAD occlusion often do not exhibit

a QS pattern from V1 to V4. In 20% of cases the ECG may even be normal.
• A thorough assessment of II, III and VF provides useful information about anteroseptal involvement in the cases of apical-anterior MI. If infarction Q waves are present in II, III and VF, the infarction of inferior wall probably equally or predominantly involves this wall with respect to the anterior wall (very long LAD). If tall R waves are present in II, III and VF, the inferior involvement is probably small or absent (short LAD).
• Sometimes there is an **rS morphology in V1–V2 with Q in other precordial leads**. This corresponds to apical-anterior infarction with more lateral than septal **involvement (R wave in V1–V2)**.

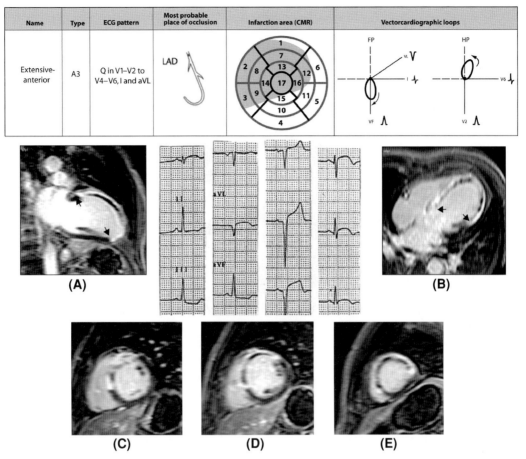

Figure 5.18 Example of an extensive anterior MI (type A-3) (Q in precordial leads and VL with qrs in I). Most probable place of occlusion, CE-CMR area and the VCG loops of this case. CE-CMR images show the extensive involvement of septal, anterior and lateral walls, less the highest part of the lateral wall. The involvement of segment 12 explains that in this MI there is a Q in VL that is not present in MI of apical-anterior type even in the presence of anteroseptal extension. (A) Oblique sagittal view. (B) Longitudinal axis view. (C–E) Transverse view. The inferior wall is the only spared. The LAD is not very large and therefore the inferior involvement is not extensive (see (A)). Due to that there is QS in aVL and R in II, III and aVF together with Q in V1–V5.

In this case, significant extensive anteroseptal involvement, especially the middle and lower portions, and also lateral involvement (mid-low wall), explains that the infarction vector is directed posteriorly rightwards and sometimes downwards (Figure 5.35), and generates a loop that usually rotates clockwise in the FP, but in HP rotates clockwise (QR in V6) (Figure 5.19) or counter-clockwise (RS in V6) (Figure 5.35). Therefore, a Q wave is seen in most of the precordial leads, V1 to V4–V6 and in VL and I, QR or RS pattern may be seen (Figures 5.19 and 5.35). The pattern of extensive anterior infarction with

RS pattern or predominant R wave in II, III and VF is observed when the LAD is not very long and does not greatly involve the inferior cardiac wall (Figures 5.18 and 5.35).

On rare occasions apical-anterior infarctions especially with anteroseptal extension that corresponds to A-2 pattern presents with an ECG of type A-3 (extensive anterior), because an abnormal pattern is recorded not only in precordial but also in leads I and VL (QS and QR patterns). The changes caused by cardiac rotation (levorotation) or the presence of LVH, among other factors, may at least partially explain it. In the levorotated and

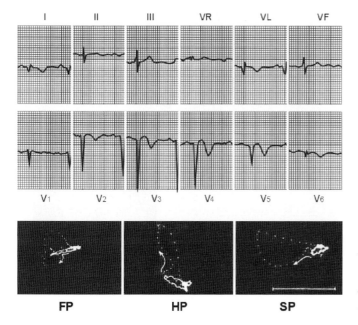

Figure 5.19 ECG and VCG of a patient with extensive anterior MI (type A-3 ECG pattern). Observe Q wave in all precordial leads and in leads I and VL. The correlation VCG loop–hemifield explains the ECG morphology.

horizontalised heart observed in very obese individuals, the LV may be more exposed to the lateral leads (I, VL and V5–V6) and, under this circumstance, the Q wave of necrosis with negative T wave may be more clearly seen in such leads. In verticalised hearts, with dextrorotation, the QS pattern with negative P and T waves is occasionally seen in VL. However, under normal conditions, in these cases, the QS pattern in VL is thin and narrow and, on the contrary, in the presence of an infarction, it frequently exhibits a lower voltage and slurrings, with the negative T wave being more symmetric and evident and without QS pattern in I (see Figures 3.27 and 5.35).

It has already been stated that in some large anterior infarctions, no Q wave is seen in I and VL. This may occur in cases of proximal occlusion of a very long LAD, which may cause an inferior infarction that counterbalances the Q wave of the infarction of the mid-anterior area (Takatsu et al., 1988; Takatsu, Osugui and Nagaya, 1986) (Figure 5.7B).

A-4. Electrocardiographic pattern type A-4 (Figure 5.9-A4): Q wave in VL and often I without abnormal 'q' in V6 and, sometimes, with a 'q' wave in V2–V3 (Figures 5.20–5.22). It corresponds to the **mid-anterior infarction.**

(a) When is this pattern recorded? Its correlation with the infarcted area and the culprit coronary artery.

It is called mid-anterior infarction because it corresponds to an infarcted area that mainly involves the mid-anterior wall with extention to mid-lateral wall and also to the basal and low-anterior and low-lateral wall. It involves segment 7 and parts of segments 13 and 12, and, on occasion, parts of segments 1 and 16 (Figures 5.20 and 5.21).

A QS or qr morphology is seen in VL in the typical cases (Figures 5.20 and 5.21), but abnormal 'q' waves are generally never present in V5–V6. A low-voltage 'r' or 'q' wave may be seen in lead I, and small 'q' or lack of increase of voltage of R wave may also be seen in V2–V3.

This is due to a **selective occlusion of first diagonal (D1), sometimes the second diagonal (D2), or to a non-complete occlusion of the LAD, involving the first diagonal branches but not the septal branches.** Since the high-lateral wall is perfused by the LCX, generally by its OM and not by the diagonal branches, the high-lateral wall is not necrosed when a Q wave develops (QS) in VL (and/or lead I) in the absence of Q in V5–V6 due to occlusion of first diagonal branch. On

Electrocardiographic pattern of extensive anterior versus apical-anterior MI (Figures 5.9A(2) and A(3))

Some limitations exist in the presence of Q waves in the precordial leads with respect to knowing the real extension of the infarction. This is especially true when distinguishing between the apical-anterior infarction (type A-2) and the extensive anterior infarction (type A-3).

• Infarctions with a Q wave in V1–V4 and sometimes qrs or qR in V5–V6 usually with a negative T wave correspond to **apical-anterior infarction** (distal occlusion of LAD) with or without anteroseptal extension, and most of the cases that in addition to having a Q wave in the precordial leads exhibit QS or QR patterns in VL (and/or lead I) corresponding to an extensive anterior infarction (proximal occlusion of LAD).

• As regards the infarcted area, **apical-anterior infarctions do not affect a large portion of the left-ventricular lateral wall**, while in extensive anterior this wall is more affected.

• **In a few cases, the electrocardiographic patterns of apical-anterior infarction (Q wave in the precordial leads, but not in leads I and aVL) correspond to extensive anterior infarctions** (Figure 5.7). Additionally, in some rare cases, electrocardiographic patterns of extensive anterior infarction (Q wave in the precordial leads and I and aVL) correspond, in fact, to apical-anterior infarctions.

Name	Type	ECG pattern	Most probable place of occlusion	Infarction area (CMR)	Vectorcardiographic loops
Mid-anterior	A4	Q (qs or qr) in aVL (I) and sometimes in V2–V3	LAD		

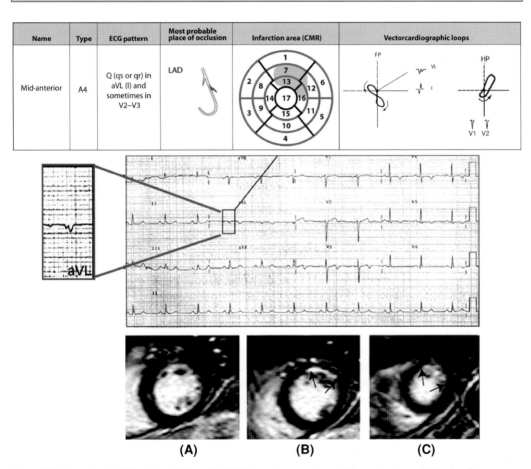

Figure 5.20 Example of mid-anterior MI (type A-4) (QS in VL without Q in V5–V6), most probable place of occlusion, CE-CMR area and the VCG loop in this case. CE-CMR images show mid-low-anterior and lateral wall involvement (B–C) but not involvement of basal part (A).

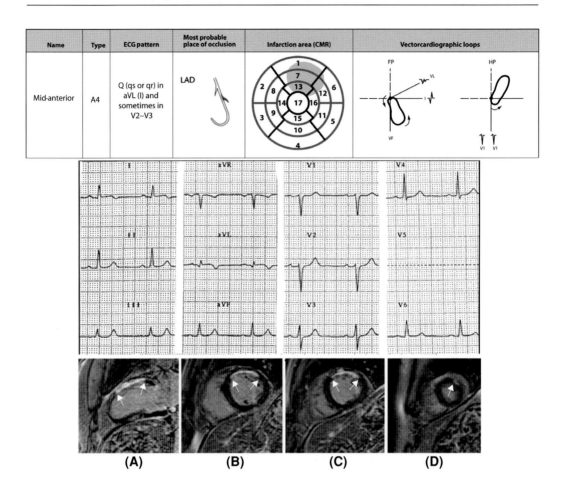

Figure 5.21 Another ECG example of mid-anterior MI (QR in VL) with small 'r' in V2. The CE-CMR shows involvement of mid-anterior (A) and part of basal (B) and mid (C) anterior wall but only small involvement of lateral wall (C–D). This explains probably that the morphology in VL is QR instead of QS.

occasions, small 'q' in V2–V3 or decrease of 'r' wave from V1 to V2 may be seen. This ECG pattern is due to D1 occlusion (Birnbaum et al., 1996a).

(b) How does the ECG pattern arise (Figure 5.22)?

The infarction vector from this infarcted area generates a loop that in FP is directed somewhat rightwards and upwards and then rotates counter-clockwise downwards and somewhat leftwards. The loop looks like folded over itself and is located in the FP slightly in the negative hemifield of VL, which explains the QS or low-voltage 'qr' pattern in VL that is seen frequently and the 'qrs' complex that may be observed in lead I (Figure 5.22). In HP often in the chronic

phase there are no significant changes in the rotation of the loop because, frequently, the ECG is nearly normal. On the contrary, in some cases in the acute phase, we have seen that a striking ST-segment upward deviation in V2, which although in some cases may become an infarction 'q' wave in the chronic phase, is often of a transient nature.

The mid-anterior infarction produced by D1 occlusion (segments 7 and 12, especially) may exhibit a QS pattern in VL. This sign is specific but not very sensitive. When the infarction is small, a Q wave is usually seen, but often with a QR pattern (QR) with normal morphology in V5–V6 (Figure 5.21). On the contrary, a **lateral infarction due to LCX occlusion** (OM) (segments 5, 6, 11 and 12 in particular) may sometimes

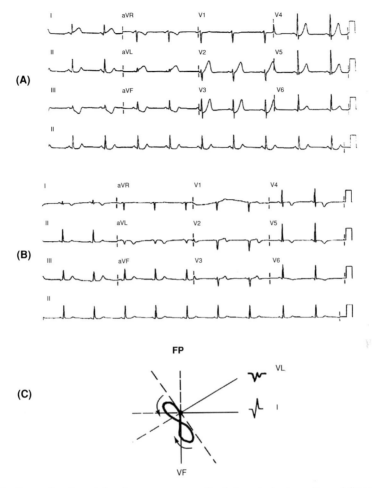

Figure 5.22 ECG patterns of acute and chronic mid-anterior MI. (A) Acute phase shows the ST-segment elevation in I and VL with in this case mild-ST-segment depression in V3 probably due to association of LCX involvement (see 'ST-segment changes in patients with active ischaemia due to multivessel disease'). (B) Chronic phase shows QS in VL and qrs in I with some reduction of 'r' wave in V2–V3 and negative T wave in left precordial leads due to involvement of LCX. (C) The VCG loop that explains the ECG pattern of VL in chronic phase.

exhibit an RS pattern in V1 and/or a low-voltage R wave in VL, or even 'qr', but generally without QS morphology, and/or a low-voltage 'qr' or 'r' pattern is seen in V5–V6 (<5–6 mm) (see Figure 5.23).

We will now remind the ECG differences in acute and chronic phase in case of D1 occlusion and OM occlusion. **During the acute phase** of infarction due to D1 occlusion (Figure 5.22A), an ST-segment elevation is seen in I and VL and frequently in several precordial leads, sometimes even from V2–V3 to V6, with, generally, an ST-segment depression in the inferior leads, since the injury vector is directed upwards. In circumflex (OM) occlusion, on the other hand, it is frequently seen that ST-segment elevation is present not only in I and/or VL, but also in II, III and VF (Figure 4.40). The reason is that the injury vector is not directed as upwards as in D1 occlusion (compare Figures 4.26 with 4.39). Furthermore, in an ACS due to OM occlusion, there is generally also a slight depression in V2–V3 (Figure 4.40), while in D1 occlusion, as we have already said, an ST-segment elevation may be seen in the

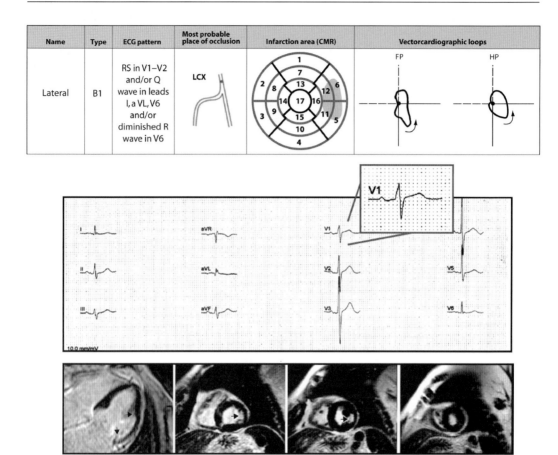

Name	Type	ECG pattern	Most probable place of occlusion	Infarction area (CMR)	Vectorcardiographic loops
Lateral	B1	RS in V1–V2 and/or Q wave in leads I, a VL, V6 and/or diminished R wave in V6	LCX		

Figure 5.23 Example of lateral MI with RS in V1 (type B-1). See the most probable place of occlusion, the CE-CMR area and the VCG loops. The CE-CMR images show that in this case the MI involves especially the basal and mid part of the lateral wall (A–C) but not the apical part (D).

precordial leads (sometimes as from V2) (Figure 4.27) that in chronic phase may or may not convert in a small 'q' in V2–V3 or a decrease of r wave (Figure 5.22). In some cases, in D1 occlusion, the injury vector may be directed somewhat posteriorly, thereby explaining the slight ST-segment depression that is sometimes seen in V2. In these cases usually there is also occlusion of LCX or RCA. **In chronic phase**, as we have already stated, in lead VL, an QS pattern is often seen in case of D1 occlusion without 'q' in V5–V6, and in OM occlusion abnormal Q wave may be seen in both leads VL and V6, but usually with 'qr' and not 'QS' pattern.

Types of infarction in the inferolateral area: presence of Q wave in II, III and VF, and/or RS pattern in V1, and/or 'qr' or 'r' wave in I, V5–V6 and/or VL (Figure 5.9B)

B-1. **Electrocardiographic pattern type B-1 (Figure 5.9-B1): tall and/or wide R wave in V1 and/or low-voltage 'qr' or 'r' pattern in V5–V6, I and/or VL** (Figures 5.23–5.26). We consider low voltage of R wave when is ≤ 7 mm, in VL and ≤ 5 mm, in V5–6. This corresponds to the so-called **lateral infarction**.

(a) **When is this pattern recorded? Its correlation with the infarcted area and the culprit coronary artery.**

Electrocardiographic pattern of the mid-anterior infarction (Figure 5.9A(4))

• **The QS or QR (qr) pattern only seen in VL**, with sometimes 'Qr or qr' in I, but with no Q wave of necrosis in V5–V6 is caused by the **occlusion of first diagonal (D1) (mid-anterior MI)** that does not perfuse the high lateral basal wall, which is perfused by the LCX (OM). Therefore, this pattern does not correspond **to a high lateral infarction.**

• In some cases a **decrease of 'r' wave from V1 to V2 or even small 'q' in V2–V3** can be seen.

• Relatively **often in chronic phase, the ECG**, in case of mid-anterior MI, is **normal** (Figure 5.9A(4)).

It is called lateral infarction, because the infarction is limited to the lateral wall, sometimes with small extension to the inferior wall. There is more or less extensive involvement of the anterior and/or inferior portion of the lateral wall. This electrocardiographic pattern is recorded especially

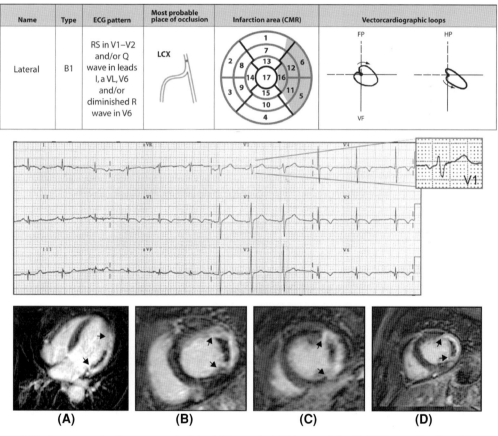

Name	Type	ECG pattern	Most probable place of occlusion	Infarction area (CMR)	Vectorcardiographic loops
Lateral	B1	RS in V1–V2 and/or Q wave in leads I, a VL, V6 and/or diminished R wave in V6	LCX		

Figure 5.24 Other example of more extensive lateral MI. There is RS in V1 and Q (qr) (in I, VL, V5 and V6). In this case the leads V5–V6 are facing the posterior part of infarction vector. See the most probable place of occlusion, the VCG loop and the CE-CMR images (A–D). In this case the MI involves more extensively the lateral wall (segments 5, 6, 11, 12 and 15) and this explains the presence of RS in V1 but also 'qr' in lateral leads.

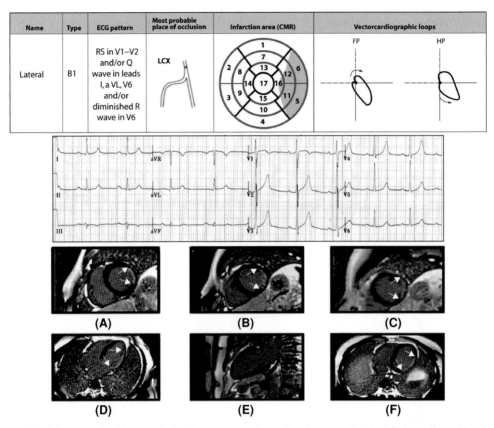

Figure 5.25 Other example of lateral MI with RS morphology in V1 but without q in V5–V6. CE-CMR images (A–F) show the involvement of lateral wall (A–D and F) without involvement of inferior wall (E). The sagittal transection (E) shows that the inferior wall is not involved. The lateral involvement is very well seen in all other transections.

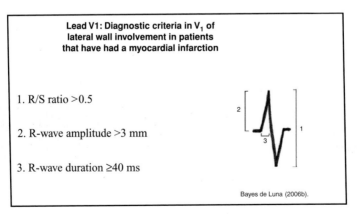

Figure 5.26 Diagnostic criteria of lateral involvement in patients that have had an MI.

when the infarction involves the mid-lateral wall (segments 11 and 12). Basal segments are often also affected and sometimes extends up to segments 15 and 16, in which case a 'q' wave may be seen in V5–V6 and II, III and VF (**inferolateral infarction**). The culprit artery is a **non-dominant LCX or**, **more frequently, occlusion of the OM or**, **in rare cases, of an intermediate artery**. The infarction has been reported (Dunn et al., 1984) to extend more frequently to the apical area (inferolateral – segments 15 and 16) when the occlusion is located in the intermediate artery.

We have already commented that the lead V6 probably faces more the apical part of inferior wall than the low-lateral wall (Warner et al., 1986) (p. 27). Probably, those cases presenting with a 'q' (qr) wave or low-voltage 'r' wave in lateral leads correspond to the predominant involvement of the most anterior segments of the lateral wall, and cases with an RS pattern and/or wide 'R' wave in V1 are usually those with a more significant involvement of the inferior segments of the lateral wall.

We have demonstrated with CE-CMR correlation that in patients who have presented an

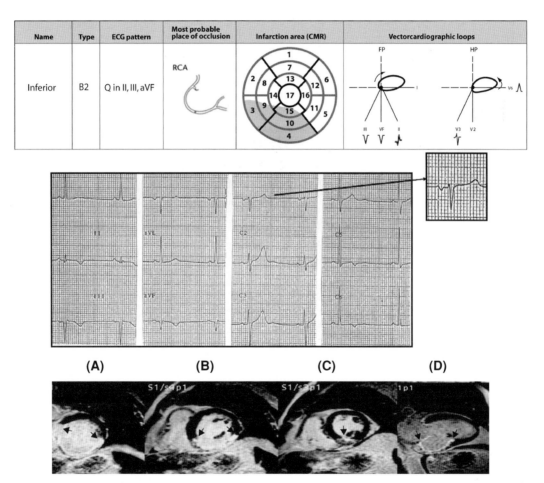

(A)   (B)   (C)   (D)

Figure 5.27 Example of inferior MI with Q in II, III and aVF and rS in V1. See the most probable place of occlusion, the CE-CMR images and the VCG loop. CE-CMR shows involvement of segments 4 and 10 and part of 15 and 3 and 9 (septal-inferior involvement) (A–C). The lateral wall is practically sparse. The most apical part of the inferior wall is not involved (D). In spite of the clear involvement of segment 4 (see (A) and (D)), the morphology of V1 is rS. Therefore, in presence of MI of segment 4 (old posterior wall) without involvement of the lateral wall, there is not RS in V1.

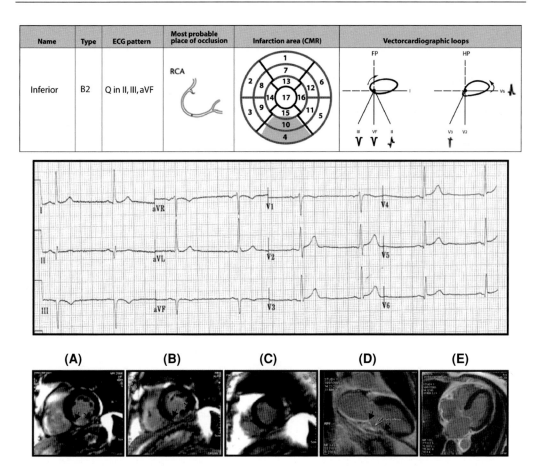

Figure 5.28 Other example of inferior MI with involvement of segments 4 and 10 (A, B and D), but not involvement in apical segment (C), rS morphology is recorded in V1. There is not lateral and septal involvement (E).

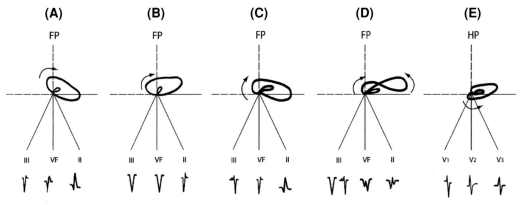

Figure 5.29 VCG loops in case of inferior MI. (A–D) FP and E: HP. Morphology (D) is seen in case of inferior MI plus superoanterior hemiblock (SAH) (see Figures 5.32, 5.54 and 5.62). The morphology QS (qrs) without terminal r in II, III and VF (although a qrs morphology may be seen) favours the presence of SAH due to special rotation of the loop in these cases (D) (see Figures 5.54, 5.58 and 5.62). In the absence of SAH, even if the entire VCG loop falls above 'x' axis (lead I), there would be terminal r at least in II, which does not happen in presence of associated SAH (B) (see Figures 5.30).

STE-ACS, the morphology in V1 with R/S ratio >50%, R-wave amplitude >3 mm and R-wave duration ≥40 milliseconds are criteria very specific of lateral MI (Bayés de Luna et al., 2006b) (Figure 5.26). However the sensitivity of these criteria is relatively low (50–60%), because this infarction does not frequently cause changes in the ECG (Figures 5.23–5.25).

As demonstrated above with CE-CMR correlation that the RS in V1 is due to lateral and not posterior MI, other papers had suggested the same, with pathological, isotopic and haemodynamic correlations (Bough et al., 1984; Dunn, Edwards and Pruitt, 1956; Levy et al., 1950), and even partially this has been suggested in some papers with CE-CMR (Hoshino et al., 2004; Moon et al., 2004). However, the impact of Perloff's paper (1964) and the statement of AHA (Surawicz et al., 1978) made that the concept that 'RS in V1 is due to posterior MI (currently inferobasal segment)' was accepted worldwide during more than 40 years.

(b) How does the ECG pattern arise (Figures 5.23–5.26)?

In cases with 'q' wave (qr) in I and VL and/or V5–V6, the infarction vector that moves away from the infarcted area (especially segments of the anterior part of the wall) is directed slightly rightwards and when segment 15 is involved also upwards (inferoapical extension). In this case a small 'q' wave in the inferior wall may also be seen (Figure 5.24). The QRS loop looks folded, initially directed rightwards and anteriorly, and after rotating usually in the counter-clockwise direction in the HP, it turns posteriorly. The loop–hemifield correlation (Figure 5.24) explains low-voltage 'qrs' or 'rs' pattern recorded in I and VL, and, in general, 'qr' found in V5–V6, and sometimes in II, III and VF and the RS pattern in V1. In other cases, the only abnormality of the loop is that it presents an important anterior part in HP, and thus the RS pattern in V1. It is explained by the fact that lateral wall infarction (especially segments of inferior part – 11) generates an infarction vector that is directed especially anteriorly, facing V1 (Figure 5.25). In this figure it can be observed that this infarction vector generates an RS pattern in V1, while in the infarction vector in case of infarction of the inferobasal segment of inferior

wall (posterior infarction in the classical nomenclature) (segment 4), there is not any abnormal infarction vector generated because it corresponds to an area of late depolarisation. Therefore in this case 'rS' morphology is recorded in V1, but never in an 'RS' pattern (see Figures 5.27 and 5.28).

Consequently, **the infarction that is presented with RS pattern in V1,** with or without small 'qr' in lateral leads, **is not the result of infarction of the most basal (posterior or inferobasal) portion of the inferior wall, but is, in fact, a lateral infarction** (Figures 5.23–5.25). Figure 5.26 shows the diagnostic criteria of lateral MI found in lead V1.

When an ACS with ST-segment elevation in lateral leads does not cause QRS changes in the chronic phase, such as **Q wave of necrosis in lateral leads** or **an R wave in V1,** this may be explained by the fact that the necrotic areas are the basal areas of late depolarisation of the lateral wall, which may not be expressed by infarction Q waves. However, in these cases, slight changes in the form of slurrings or notches in the final portion of the QRS complex (**fractioned QRS**) may be found (Figures 9.3 and 2.56). Occasionally, the **QRS complex is absolutely normal, but certain aspects of repolarisation may be suggestive.** Note in Figure 10.2 how the slight ST-segment depression in V1–V2 and the tall and symmetric T wave in these leads may suggest the suspicion of a lateral infarction, which was later confirmed via CMR (especially in segment 11).

B-2. **Electrocardiographic pattern type B-2 (Figure 5.9-B2): Q wave in at least 2 contiguous inferior leads (II, III, VF)** (Figures 5.27–5.30). This corresponds to the **inferior infarction.**

(a) When is this pattern recorded? Its correlation with the infarcted area and the most probable culprit coronary artery.

It is called inferior infarction though it usually also involves part of the inferior septum. Thus, when a Q wave is present in at least two contiguous inferior leads (see Table 5.1), as the sole electrocardiographic abnormality, the involvement of part of the inferior septum is frequently associated with an inferior wall infarction that also very often includes the inferobasal segment (segment 4) of the inferior wall, classically named 'posterior wall'

Electrocardiographic pattern of the lateral infarction (Figure 5.9B(1))

- **The electrocardiographic changes induced by lateral infarction, caused by OM or non-dominant LCX occlusion, consist in the following:**
  – **I, VL and V5–V6** 'qr' pattern and/or low-voltage complexes (r, or rs, qrs) – fractioned QRS – in leads I, VL, V5-V6
  – **Lead V1** having an RS ratio >50% and/or wide

–R waves ≥40 milliseconds and/or R-wave amplitude >3 mm in V1 (Figure 5.26)
- **Frequently, the ECG presents changes in mid-late QRS (fractioned QRS) or even is normal or near to normal,** especially when the infarction is small or, in case of transmural MI, when principally involves areas of delayed depolarisation, as the basal areas.

(Figures 5.27 and 5.28). These infarcts are generally due to proximal **non-dominant RCA occlusion or distal dominant LCX occlusion.** When the LAD is short, this infarction may also involve entire segment 15 and very rarely part of segments 16 and 17. In the last situation, a Q wave of necrosis would be recorded in V5–V6 (**inferolateral apical infarction**).

(b) How is the ECG pattern explained (Figures 5.27–5.30)?

The infarction vector generated in the infarcted area is directed upwards, and somewhat rightward, explaining the change of the loop, which is also directed upwards and somewhat rightwards in the beginning, in the clockwise direction and then suddenly turns leftwards, at least 25 milliseconds

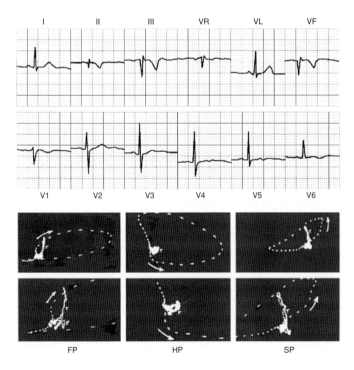

Figure 5.30 Typical example of inferior myocardial infarction (Qr in II, III and VF) with leftward ÂQRS. Nevertheless, the left-deviated ÂQRS (-35°) is not explained by an added superoanterior hemiblock (SAH), but simply by the inferior necrosis, because although the majority of the QRS loop in the frontal plane is above 0°, as it completely rotates in the clockwise sense, a small terminal r (Qr morphology) in II, III and VF is recorded. If an added SAH exists, the first part of the loop would be the same, but would later rotate in the counter-clockwise direction and would generate QS with notches but without the final 'r' wave in inferior leads.

above the *x*-axis and, later, usually downwards (Figure 5.29A). Rarely, the entire loop remains above the axis of the orthogonal lead 'x' (Figures 5.29B and 5.30). The inferior lead that most specifically detects infarction is lead II (Q wave ≥30 ms), though an abnormal Q wave may be seen in all three leads. In an isolated and not very large inferior infarction, the Q wave (QR or QS) is mainly seen in III and VF, and less in II, which generally exhibits a qR or qr morphology. The T wave may be positive, though it is most frequently negative and symmetric, especially in III.

When **the location of the occlusion is distal RCA, the infarction is small**, involving basically the low inferior wall (segments 10 and 15), and if the RCA is dominant, the low-lateral wall (part of segment 16). According to the predominance of the lateral involvement (segment 16), **the infarction vector is directed upwards and somewhat rightwards**, thus usually generating an 'r' wave ≥1 mm in VR. In cases of small infarction, the Q wave may not be very evident and sometimes presents a qR pattern, but with the characteristics of Q wave of necrosis (duration >30 ms), and is usually only visible in one or two leads. **In some small inferior infarctions** the beginning of the loop may be directed downwards before it rotates upwards in the clockwise direction. In this situation a small 'r' wave may be recorded in the inferior leads, especially III (Figure 5.29C). When the Q wave is not definitely abnormal, small details in the ECG may be of help. In an inferior infarction, the recording of the QRS complex begins earlier in II than that in III (Figure 5.7A(2)).

The diagnosis of the association of inferior infarction with a superoanterior hemiblock (SAH) may usually be easily performed. The presence of a Qr morphology in the inferior leads (at least in lead II) suggests an isolated inferior infarction, without SAH (Figure 5.29D and 5.30), while the presence of QS (ᐯ) in the same lead II supports the association of SAH (Figure 5.54). The changes of QRS loop due to SAH (Figure 5.29D) explain, by diagnostic point of view, these subtle but important changes in morphology. Sometimes the diagnosis is more difficult, since small inferior infarctions may be masked by SAH. However, the presence of slurrings in 'r' wave of inferior leads and of 'r' in III > II (Figure 5.7A(1)) may be of help in the case

of a doubtful inferior infarction associated with an SAH. All the aspects related with the association of inferior MI and both types of hemiblocks superoanterior (SAH) and inferoposterior (IPH) are explained in detail in the section 'Hemiblocks' (p. 174).

Examples of an isolated inferior infarction are seen in Figures 5.27 and 5.28. The ECG recordings of these figures are similar (QR or Qr in III and VF, qR or QR in II and rS in V1). However, the pattern in VR is 'rS' in Figure 5.28, with 'r' wave >1 mm, while in Figure 5.27, QS pattern is seen. CE-CMR reveals that, in general, in the presence of a QS pattern in VR, the infarction extends to the inferior septal portions (Figure 5.27), while in cases of isolated inferior infarction without septal involvement and often with low-lateral involvement VR may exhibit an 'r' wave >1 mm. This may be explained, according to our experience, because the infarction vector may be addressed more to the left when septal involvement exists and therefore fails less in the positive hemifield of VR, and more to the right when low-lateral involvement is present without important septal involvement. This has to be demonstrated in a larger series. The involvement of segment 4 does not generate changes in the first part of QRS because this segment depolarises after 40 milliseconds (Durrer et al., 1970) (see Figure 9.5). We have already commented that the presence of pathologic RS morphology in V1 (R/S >50%, R amplitude >3 mm and R duration ≥40 ms) is due to lateral MI and has not any relation with MI of segment 4 (Figure 5.26).

B-3. **Electrocardiographic pattern type B-3** (Figure 5.9-B3): Q wave in II, III and VF, and tall R wave in V1 and/or abnormal 'q' wave in V5–V6 and/or I, VL and/or low R wave in V6 (Figures 5.31–5.34): This corresponds to an **infarction that involves the inferolateral region** (**inferior and lateral walls**).

(a) **When is this pattern recorded? Its correlation with the infarcted area and the culprit coronary artery.**

It is thus called inferolateral MI, because it involves part of the inferior wall (B-2) plus part of the lateral wall (B-1). The typical pattern is recorded because large areas of the inferior and lateral walls are involved, which is due to **occlusion of a dominant RCA or a very dominant LCX. In the first case**

Electrocardiographic pattern of the inferior infarction (Figure 5.9B(2))

The ECG pattern of inferior MI includes the following:

• **Q wave of necrosis** (QS, Qr, QR and qR) that **may be seen in all three inferior leads, but never in lead II with QS pattern except in the presence of SAH.** In the latter case, a QS with notches ( ) is recorded (see Figure 5.54).

• **In patients with an inferior infarction,** which very frequently involves segment 4 (classically known as the posterior wall), **the pattern in V1 is** **always rS** being RS ratio always <50% and always with R wave width <40 ms (see Figures 5.27 and 5.28).

• The presence of **r wave ≥1 mm in VR suggests that the involvement of septal wall is probably scarce** or inexistent and supports the involvement of low-lateral wall.

• The association of hemiblocks to inferior MI are fully discussed in section 'Hemiblocks' (p. 174).

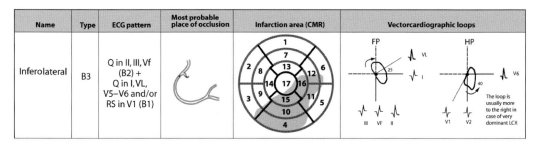

Name	Type	ECG pattern	Most probable place of occlusion	Infarction area (CMR)	Vectorcardiographic loops
Inferolateral	B3	Q in II, III, Vf (B2) + Q in I, VL, V5–V6 and/or RS in V1 (B1)			The loop is usually more to the right in case of very dominant LCX

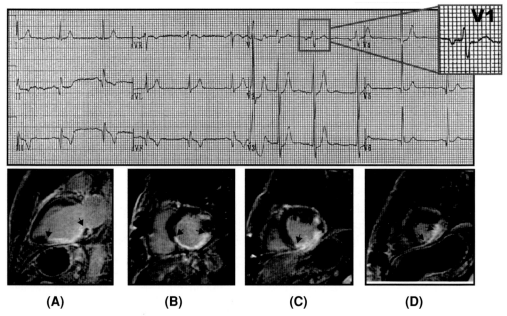

(A)   **(B)**   **(C)**   **(D)**

Figure 5.31 Example of inferolateral MI (Q in II, III and VF, and RS in V1). The most probable place of occlusion (RCA), the CE-CMR images and the corresponding VCG loops. The CMR shows the involvement of inferior wall and also part of lateral wall. (A) Sagittal-like transection showing the involvement of inferior wall. (B–D) Transverse transections at basal, mid and apical level showing also the lateral involvement especially seen on mid and apical level.

Electrocardiographic pattern of the inferolateral infarction (Figure 5.9B(3)): diagnostic criteria supporting the RCA or the LCX being the culprit arteries

RCA occlusion (Figure 5.33)

1. Q wave in II, III and VF (QIII always > QII)
2. rS or RS pattern in V1 (see Figure 5.26)
3. Sometimes, a Q wave (generally qR or qr) in V5–V6
4. An r wave ≥1 mm may be seen in VR, but it is generally <2 mm

LCX occlusion (Figure 5.34)

1. Q wave in II, III and VF (QII sometimes > QIII)
2. Rs or R > S in V1 (see Figure 5.26)
3. QR pattern in V5, V6, I and VL
4. Generally, an r wave ≥1 mm in VR with even R wave ≥ S wave

Name	Type	ECG pattern	Most probable place of occlusion	Infarction area (CMR)	Vectorcardiographic loops
Inferolateral	B3	Q in II, III, Vf (B2) + Q in I, VL, V5–V6 and/or RS in V1 (B1)			

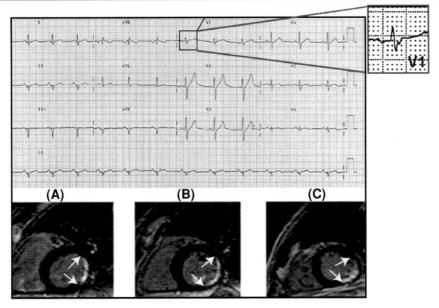

Figure 5.32 Other example of inferolateral MI (RS in V1 and ECG criteria of inferior involvement; small 'r' or qrS in II, III and VF). There is probably SAH associated (no r' in II, III and VF). The most probable place of occlusion, the CE-CMR area and the most probably VCG loops. Transverse transections of CMR shown in different levels, the lateral wall involvement (A–C) and extension to inferior wall at mid and apical level (B and C).

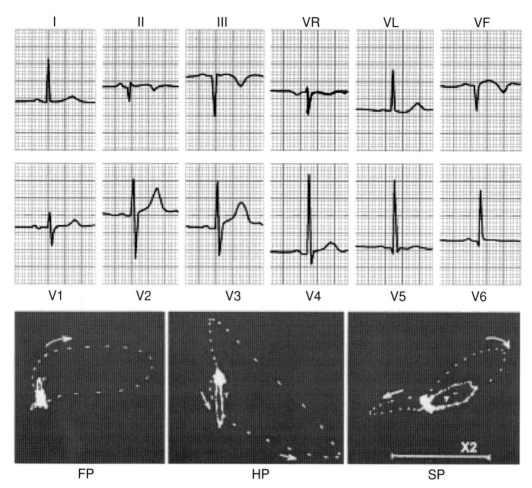

FP   HP   SP

Figure 5.33 ECG of inferolateral wall MI due to occlusion of dominant RCA (Q in II, III and VF (III > II), and RS in V1). The VCG loop in FP is only clockwise but all above axis *x*. The absence of associated SAH explains the Qr morphology in lead II, because the last part of the loop falls in the positive hemifield of lead II but as it falls in the negative hemifield of lead III and VF, there is not terminal 'r' in III and VF (see Figure 5.29B).

(RCA occlusion) **more involvement of the inferior portions of the septum and less involvement of the lateral portions will be seen. The opposite occurs in the second case.** This explains the segments that are compromised when infarction is due to RCA or LCX occlusion.

(b) How does the ECG pattern arise (Figures 5.33 and 5.34)

The inferolateral infarction due to an RCA occlusion generates an infarction vector that points upwards and a little rightwards, and anteriorly.

This modifies the QRS loop, which in the FP rotates in the clockwise direction, after being directing upwards, to end up being usually directed somewhat downwards. In the HP the loop is initially directed anteriorly and somewhat rightwards. Afterwards, its maximum vector is directed anteriorly and leftwards, to end up generally running posteriorly. The loop–hemifield correlation explains the ECG morphology that includes ECG criteria of inferior MI (abnormal 'q' in II, III and VF) plus ECG criteria of lateral MI (Q in I, VL and/or

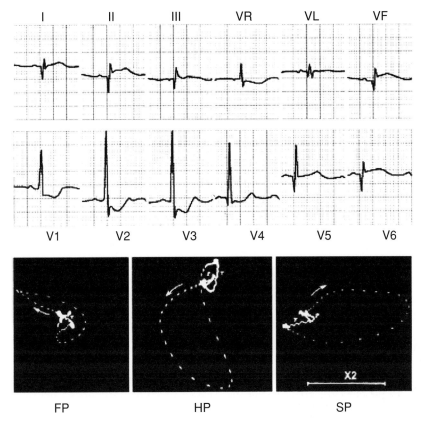

Figure 5.34 ECG of inferolateral MI due to occlusion of dominant LCX (Q in II, III and VF (II > III), R in V1 and Q in V5–V6 and I, VL). The VCG loop of this case – correlation loop–hemifields – explains this morphology. For example the exclusive R in V1 is clearly understood observing the loop in HP as the same happens with the QRS pattern in I and VL if we correlate with the loop in FP.

V5–V6 and/or pathologic R wave in V1 (see above).

In inferolateral infarction due to RCA occlusion, there are more signs of inferior than of lateral infarction, and, in any case, the latter may be manifested by an RS in V1 and in some cases by abnormal 'q' wave in the left precordial leads, but not by 'q' wave in leads I and VL (Figure 5.33). In turn, in **inferolateral infarction due to LCX occlusion**, the lateral wall is more involved than the inferior wall, and this explains why a Q wave may be recorded in I, VL, V5 and V6, though usually a QR, instead of a QS, pattern is seen. Also, according to the loop–hemifield correlation, the Q wave in II, III and VF may be more important in II than in III (QII > QIII) (a specific but not very sensitive sign). Sometimes lateral involvement is more evident (R in V1 and R ≥3 mm in VR) (Figure 5.34).

In some cases of inferolateral involvement, especially due to RCA occlusion, there is a clear sign of inferior infarction but no evidence of lateral infarction (no 'q' in lateral leads and/or R in V1). In our experience the contrary inferolateral involvement with only ECG evidence of lateral infarction occurs less frequently.

In front of an isolated ECG everyone should imagine how the ECG pattern is explained by the correlation with the way that the electric stimulus follows in the heart (VCG loop) and the projection

Changes of QRS due to MI: Q-wave and fractioned QRS

(a) The presence of pathological Q waves (Q waves of necrosis) or their equivalent in different leads reveals what area is affected by an infarction. In fact, they correspond to two zones of the LV **according to coronary artery circulation** (**Figure 5.4**): (1) anteroseptal (**four patterns**) and (2) inferolateral (**three patterns**).

- **Anteroseptal zone: Q wave especially in precordial leads and/or I and VL**
  – This infarction is secondary to the occlusion of the **LAD** or its branches. This corresponds to MI of types A-1 to A-4 of Figure 5.9.

  – The QS morphology in VL without Q in V5–V6 is due to a mid-anterior infarction with mid-low lateral wall extension (first diagonal branch occlusion or LAD non-complete occlusion, proximal to D1).

- **Inferolateral zone: Q wave in II, III, VF and V5–V6 and/or I and VL (qr or low-voltage R wave) and/or RS in V1**
  – This infarction is due to **RCA or LCX occlusion.**
  – This corresponds to an **inferior and/or lateral wall infarction** (Figure 5.9B(1–3)). In this book, segment 4, which was traditionally known as the posterior portion of the inferoposterior wall, is named inferobasal segment of the inferior wall. The RS morphology in V1 is due to an infarction of the lateral wall.

(b) **The presence of abnormalities in the second part of QRS as low R wave in lateral leads (Figure 5.9B(1)), motches/slurrings, etc. (fractioned QRS) are frequently found.**

---

of this loop in different hemifields. With this aim, one should draw the loop that might potentially explain the ECG findings and the polar map of the area of the LV involved (see example in Figures 5.35 and 5.36).

The ECG in two or more infarctions (Figures 5.37–5.40)

So far, we have dealt with the ECG's usefulness in locating the infarcted area in the chronic phase of first infarction, though in many of these cases two or more coronary arteries were involved. **The ECG may locate more than one Q-wave infarction when Q waves are found in different territories (e.g. Q wave in II, III and VF and in the precordial leads V1–V4)** (Figure 5.37). However, on other occasions, the Q wave seen in case of double infarction could be explained by a single one (Figure 5.40). On occasions, some patients may present a normal ECG without Q waves in presence of than more than one transmural MI due to a cancellation of vectors (Figure 5.38). However, often at least signs of equivalents of Q (RS in V1) morphology of fractioned QRS (p. 129) or abnormal ST/T changes (Figure 5.39) are frequently seen.

The VCG has been used to locate the presence of multiple infarctions. However, this technique is rarely used in daily practice. Furthermore, as we have already stated, it has been demonstrated that practically the same information may be obtained if the ECG–VCG correlation is used to understand ECG morphologies, as is done in this book (Warner et al., 1982). We need to also have in mind that, in some cases of single infarction, Q waves in leads of different areas may be seen, e.g. in an apical infarction due to a distal LAD occlusion, in addition to Q waves in the precordial leads; these may also be seen in the inferior wall when the LAD is very long and there is infarction of the inferior wall that may be even greater than the anterior involvement (Figure 5.16).

The ECG signs that most accurately suggest the diagnosis of a new infarction are as follows:

1. New onset Q waves are recorded.
2. Patterns suggesting involvement of the inferolateral and anteroseptal areas, such as QR or qR patterns in II, III or VF, and QS or QR in some precordial leads (Figure 5.37). However, we have to remind that in MI due to distal LAD occlusion Q

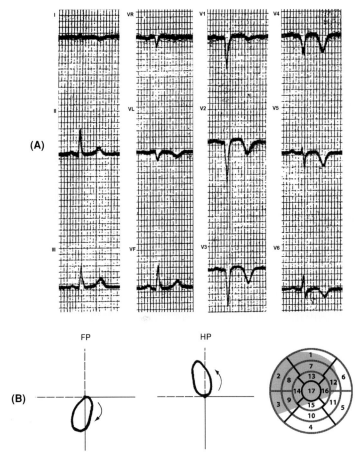

Figure 5.35 (A) The ECG shows QS in V1–V4, and VL, and rS in V5–V6. This corresponds to an extensive MI (type A3). The VCG loops that explain the ECG and the left ventricle area involved are shown in (B). The counter-clockwise rotation in HP explains the rs pattern in V5–V6 (see Figure 5.6-A3-B) but in FP presents a clockwise rotation with the loop directed downwards and a little bit to the right. This morphology explains the rs in I, the QS in VL and R in II, III and VF. The presence of dominant R in inferior leads favours that the inferior wall is not involved because the LAD is not long (see Figure 5.18).

waves are often present in precordial and inferior leads (see Figure 5.14).

3. A new infarcted area suddenly masks totally or partially previous Q waves (Madias and Win, 2000) (Figure 5.39). The ECG may seem even normal or nearly normal due to cancellation of vectors. It should be ruled out that the disappearance or decrease of the Q wave is not secondary to the development of a new intraventricular block. Also ischaemia induced by exercise may mask transiently, due to ischaemia in the opposite sites, the Q wave of necrosis (Madias et al., 1997).

The presence of two or more true Q-wave MI may be suggested by the criteria mentioned above. However, in clinical practice nowadays, after the consensus of ESC/ACC (Alpert et al., 2000), there are more patients that present two or more infarctions. Very often some of them are small non-Q-wave MI infarctions that correspond frequently to 'necrossete type'. The CE-CMR can allow us to detect with great accuracy the presence of two or more infarctions (Figure 5.40), although, as we have already pointed, sometimes the vector of infarction of two MIs may cancel each other (Figure 5.38). It is

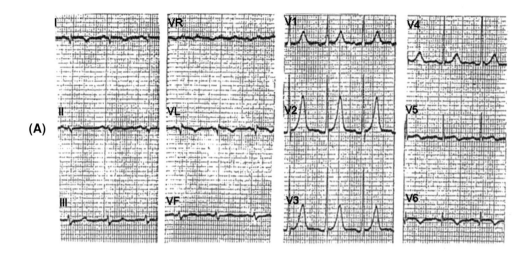

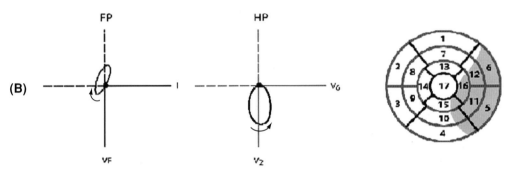

Figure 5.36 (A) The ECG corresponds to extensive MI of lateral wall due to LCX occlusion (R in V1, Qr in I and qr in VL and V6) with some inferior wall involvement especially the apical part (slurred 'r' in inferior leads, 'qr' in V6 and 'r' in VR). The VCG loops that explain the ECG are shown in (B). The VCG in HP is similar to the Figure 5.6-B1, but in FP it has to be different (small and with clockwise rotation) to match with the ECG morphologies. The area involved includes all lateral wall (R in V1 and q in lateral leads) and some part of inferior wall.

important to point that the late enhancement due to infarcted area has to be differentiated from other causes that may also induce hyperenhancement (see Figure 1.5).

Differential diagnosis of an infarction Q wave: Q wave or equivalent without MI (Figures 5.41–5.43)

Despite the high specificity of the abnormal Q wave for the diagnosis of an MI, it should be borne in mind that similar Q waves may be found in other situations. Furthermore, the diagnosis of an acute infarction is not exclusively based on ECG changes, but also on clinical and enzymatic assessment. The pattern of ischaemia or injury accompanying an abnormal Q wave favours the possibility that the Q wave is caused by coronary heart disease.

In a recent study (MacAlpin, 2006) it was demonstrated that the presence of Q wave according to parameters similar to Table 5.3 was strong predictor of organic heart disease (>90%) but its utility to diagnose MI was age dependent. In the group of less than 40 years the MI was present in only 15% of the cases with abnormal Q wave; on the contrary, in the older group it was present in 70% of the cases. Therefore, the Q wave has low specificity for MI in young and higher in older patients. In a group of

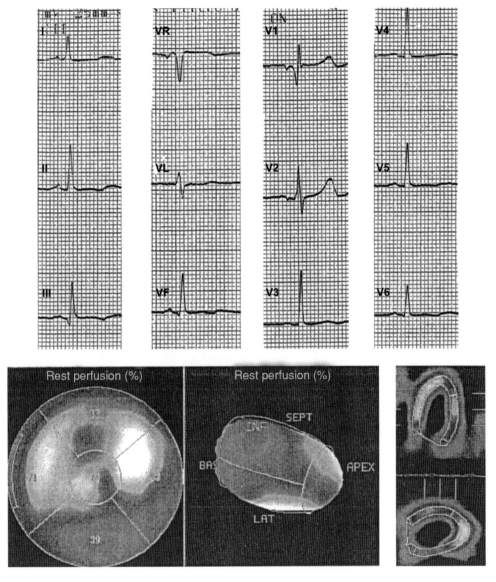

Figure 5.37 ECG of a patient with two MIs, one apical and the other inferolateral. The presence of QR in V1, RS in V2 and qR with wide q in III is the abnormal QRS change. The QR pattern of V1 is explained by double infarction (apical + inferolateral). However, there are not many leads with Q wave in spite of clinical and isotopic evidence of double infarction, probably due to partial cancellation of infarction vectors. The final R in V1 and the R in V2–V3 are explained because the inferolateral infarction is more important than the apical infarction. The nuclear study shows clearly the presence of double infarction of inferolateral zone and smaller apical area.

patients who have suffered an STE-ACS the specificity of the presence of Q wave for MI is even greater (>95%) (Bayés de Luna, 2006a).

In Table 5.5 the main causes of Q waves or equivalent not secondary to an MI are listed, which include the following:

1. Transient Q waves in the course of an acute disease. Sometimes in the course of typical ACS a generally transient Q wave appears. This results in the clinical setting of aborted MI and also happened in the coronary spasm (Prinzmetal angina) (atypical ACS). As has already been commented on

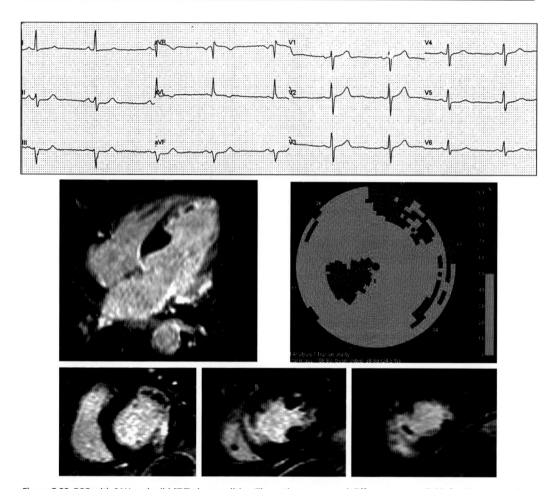

Figure 5.38 ECG with SAH and mild ST/T abnormalities. The patient presented different myocardial infarctions – septal, anterior and lateral detected by CE-CMR that masked each other. This figure can be seen in colour, Plate 4.

(see 'Changes of QRS due to MI'), (p. 129) the development of a Q wave implies the presence of an overt diastolic depolarisation in the involved area, which makes it non-excitable, but not necessarily already dead. Also in the course of some non-ischaemic acute disease as myocarditis (Figure 5.43) and pulmonary embolism, a transient Q wave may be recorded.

2. Persistent (chronic) Q wave. Recording artefacts, normal variants (Figure 5.42) and different types of heart diseases (among them, hypertrophic cardiomyopathy (Figure 5.41) and congenital heart diseases) are included in this group. It is important to emphasise that often the duration of the Q wave is normal but its amplitude is

pathologic (see Figure 5.41). CE-CMR may detect in some of these cases the presence of fibrosis localised in specific area of myocardium (Figure 1.5). The presence of this localised area of fibrosis in cases of non-ischemic heart diseases may have prognostic implications.

Diagnosis of the Q-wave infarction in the presence of intraventricular conduction disturbances

In this first part the electrocardiographic diagnosis of Q-wave infarction associated with intraventricular conduction disturbances will be discussed. We consider that there are electrophysiological

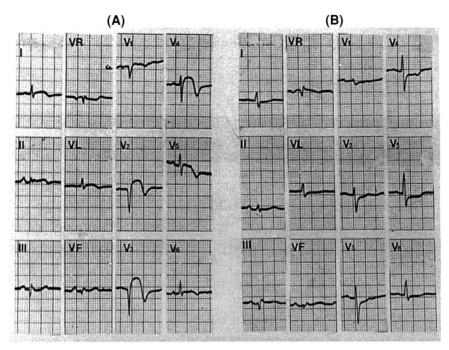

Figure 5.39 (A) Apical-anterior infarction in subacute phase. Observe QS in V2–V3 with ST-segment elevation and small ST-segment elevation in II (occlusion distal to S1 and D1) (see p. 1.80). (B) Six months later another infarction occurs with appearance of 'r' in V1–V3 and mild ST-segment depression in the same leads. This false improvement of the ECG is due to a lateral infarction, which was confirmed later in the post-mortem examination.

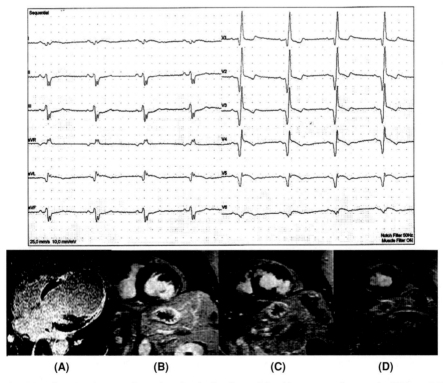

Figure 5.40 ECG and CE-CMR images of a patient that had double infarction (A and C), one lateral with some inferior extension present in segments 4, 5, 11 and 12 (B and C), and the other septal that affects especially segments 8, 13 and 14 (C and D). The ECG shows RBBB and signs that may be explained by an extensive anterior MI (type A-3) with Q in I, VL and precordial leads but that in this case are due to the sum of Q waves of septal (V1–V2 and V3) + lateral (V5–V6 and I–VL) infarctions with some inferior extension.

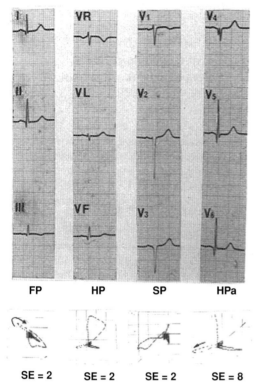

FP   HP   SP   HPa

SE = 2   SE = 2   SE = 2   SE = 8

Figure 5.41 Typical, although not frequent, ECG pattern in a 25-year-old patient with obstructive hypertrophic cardiomyopathy. There are no voltage criteria for left ventricular enlargement. Nevertheless, a deep but not wide 'q' wave in precordial leads, with QS in V2–V4, probably due to a important septal vector of hypertrophied basal septum, in the absence of repolarisation alterations in the leads with a pathological 'q' wave, suggest this diagnosis, which was confirmed by echocardiography. The correlation with VCG loops (below) explains the ECG patterns.

and pathological evidences that the intraventricular conduction system (ICS) is usually quadrifascicular (Uhley 1964, 1973): the right bundle branch (RBB), the supero anterior (SA) and inferoposterior fascicles of the left bundle branch (LBB) and the middle fibers of the LBB (Fig 9.5). These fibers, that exist in the majority of cases, may present different morphological aspects (Bayes de Luna 1977, Demoulins J, Kulbertus H 1972). The diagnosis of RBB block – LBB block and the block of superoanterior (SA) and inferoposterior (IP) divisions of LBB (the hemiblocks) are well known (Sodi D, Bisteni A, Medrano G 1960) (Rosenbaum M, Elizari M, Lazzari J 1968). The diagnosis of block of the middle fibers of the

LBB is not so well known and defined. Currently the Brazilian school (Moffa, Perez Riera, Pastore, etc) have systematized the ECG – VCG criteria of this diagnosis (see p. 193).

Clinical and prognostic issues in patients with Q-wave MI and wide QRS will be commented in the second part of the book (p. 247 and 287).

Complete right bundle branch block
(Figures 5.44–5.47)

The beginning of the cardiac activation is normal in the presence of a complete RBBB and, consequently, in the course of an infarction change occurring in the first part of the QRS complex, as in normal conditions. This causes an infarction Q wave that usually makes a distortion in the general morphology of the bundle branch block. For example, in the course of an anteroseptal infarction not only a Q wave appears but also it decreases the amplitude of R wave from V1 to V3 because of the large infarcted area (Rosenbaum et al., 1982). Also, the ST segment may be more or less elevated, instead of depressed as it is in isolated RBBB (Figure 5.45). When the MI involves the inferolateral wall Q in inferior leads, an R wave in V1–V2 with positive T wave may be present (Figure 5.46).

Gadolinium MRI allows for the accurate identification of the infarcted area and its correlation with the ECG morphology (Q waves). An extensive anterior infarction (Q in precordial leads and VL) is shown in Figure 5.47. The basal segments, especially of the lateral area, are spared. However, despite the lack of high lateral infarction, a QS morphology is seen in VL (and almost in lead I), due to the large mid-low anterior infarction with mid-low lateral extension. It has already been discussed that the QS morphology in VL is not caused by high lateral infarction (OM occlusion) but especially by mid-anterior infarction (diagonal occlusion). As the LAD is not very long, the infarcted inferior area is small – see A and D – and therefore, the Q wave of inferior infarction is not recorded (see also Figure 5.16C).

Complete left bundle branch block
(Figures 5.48–5.52)

In the presence of complete LBBB, even when large ventricular areas are infarcted, the general direction of the depolarisation usually does not change. This

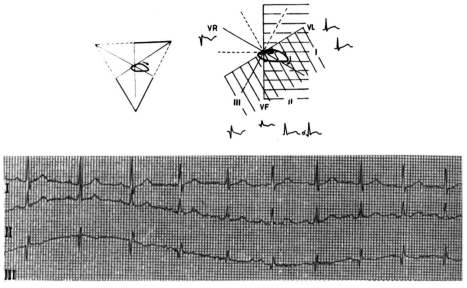

Figure 5.42 Positional Qr morphology that disappears with deep inspiration changing into rsr' pattern. It is usually accompanied by S in I lead (SI and QIII) and corresponds to normal horizontalised and dextrorotated heart.

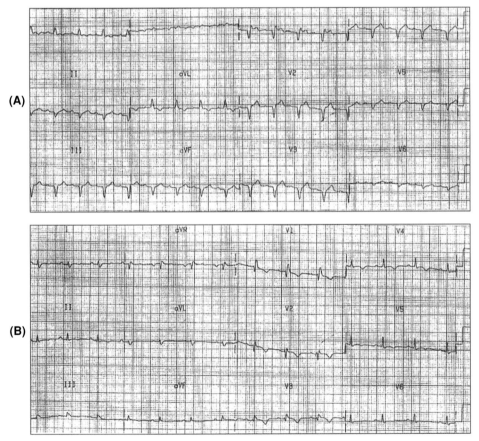

Figure 5.43 (A) Patient with acute myocarditis and ECG with signs of RBBB plus SAH and Q wave of necrosis in many leads. After the acute phase (B), the Q waves practically disappear and also the superoanterior hemiblock. In many leads a mild and diffuse pattern of subepicardial ischaemia is still present. Observe the low voltage in both ECG.

occurs because the vectors are still directed from right to left and frequently, in general, infarction Q waves are not recorded (Figure 5.48).

VCG may be useful in suspecting the presence of an associated infarction when a Q wave is not recorded. For example, the QRS loop that is normally directed initially somewhat anteriorly and leftwards, and then posteriorly it may be directed exclusively posteriorly and/or with an anomalous rotation (Figures 5.49 and 5.50). However, if we look with great detail the ECG we may find small changes that may suggest an associated infarction. For example, an 'r' wave in V1 > 1 mm (Figure 5.49) should not be recorded in the isolated LBBB. In Figure 5.50 the morphology from V3 to V5 is suspicious of an associated infarction. The Mexican School described in the 1950s the electrocardiographic signs based on the changes of the QRS morphology with or without the development of Q waves (Cabrera, 1958; Sodi, Pallares and Rodríguez, 1952).

Studies assessing the ECG–scintigraphy correlation have proven that most of these signs were not very sensitive, even though they were specific (Wackers, 1978) (Table 5.6). **The most specific QRS criteria ($\cong$90%), even though they show a low sensitivity (30%), are the following (Figures 5.51 and 5.52, and Table 5.6):**
1. An abnormal Q wave (QS or QR morphology) in leads I, VL, V4–V6, III and VF
2. Notches in the ascendent limb of R wave in I, VL, V5 and V6 (Chapman's criterion)
3. Notches in the ascending limb of the S wave in the intermediate precordial leads V2–V4 (Cabrera's criterion)
4. Presence of an R wave (rS and RS) in V1 and RS in V6

Gadolinium MRI confirms that in the presence of abnormal intraventricular conduction, such as LBBBs, the presence of a Q wave in VL (along with a Q wave in I and sometimes in precordial leads) means that the infarction caused by a proximal occlusion of LAD above the diagonal branches involves all the anterior and septal walls, with also mid-lateral wall involvement (Figure 5.52).

In some cases of LBBB due to block of SA + IP divisions (see Fig 5.53), a small and narrow "q" wave in I, VL, V6 may be present if the activation of the LV

starts through the middle fibers that are not blocked (Medrano, Brenes, de Micheli 1973).

With respect to **chronic repolarisation abnormalities**, the negative T wave is more symmetric than that in the isolated complete LBBB (Figures 3.40 and 1.58). In clinical practice positive T wave in V5 and V6 is usually seen when the LBBB is not too advanced, and septal repolarisation does not predominate completely over left-ventricular repolarisation. In some cases it may be the expression of changes of repolarisation polarity induced by ischaemia.

Hemiblocks

Figure 5.53 shows the location of two classical divisions of left bundle superoanterior and inferoposterior with the middle fibers that are also usually present in sagittal view and in the LV cone. We will now examine the following aspects of the associations of MI to block of two classical divisions of left bundle (hemiblocks) (Rosenbaum, Elizari and Lazzari 1968).

Diagnosis of Q-wave infarction associated with hemiblocks

We will refer to the diagnosis in the chronic phase. The hemiblocks do not alter the repolarisation changes that can be observed in the acute phase of MI.

The late activation of some areas of the LV due to delay in activation of this area explains the late QRS complex forces opposed to the infarction Q wave. This was related for many years as 'peri-infarction block'. Currently, the combination of an infarction with some intraventricular zonal blocks is based on the concept of the hemiblocks, defined by Rosenbaum, Elizari and Lazzari (1968). Because hemiblocks are diagnosed mainly by the changes in the vector's direction in the FP, the electrocardiographic changes secondary to the association with MI will be evidenced also specially in the FP leads.

Furthermore, the hemiblocks do not modify the diagnosis of MI of anteroseptal zone in precordial leads (HP), but may modify the presence or appearance of Q waves in inferior leads (inferior MI) and in VL (mid-anterior MI or extensive MI involving mid-anterior area).

Table 5.5 Pathologic Q wave or equivalent – R wave in V1 – not due to myocardial infarction

A **Transient Q wave pattern appearing during the evolution of an acute disease – ischemic or not – involving the heart**
1   Acute coronary syndrome with an aborted infarction
2   Transient apical ballooning: Recently has been suggested that it is the expression of spontaneous aborted infarction (Ibañez, et al. 2006)
3   Coronary spasm (Prinzmetal angina)
4   Acute myocarditis. (Figure 5.43)
5   Pulmonary embolism
6   Miscellaneous: Toxic agents, etc.

B **Chronic Q wave pattern**
1   Recording artefacts
2   Normal variants. Q wave may be seen in VL in the vertical heart and in III in the dextrorotated and horizontalised heart and in some positional or respiratory changes (Figure 5.42)
3   QS pattern in V1 and even in V2 in septal fibrosis, emphysema, the elderly, chest abnormalities, etc. Low progression of 'r' wave from V1 to V3
4   Some types of right-ventricular hypertrophy (chronic cor pulmonale) or left-ventricular hypertrophy (QS in V1–V2, or slow increase in R wave in precordial leads, or abnormal 'q' wave in hypertrophic cardiomyopathy) (Figure 5.41).
5   Left bundle branch block
6   Infiltrative processes (amyloidosis, sarcoidosis, Duchenne's dystrophy, tumours, chronic myocarditis, dilated cardiomyopathy and others)
7   Wolff–Parkinson–White syndrome
8   Congenital heart diseases (coronary artery abnormalities, dextrocardia, transposition of the great vessels, ostium primum, etc.)
9   Miscellaneous: pheochromocytoma, etc.
C. **Prominent R in V1 not due to lateral MI (Bayes de Luna 2006)**
1. Normal variants. The R is prominent but of low voltage. These include (Bayés de Luna 1977).
    a) Post term newborns: The pattern with dominant R due to RV overload, as a consequence of prolonged pregnancy, may remain till the adulthood
    b) Less number of Purkinje fibers in anteroseptal area may generates a delay in depolarization in this area that explains the more anterior QRS loop.
2. Right ventricle hypertrophy (negative T wave in V1) or septal hypertrophy as in hypertrophic cardiomyopathy.
3. Right bundle branch block (negative T wave in V1)
4. WPW syndrome (δ wave and negative T wave in V1)
5. Cardiomyopathies with predominant fibrosis in lateral wall (Duchene's cardiomyopathy, etc.).
6. Dextroposicion (not dextrocardia) due to location of the heart in the right side of the thorax (lung diseases).
7. Block of middle fibers of LBB (fig 5.64 and p. 172 and 193). The T wave in V1 is usually negative, on the contrary that in case of lateral MI.

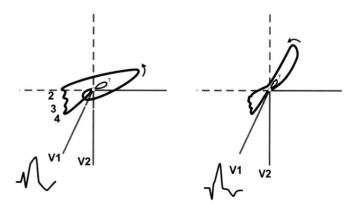

Figure 5.44 ECG–VCG correlation in case of isolated RBBB (left) and RBBB plus anteroseptal MI (right).

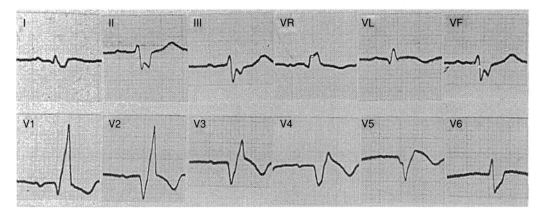

Figure 5.45 A 71-year-old patient with chronic obstructive pulmonary disease and wide QRS complex secondary to complete right bundle branch block. The qR morphology in V1–V2, with pointed R wave, QR in V3 and V4, or in V5 and RS in V6, qr in VL with small r in lead I is explained by an associated anterior myocardial infarction.

(A)   **(B)**

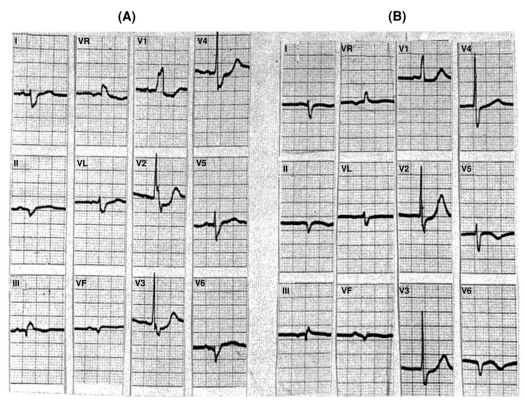

Figure 5.46 (A) Patient with complete right bundle branch block in acute phase of inferolateral infarction. ST-segment depression is seen in V1, V2 and V3 with final positive T wave and Q wave in inferior leads. The high localisation of the 'notch' on the upward slope of the R wave supports the involvement of lateral wall. This diagnosis of inferolateral infarction is confirmed when the right bundle branch block resolves after a few days (Q in II, III, VF and R in V1, and QS in V6) (B).

(a) Infarction of inferior wall associated with an SAH (Figures 5.54A and B) or **an IPH** (Figures 5.55A and B)

In first case (SAH), when the infarction is large and involves the entire or most of the area where ventricular depolarisation begins (point C and A) (Figure 5.54A), the vector of infarction counteract the first vector and is directed upwards, as in an isolated inferior infarction, as well as in the QRS loop. However, instead of rotating the entire loop in the clockwise direction, due to the SAH, its second portion rotates in the counter-clockwise sense. Thus, the entire loop lies above the axis of lead X (Lemberg, Castellanos and Arceba, 1971). This explains why a QS morphology usually with notches (ᵂ) is recorded in III and VF in case as associated SAH (Figure 5.54), while a Qr morphology is frequently recorded in isolated inferior infarction (Figures 5.29 and 5.30).

In IPH associated with an inferior infarction, in case of a large infarction, the first vector moves away from the inferior wall leads (II, III and AVF), more so than in the isolated inferior infarction, and consequently more evident Q wave will be seen due to the association of a vector of infarction with the initial depolarisation vector due to IPH (IV +1 in Figure 5.55A). However the second vector of depolarisation (2 in Figure 5.55A) explains the presence of an evident final R wave (QR morphology) in II, III and VF. Therefore, since the final forces in the IPH are directed downwards, QS morphology is not seen and, to some extent, the IPH masks the infarction, because instead of QS or Qr morphology, a QR morphology appears (see Figure 5.55).

(b) Anterior infarction associated with an SAH (Figure 5.56) or **IPH** (Figure 5.57). In the first case, the first vector of ventricular activation (sum of the mid-anterior vector of infarction plus the normal activation vector in case of an SAH) (1 + vector of infarction in Figure 5.56A) moves away from I and VL and generates an infarction Q wave followed by an R wave due to the late activation of the non-infarcted area consequence of SAH. To some extent, the SAH somewhat masks the infarction morphology, since in its absence a QS morphology would perhaps be recorded in I and VL, instead of a QR morphology.

In case of IPH associated with an extensive anterior infarction including mid-anterior wall, the vector of infarction (B) counteracts the initial depolarisation vector (1) (Figure 5.57) and generates a change in the QRS loop that is directed rightwards and downwards. Thus, it explains the QS morphology in I and VL (Figure 5.57).

Hemiblocks masking Q waves

In addition, the presence of a hemiblock can mask the presence of a coexistent infarction. We will briefly discuss some examples.

(a) An SAH may mask the Q wave of infarction.

1. In case of a small inferior infarction (Figure 5.58) we can observe how the loop rotation in the FP, first in the clockwise direction and then in the counter-clockwise, confirms the presence of the SAH associated with an inferior infarction. The beginning of the loop is directed downwards because the beginning of the ventricular activation that occurs in (C) (Figure 5.58A) due to the SAH is spared. The vector originated at least partly in this area (1) counteracts the inferior vector of infarction and permits the loop to move first somewhat rightwards and downwards and then rapidly upwards (due to the inferior infarction), and ends up rotating in the counter-clockwise direction and directed upwards (due to the SAH). All this explains the initial and sometimes slurred 'r'-wave morphology in II, III and VF that masks the inferior infarction (Figure 5.58B). If no SAH existed, the entire loop would rotate in clockwise, first above and, generally, later below the axis of lead X, and would almost certainly be recorded as a Qr complex in the inferior leads (Figure 5.29A). The 'r' wave in III being higher than the 'r' wave in II supports the diagnosis of added inferior infarction (Figure 5.7A) (p. 140).

2. In case of a small septal infarction, the SAH may mask the infarction in horizontalised hearts (Figure 5.59). In that figure it is seen that a high positioning of the leads V1–V2 in the third intercostal space may be necessary in obese patients to check for a QS morphology, which would suggest the presence of an associated septal infarction (p. 188).

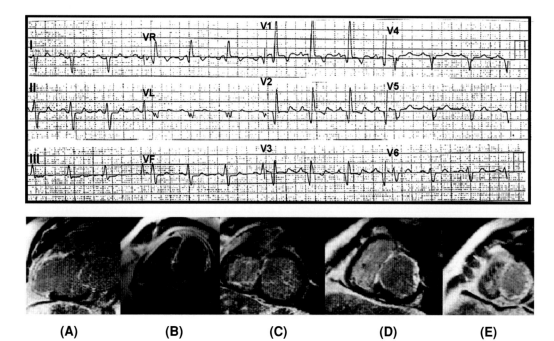

(A)   **(B)**   **(C)**   **(D)**   **(E)**

Figure 5.47 Patient with complete RBBB and myocardial infarction type A-3 (extensive anterior MI). Observe the Q wave in precordial leads and the QS morphology in VL. In CE-CMR images (A–E) show important involvement of lateral, anterior and septal walls, and even the lower part of inferior wall (E). The lateral involvement (B, D and E in white) is more important than in the apical-anterior MI even when there is an anteroseptal extension (see Figures 5.15 and 5.16).

(b) An IPH may mask a Q wave of infarction.

1. **In case of a small mid-anterior infarction**, the area where the depolarisation begins in the IPH (B in Figure 5.60) is spared. This initial depolarisation vector (1 in Figure 5.60) partly counteracts the vector of infarction and gives rise to an initial sometimes slurred 'r' wave in I and VL that masks the mid-anterior infarction.

2. **In case of a small infarction of septal area**, the IPH may mask the infarction in vertical hearts (Figure 5.61B). In this figure it is seen that in case of IPH, the first vector in vertical heart, the beginning of QRS, is recorded as positive (rS pattern) in the fourth intercostal space (Figure 5.61B), because these leads are higher than that in the normal heart (Figure 5.61A). They should be positioned in the fifth intercostal space to record a QS morphology in V1–V2 so that the diagnosis may be confirmed (Figure 5.61B).

3. **In case of large inferior infarction**, the association of an IPH may convert the morphology QS or Qr in inferior leads in QR and therefore the IPH may partially mask the inferior MI (Figure 5.55).

Q waves of infarction masking hemiblocks

Q wave of infarction masking an SAH. On certain occasions, large inferior infarctions may make the diagnosis of hemiblock difficult. This occurs because the rS morphology disappears and a QS morphology is seen in all the inferior wall leads (Figure 5.54B). In a mid-anterior infarction the RS morphology in the inferior wall may make the diagnosis of SAH more difficult (Figure 5.56B).

Q wave of infarction masking an IPH. In large anterior infarctions associated with an IPH, a QS morphology is seen in VL (instead of an rs morphology in the isolated IPH) (Figure 5.57B) and in inferior infarctions a QR morphology (instead of qR morphology) (Figure 5.55B). In these cases the hemiblocks may be masked to some degree because the typical IPH morphology has changed due to the infarction.

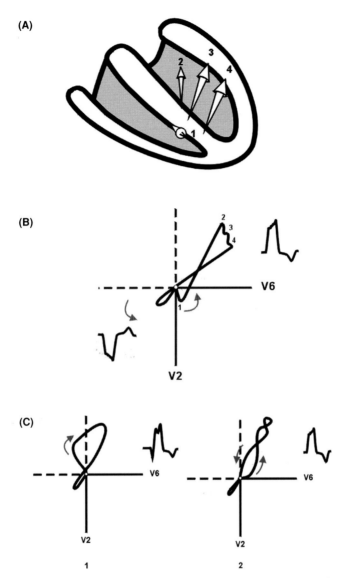

Figure 5.48 (A, B) Ventricular activation in case of LBBB and how this activation explains the LBBB morphology according to the ECG–VCG correlation. (C) The association of infarction frequently originates changes in the QRS loop that usually do not modify the ECG pattern of chronic infarction (C(2)). However, when the infarcted area is extensive, it may produce changes in the direction of the vectors and in the morphology of the loop that explains the appearance of Q waves in the ECG (C(1)).

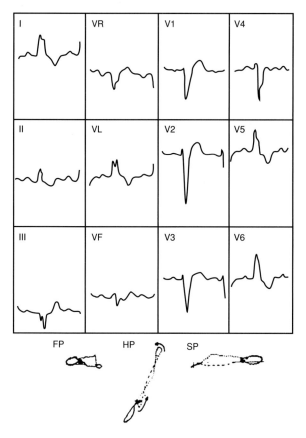

Figure 5.49 Example of the usefulness of VCG to diagnose associated necrosis. The loop presents double-eight morphology (see Figure 5.48C(2)) in the horizontal plane that is abnormal and suggests the presence of associated necrosis in a patient with ischaemic heart disease. The ECG does not suggest evident signs of necrosis, as the QRS is practically normal, although the presence of r ≥ 1 mm in V1 and symmetric T wave in I, VL and V5 is not usually seen in isolated LBBB.

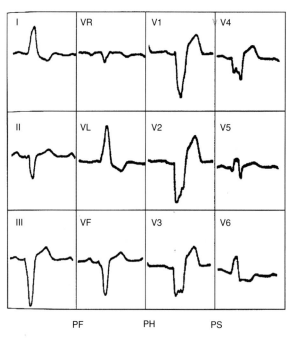

Figure 5.50 ECG–VCG of complete LBBB with signs suggesting associated infarction. It might be suspected from the morphology in V5 (qrs) and evident slurrings in V2–V4 (Cabrera's sign). Also the initial forces are posterior in the VCG, which is abnormal and clearly suggests associated myocardial infarction.

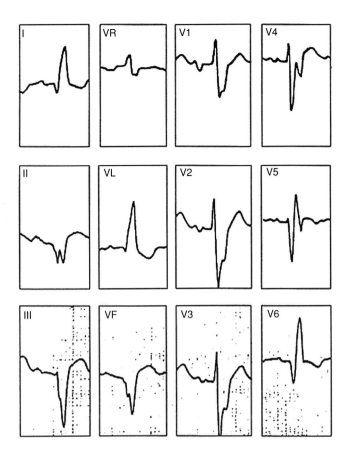

Figure 5.51 A 65-year-old patient, with severe ischaemic heart disease and high blood pressure, who has suffered an acute myocardial infarction 2 months ago and presents an ECG with complete LBBB pattern. The ECG is quite pathological and shows the classic signs of an extensive infarction associated to an LBBB (Q wave in I, VL and V6, rS in V1 with 'r' wave of 5 mm and S wave with significant slurrings in the ascending slope and poliphasic rSR's' complexes in V5).

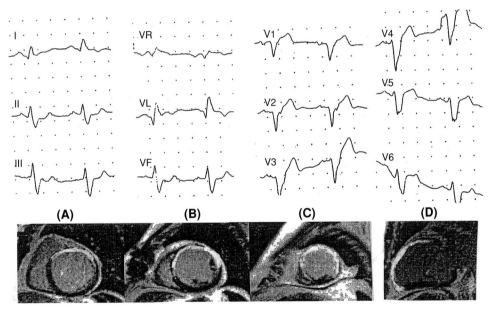

Figure 5.52 The ECG of a patient with complete LBBB and associated infarction. There are ECG criteria suggestive of extensive anterior myocardial infarction (qR in I, QR in VL and low voltage of S in V3). The CMR images (A–D) demonstrated the presence of an extensive infarction of anteroseptal zone (type A-3) (proximal LAD occlusion). The inferolateral wall is free of necrosis (see (D)), because the LAD does not wrap the apex. In the transverse transection in CMR (A–C) is well seen that the MI involves the greatest part of anterior and septal walls with also lateral extension but preserving the high lateral wall (A), because it is perfused by LCX, and the inferior wall because the LAD is not long.

Table 5.6 Sensitivity, specificity and predictive accuracy of various electrocardiographic criteria* for patients with complete LBBB and myocardial infarction, in relation to the specific location of infarction detected by 201-thallium scintigraphy.

ECG criterion	Sensitivity %				Specificity %	Predictive accuracy (%)			
	All AMI	AS	A	I	All controls	All AMI	AS	A	I
Cabrera's sign[†]	27	47		20	87	76	47	12	18
Chapman's sign[‡]	21	23	34	—	91	75	33	41	—
Initial (0.04 s) notching of QRS in II, III or precordial leads	19	12	13	27	88	67	17	17	34
RS in V6	8	18		—	91	50	50		
Abnormal Q in I, VL, III, VF and V6	31	53	27	13	91	83	50	22	11
QV6, RV1	—	20			100	—	100		—
ST ↑[§]	54	76	40	47	97	96	48	22	26
Positive T in leads with positive QRS	8		7	20	76	33		8	25

* Positive response for at least two observers.
[†] Notching of 0.05 s in duration in the ascendant limb of the S wave in V3–V4.
[‡] Notching of ascendant limb of R wave in I, VL, V5 or V6.
[§] >2 mm concordant with main QRS deflection or >7 mm discordant with main deflection.
AMI, acute myocardial infarction; AS, anteroseptal infarction; A, antero(lateral) infarction; I, infero(posterior) infarction.
Adapted from Wackers et al. (1978).

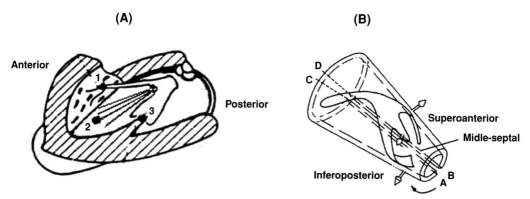

Figure 5.53 (A) Lateral view of superoanterior 1 and inferoposterior 3 divisions of left bundle. The middle-septal fibers are seen (2). (B) Situation of two divisions and middle-septal fibers in the left ventricle cone.

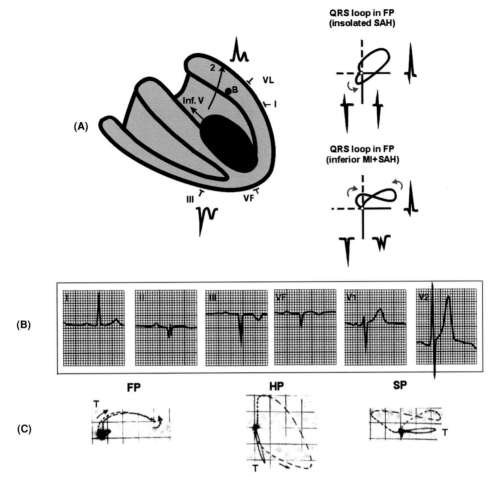

Figure 5.54 Inferior infarction associated with an SAH: (A) When the necrosis is rather large and comprises the area where ventricular depolarisation is initiated in case of SAH (point A + C), the first vector of ventricular depolarisation (1), is neutralised by the infarction vector (Inf. V.) and the loop first goes directly upwards and then, due to the SAH (see lower FP image) instead of rotating in the clockwise direction downward, it rotates in the counter-clockwise direction upward (2). Consequently, a QS morphology develops often with slurrings and generally with a negative T wave in III, VF and even lead II, but without a terminal 'r' wave because the final portion of the loop falls in the negative hemifield of these leads. In the isolated inferior infarction, there is a terminal 'r' wave (at least in II), because the final part of the loop that rotates in the clockwise direction is usually in the positive hemifield of inferior leads (at least of lead II). (B, C) ECG–VCG example of the inferior infarction in the presence of SAH.

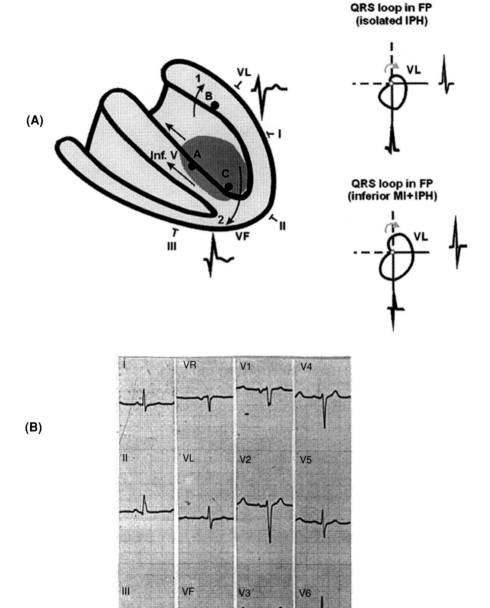

Figure 5.55 Inferior infarction associated with an IPH: (A) the vector of the first part of the activation (the sum of the normal activation initiating vector in the case of an IPH – see B(I) plus the infarction vector – Inf. V) moves away from the inferior wall more than that would be seen in an isolated IPH and is opposite to the final vector of ventricular depolarisation that is directed downwards because of the IPH (vector 2). This explains why the QRS loop is moving further upwards and opens more than normal, generating the qR (QR) morphology in III and VF and RS in I and Rs in VL (see ECG–VCG drawings of isolated IPH and IPH associated with inferior MI on the right part of (A). (B,C) ECG–VCG correlation of inferior infarction plus IPH.

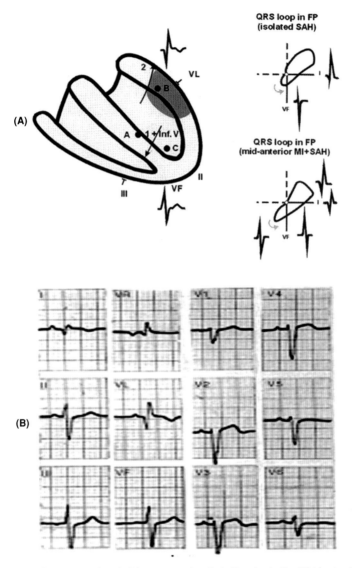

Figure 5.56 Mid-anterior infarction associated with an SAH: (A) the vector of the first part of the activation (that is the sum of vector 1 – which is generated in A + C areas – plus the infarction vector (Inf. V) (which moves away from VL) is opposite to the final vector of the ventricular depolarisation due to the SAH (vector 2). This explains that the initial part of the QRS loop moves more rightwards and downwards and generates an RS morphology in II, III and VF with RIII > RII and QR in VL and I. (B) ECG example of mid-anterior infarction (type A-4) plus an SAH.

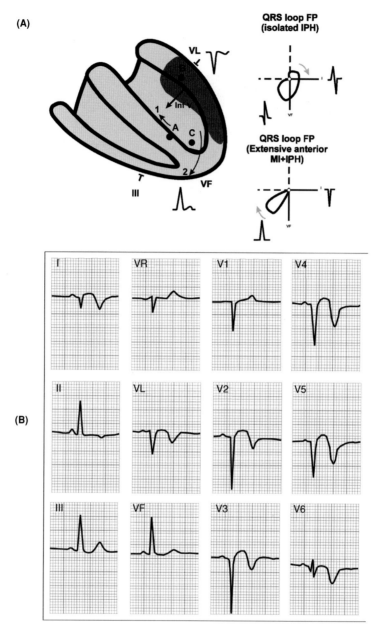

Figure 5.57 Extensive anterior infarction including mid-anterior wall associated with IPH: (A) the first ventricular depolarisation vector (1) generated in A + B areas in case of isolated IPH is directed upwards. However in case of extensive anterior infarction plus IPH, the infarction vector (Inf. V) is more important than the first depolarisation vector and all the loops move away from the infarcted area in the same direction of the second vector of depolarisation (2). Consequently, all the activation (loop) is moving away from VL and I, which explains the QS morphologies in VL and sometimes I, with a dominant R wave, generally pure R wave in II, III and VF (see the drawings of isolated IPH and IPH + associated anterior MI). (B) ECG of extensive anterior infarction, associated with an IPH.

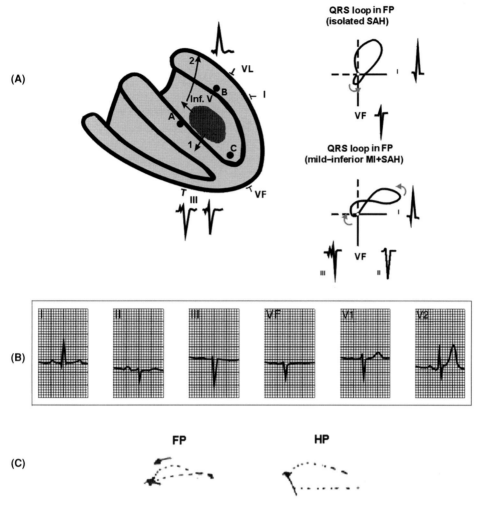

Figure 5.58 SAH may mask small inferior infarction. (A) In this situation, when in the presence of an SAH the area initiating the ventricular depolarisation (A + C) is spared by the necrosis, vector 1 that is directed downwards and rightwards can be only partially counterbalanced by the relatively small infarction vector (Inf. V). This allows the loop to initiate its movement downwards and rightwards, and then rotates immediately upwards. The loop (see the low-right side of (A)) can mask the inferior infarction pattern (QS in III and VF) and may present slurred rS morphology and often rIII > rII. (B) ECG–VCG of small inferior infarction plus SAH (see the rotation of QRS loop in FP and rIII > rII) (Figure 5.7).

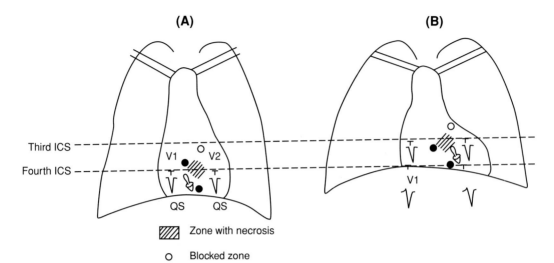

Figure 5.59 (A) Normal habitus. In the presence of small septal infarction with SAH, the infarction vector is directed newly backwards for the necrosis and downwards for the SAH, and in V1 and V2, as in patients without SAH, a QS pattern is recorded. (B) In an obese patient the same area of necrosis with SAH can produce an rS morphology in V1 and V2, because although the vector is oriented backwards and downwards, since it is above the normal V1 and V2 due to obesity, these leads at this place record the head of the first vector as positive. In this case, a higher V1–V2 lead (third intercostal space) records the tail of the first vector as QS and confirms the diagnosis of small septal infarction associated with SAH. The two black points represent the onset of depolarisation.

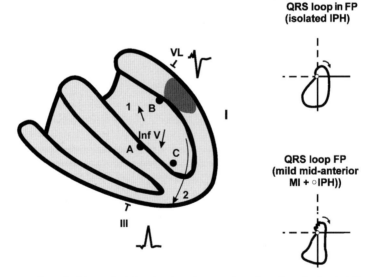

Figure 5.60 IPH may mask small mid-anterior infarction. In this situation, when in presence of an IPH, the ventricular depolarisation initiating area (A + B) is spared by the small necrosis, the first vector of depolarisation vector 1, which is directed upwards, can counteract the relatively small infarction vector (Inf. V). This allows the initial part of the loop to show slurred conduction but directed as in the isolated IPH. This loop (see the right side of the figure) can mask the mid-anterior infarction pattern (QS in VL and sometimes in lead I) and explain slurred 'r' S morphology in VL with slurred qR pattern in inferior leads.

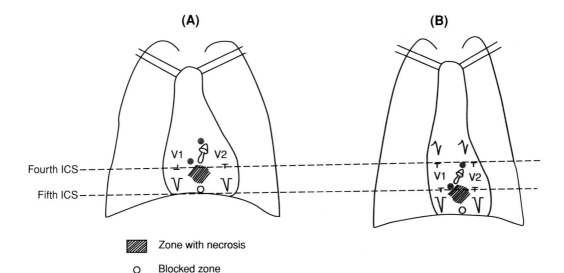

Figure 5.61 (A) normal habitus. In the presence of small septal infarction with IPH, the infarction vector is directed backwards for the necrosis and upwards for IPH, and in V1 and V2, as in patients without IPH, a QS pattern is recorded. (B) In a very lean patient the same area of necrosis in the presence of IPH can generate an rS morphology in V1 and V2, in spite of the backward and upward direction of the vector. These leads record the head of first vector as positive because they are in upper position than the normal V1 and V2 due to lean body habitus. In this case, a lower V1–V2 (fifth interspace) records the tail of first vector as QS and confirms the diagnosis of small septal infarction associated with IPH. The two black points represent the onset of depolarisation.

False Q wave patterns due to hemiblocks

When the V1–V2 electrodes are positioned very high, an initial 'Q' wave may be recorded in SAH, due to the first activation vector, which is directed downwards. This suggests the false pattern of septal infarction that disappears when the electrodes are located more inferiorly. It has already been stated that in obese or very lean individuals the higher or lower positioning of electrodes V1–V2 may be required to find patterns of added true septal infarction (Figures 5.59 and 5.61) (see 'Hemiblocks masking Q waves') (p. 181).

Q wave in case of left-deviated ÂQRS without no SAH (Figures 5.62 and 5.63)

In spite of the left-deviated ÂQRS, Figure 5.30 shows that there is no SAH associated with the inferior infarction, since the QRS loop is always rotating in the clockwise direction. With the surface ECG we can suspect that there is no coexisting SAH because a Qr morphology is seen in the inferior leads (see Figure 5.30). The final 'r' wave is explained by the fact that as the loop rotates only in the clockwise direction, the final portion is in the positive side of lead II (Figure 5.29B). Occasionally, in the case of an inferior infarction without the coexistence of SAH, the loop that makes an entire clockwise rotation is completely above the axis of lead X (Figure 5.30). In this situation, a QS morphology can be seen, but at least a terminal small 'r' wave generally exists in II. In case of associated SAH the final part of the loop rotates counter-clockwise and explains that in lead II a QS or qrs morphology may be seen (Figures 5.29D, 5.54 and 5.62). In isolated inferior MI, the loop is only clockwise and the morphology in II is qR but not qrS (Figures 5.29A–C and 5.63). Thus, though the VCG is the only technique that can assure the presence or not of an associated SAH, the correct incorporation of this information to ECG curves virtually allows to

> The presence of Qr in the inferior leads, at least in II, virtually excludes an associated SAH, while the QS morphology, in turn, supports it (Figures 5.29, 5.62 and 5.63).

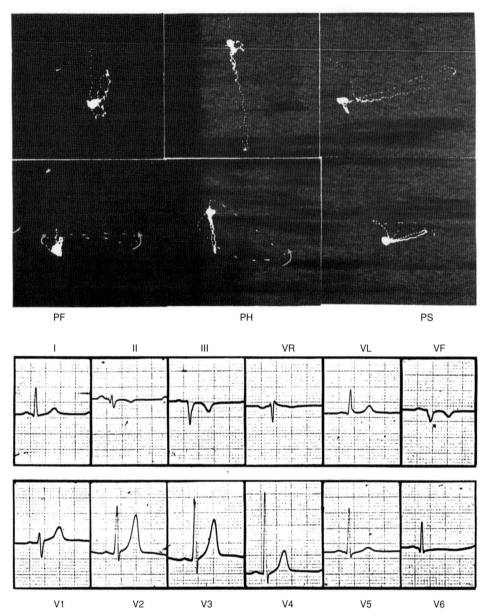

Figure 5.62 ECG–VCG example of inferior MI + SAH. There is q wave in II, III and aVF without terminal r wave (qrs in II and QS in III and VF). VCG loop in frontal plane rotates first clockwise and then counter-clockwise.

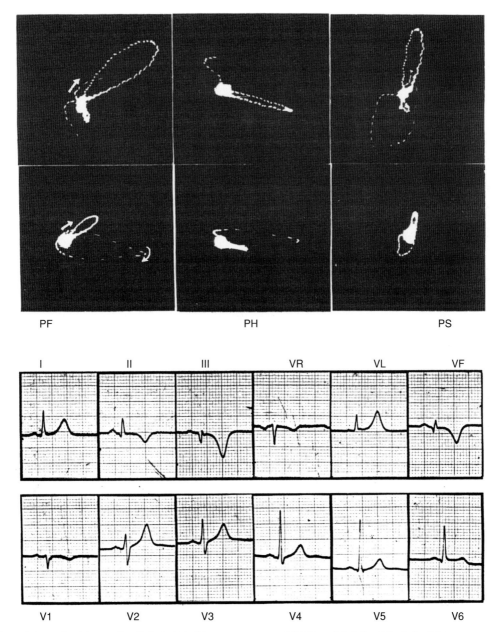

Figure 5.63 ECG–VCG example of inferior MI without SAH. There is qR in II, and qr in III and aVF. VCG loop in frontal plane rotates always clockwise but is directed a little bit more downwards than in Figure 5.33. (The last part of QRS loop fails below '*x*'-axis; lead X is an orthogonal lead, equivalent to lead I.) When all the loop rotating clockwise is above *x*-axis (Figure 5.33), the ECG pattern in lead II is qr and not qR as happens in this figure.

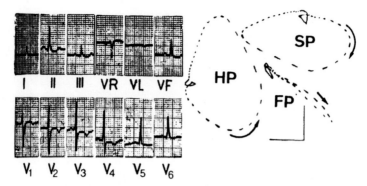

Figure 5.64 An example of ECG and VCG of the block of midle fibers in a coronary patient with affectation of the anterior descending coronary artery and no abnormalities in posterior descending artery. Observe R = S in V2 and r = 5 mm in V1 without q in V6, and the anterior orientation of approximately 50% of the loop in HP (from Moffa et al., 1982).

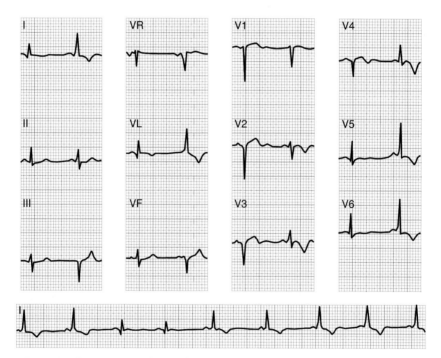

Figure 5.65 Above: ECG of a patient with an intermittent Wolff–Parkinson–White syndrome. In all the leads, the first complex shows no pre-excitation, while the second complex does. In the ECG without pre-excitation, the existence of an apical myocardial infarction can be observed, while in the ECG with pre-excitation the primary characteristics of repolarisation can be seen (symmetric T wave from V2 to V4). Observe how the ischaemic T wave in the absence of pre-excitation is flat or negative in I and VL, the contrary of what happens in the absence of ischaemic heart disease (Figure 3.35 and p. 52). Below: Lead I with progressively pre-excitation activation (concertina effect).

(A)   **(B)**

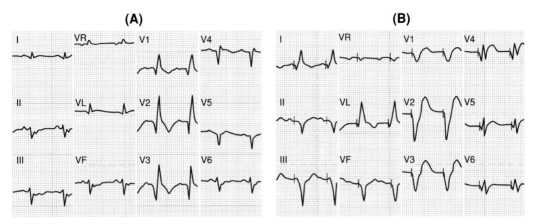

Figure 5.66 (A) Acute anterior myocardial infarction plus complete RBBB. (B) The implanted pacemaker still allows for the visualisation of the necrosis (ST-Q in I, VL and V4–V6).

rule out this association due to the presence of a final 'r' wave (Qr) in the inferior leads, at least in II. In turn, the absence of a terminal 'r' wave (slurred QS or sometimes qrs morphology) in II, III and AVF virtually confirms the presence of an SAH associated with the inferior infarction (compare Figures 5.62 and 5.63).

Block of the middle fibers of LBB

This block may generates a delay in depolarization in anteroseptal part of the septum. This explains a prominent anterior forces of QRS loop and the RS pattern in V1, V2 or at least R wave greater then normal (Figure 5.64) (Hoffman I, Metha J, Hilserath J 1976; Moffa P, Del Nero N, Tobias et al., 1982, Reiffel J, Bigger T, 1978; Bayes de Luna A 1977). Recently the Brazilian school have defined the ECG-VCG criteria for this diagnosis (Guidelines for interpreting rest ECG 2003).

The block of middle fibers of LBB has to be included in the differential diagnosis of prominent R wave in V1 (see Table 5.5). To make this diagnosis in patients with ischemic heart disease the involvement (ischaemia or necrosis) of lateral wall has to be rule out (coronary angiography and/or cardiovascular magnetic resonance –CMR-) (Fig. 5.64). In the case of lateral MI a positive T wave in V1 is seen, and in case of block of middle fibers the T wave in V1 is usually negative.

The evidence that the pattern is transient assure the diagnosis of the block of middle fibers of LBB

(Uchida A, Moffa P, Pérez-Riera A et al., 2006). On the other hand in patients without heart disease the presence of prominent R wave inV1, especially if the voltage of R is low, is much probably due to a normal variant (see Table 5.5).

Wolff–Parkinson–White-type pre-excitation (Figure 5.65)

It is difficult, and sometimes impossible, to confirm the association of a Q-wave infarction in the presence of a Wolff–Parkinson–White-type (WPW-type) pre-excitation. In Figure 5.65 we observe that no Q wave is seen in the complexes with pre-excitation, despite the existence of an apical infarction (second QRS in each lead). When the pre-excitation disappears (first complex in each lead), the presence of Q wave from V1 to V4 is clear. However, during the pre-excitation, the presence of evident repolarisation abnormalities can suggest the coexistence of IHD (symmetric and negative T wave from V2 to V6). We need to remind as well that intermittent conduction by the right anomalous bypass tract, intermittent complete LBBB and intermittent right-ventricular stimulation (Figures 3.34 and 3.35) can be accompanied by a negative T wave when the conduction is made via the normal pathway, which can be explained by a 'cardiac memory' phenomenon (Rosenbaum et al., 1982).

The possibility that a WPW-type pre-excitation may mask the infarction depends on the type of WPW. When the infarct is located contralaterally

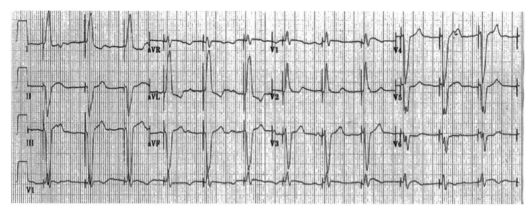

Figure 5.67 A 72-year-old man with previous apical-anterior MI with anteroseptal extension with an implanted pacemaker due to paroxysmal AV block. There is a clear latency between the stimulus of pacemaker and the QRS complex.

to the anomalous path, it is most probable that the infarction is masked. However, when the infarction is located ipsilaterally, it is most probably detected (Wellens, 2006).

Pacemakers (Figures 5.66 and 5.67)

In the chronic phase, the presence of a qR morphology after the pacemaker spike (St-qR) from V4 to V6, I and VL (Figure 5.66) is quite useful, being highly specific, but less sensitive for the diagnosis of associated MI (Barold et al., 1987; Brandt et al., 1998; Castellanos et al., 1973). Besides, the presence of St-rS morphology in VR has been described as a quite sensitive sign, but with a low specificity, for the diagnosis of an inferior infarction. Finally, an interval between the pacemaker stimulus and the beginning of the QRS complex has also been described

in patients with associated MI (Figure 5.67). This occurs when the pacemaker stimulates the fibrotic infarcted area (latency) (Wellens, Gorgels and Doevendans, 2003).

As we have discussed previously ('cardiac memory' in the intermittent LBBB and WPW syndrome), patients with intermittent right-ventricular stimulation, when the stimulus is conducted via the normal path (Figure 3.35), can show a 'cardiac memory' phenomenon (lack of adequacy of the repolarisation to the depolarisation changes), which explains the anomalous repolarisation (negative T wave) that is sometimes observed, in sinus rhythm in the absence of IHD. It has been demonstrated that in this situation, the T wave is negative in precordial lead but is positive in I and VL (see Figure 3.35, p. 52).

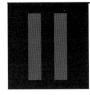

PART II

The ECG in different clinical settings of ischaemic heart disease: correlations and prognostic implications

This second part deals with ECG characteristics in different clinical situations of ischaemic heart disease (IHD) and their, clinical, coronariographic, haemodynamic and imaging correlations, especially related to prognostic implications and risk stratification. This includes different types of **ACS** with or without evolving Q-wave infarction and the specific characteristics of atypical ACS. This part also includes different types of myocardial infarction without Q waves and different clinical settings of chronic IHD including chronic Q-wave infarction and other clinical situations presenting with anginal pain in a stable phase but without necessarily previous Q-wave MI. Finally, the aspects related with the ECG changes in silent ischaemia and the role of ECG as a predictor of future IHD will be discussed.

6 CHAPTER 6

Acute and chronic ischaemic heart disease: definition of concepts and classification

The term **acute coronary syndrome** (ACS) encompasses all the clinical situations with acute myocardial ischaemia expressed by chest pain, discomfort or equivalent, which appears suddenly at rest (de novo) or has increased with regard to prior anginal (in crescendo angina). All this leads the patient to seek urgent medical care. However, occasionally the patient may underestimate the symptoms or the physician may not interpret them properly. In addition, the ACS may occur with no anginal pain, or the pain may be atypical or may present other symptoms, such as dyspnoea. Also, an ACS may be clinically silent. **In its classic or typical form**, ACS occurs in patients presenting a **coronary atherothrombosis**, generally related with the rupture or erosion of a vulnerable plaque (Figure 6.1B–D). However, rarely, there are **other causes** that could explain the presentation of the **atypical ACS** (Table 6.1-1).

In **ACS** the clinical situation can be controlled and the ACS might not evolve, **whereby it is unstable angina** (UA) or may well progress towards an **acute myocardial infarction** that may or may not present Q wave of necrosis (chronic MI). We should recall that cases presenting with troponin elevation, along with any of the characteristics shown in Table 6.2, are recognised as infarctions according to

Table 6.1 Classification of clinical settings due to myocardial ischemia.

1. **Acute coronary syndromes**
   - **Due to coronary atherothrombosis ("classical" or "typical")**
   - **Not due to coronary atherothrombosis ("atypical")**
     - Hypercoagulability
     - Tachyarrhythmia
     - Coronary dissection
     - Transient apical LV ballooning (Tako-Tsubo syndrome)
     - Congenital abnormalities
     - Bypass surgery
     - Percutaneous coronary intervention (PCI)
     - Coronary spasm (Prinzmetal angina)
     - Miscellaneous (cocaine, CO, anaphylaxis, acute anaemia, others, etc)
2. **Clinical settings with angina outside the ACS.**
     - Classical exercise angina
     - Syndrome X
     - Myocardial bridging
     - Miscellaneous: pulmonary hypertension, chronic anaemia, etc.

Table 6.2 Proposal for new diagnostic criteria for MI (consensus ESC/ACC, 2000).

Any of these two criteria will be sufficient to approve a MI diagnosis, in evolution or recent.

1) Typical elevation and gradual descent of troponin[1] or other typical markers of myocardial necrosis (CK-MB), in the presence, of at least, one of the following factors:
   • Symptoms of isquemia (angina or equivalent)
   • Pathologic Q-waves in the ECG (see table 5.3)
   • Electrocardiographic changes indicating isquemia (ST / T changes)
   • PCI and surgery-related acute coronary syndrome.
2) Pathologic changes, related to acute MI

[1] It is important to remember other reasons for troponin elevation without MI – heart or kidney failure, hypertensive crises, etc.)

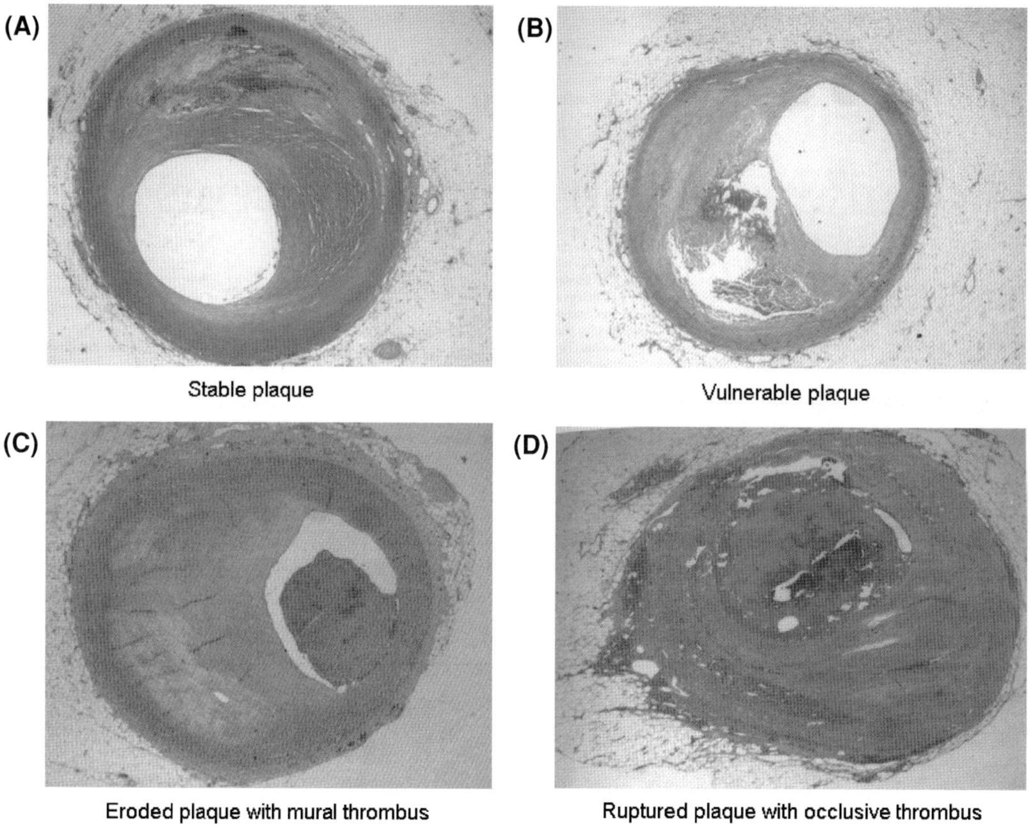

(A) Stable plaque

(B) Vulnerable plaque

(C) Eroded plaque with mural thrombus

(D) Ruptured plaque with occlusive thrombus

Figure 6.1 Different examples of (A) stable plaque, (B) vulnerable plaque, (C) eroded plaque with small thrombus and (D) ruptured plaque with occlusive thrombus. This figure can be seen in colour, Plate 5.

the ESC/ACC task force (Alpert et al., 2000). This extends the myocardial infarction spectrum, since many UAs now become 'small infarctions' (**enzymatic infarction or necrosette**).

There are also **cases of anginal pain that do not require urgent medical assistance in emergency department**. These will also be discussed later (see Table 6.1-2 and p. 296).

CHAPTER 7

Patients with acute chest pain: role of the ECG and its correlations

Patients looking for urgent medical attention and presenting with new onset chest pain or with any change in duration, intensity or characteristics of a prior chest pain or equivalent symptoms (dyspnoea, thoracic discomfort, etc.) are considered suspicious to present an ACS. In these cases the ischaemic aetiology should be confirmed. Special mention will be made of the usefulness of the ECG in those cases even before the patient arrives to the hospital. The recording of a pre-hospital ECG by emergency medical services may be an effective method of reducing time to reperfusion. However, pre-hospital ECG is not always used, and when used the information provided often is not being translated into action (Curtis et al., 2006). Increased experience and the development of more reliable methods of performing and communicating results of pre-hospital ECG may lead to dramatic system-wide reduction in time to reperfusion and ultimately reductions in morbidity and mortality for ACS patients.

Firstly, one should bear in mind that it is always **necessary to consider the possibility of heart diseases other than IHD that could explain one abnormal ECG recording**. These changes may include abnormal ST segment or T wave and/or an abnormal Q wave. These changes may be chronic, as occurs in dilated cardiomyopathy (DCM), hypertrophic cardiomyopathy (HCM), aortic stenosis (AS), hypertension, dissecting aneurysm, etc. In other cases there may be new changes, such as in pericarditis, acute myocarditis (perimyocarditis) or pulmonary embolism, among others. However, not all electrocardiographic abnormalities occurring in a patient with chest pain must be explained by myocardial ischaemia. Although heart disease other than IHD exists, the ECG changes can be partly or completely due to an associated IHD. The clinical–electrocardiographic correlation will allow for iden-

tifying the cause or causes that could have altered the ECG.

Types of pain

Patients can be divided into **three groups** according to type of chest pain: **non-ischaemic chest pain**, **ischaemic chest pain** and **doubtful chest pain**. Each of these groups accounts for approximately 20–40% of all patients arriving at the emergency department with chest pain (Erhardt et al., 2002; Santalo, 2003) (Figure 7.1).

Obviously, most patients presenting with a doubtful chest pain on arrival at the emergency department correspond to either the non-ischaemic or the ischaemic chest pain group, since just a few cases with an unclear diagnosis remain. In the end, ischaemic chest pain accounts for 40–50% of all cases and non-ischaemic chest pain for a somewhat higher percentage. Non-ischaemic cardiovascular pain is not frequent, but includes cases that may need urgent treatment (Erhardt et al., 2002; Figure 7.1). Additionally, in a review of the diagnoses made in patients with chest pain who were seen by general practitioners in Europe somewhat different figures have been obtained. These are higher for pain of bone or musculoskeletal origin (50% of all cases) and lower for ischaemic chest pain (20–25% of all cases) (Hasdai et al., 2002).

Non-ischaemic pain
The diagnosis of non-ischaemic chest pain is made on the basis of its characteristics (atypical localisation, with no radiation, non-oppressive and with no vegetative symptoms) **and other circumstances** (age, lack of risk factors, prior history, concomitant findings, complementary tests, etc.) (Figure 7.1). Occasionally, the diagnosis of non-ischaemic chest pain is clear, as it occurs with radicular pain (patient

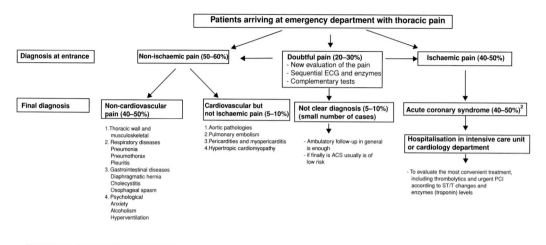

1 X-ray, exercise testing and if necessary, echocardiography, other imaging techniques and coronary angiography
2. Clinical, ECG and enzymatic characteristics

Figure 7.1 Patients who present at the emergency department with thoracic pain: types of thoracic pains and their etiology.

history and physical examination), pneumonia (clinical history, auscultation and X-ray), pneumothorax, the diagnosis of which is clearly made by history taking, physical examination and, especially, X-ray studies. However, **in any case of chest pain, located in the precordium or even in any pain originated from the level of the navel or above, including head and arms and, especially, if it is associated with physical exertion, an ECG, and if necessary, an enzyme test should always be performed** to recognise whether the pain is of ischaemic origin or not. When doubts exist, cardiac enzyme levels and the ECG should be repeated (if possible, electrocardiographic monitoring should preferably be employed). Enzymatic tests should be preferably performed at 6–12 hours after the onset of symptoms. Additionally, complementary techniques should be utilised (X-ray, echocardiography, exercise stress test, TAC-multislice, etc.).

Non-ischaemic pain may or may not be cardiovascular. Most frequently, non-cardiovascular thoracic pain is of radicular and/or musculoskeletal origin (approximately one-third of all thoracic pains – Figure 7.1). This type of pain does not exhibit visceral characteristics and it occurs in relation to bone movement and/or pressure to the thoracic wall, and it is not related to exercise. Other kinds of pain in this group include those of **gastrointestinal origin** (5–10%: oesophageal disease, chole-

cystitis, etc.), **pulmonary origin** (5–10%: pneumothorax, pneumonia and pleuritic pain) **or even psychological origin** (5–10%).

Among the **non-ischaemic cardiovascular causes of thoracic pain** that should be ruled out, **some present a benign prognosis** as pericarditis, **while others, in turn, point to a much serious prognosis**, such as an acute aortic syndrome (**dissecting aneurysm or other aortic pathologies**) and a **pulmonary embolism**. On the whole, these account for 5–10% of all cases of thoracic pain.

Acute pericarditis may show a clear clinical picture with a history of upper airway infection and chest pain that, though may appear to be of ischaemic origin, often has special characteristics. (It radiates to the left shoulder, increases with respiratory movements, etc.). Furthermore, troponin levels may increase even in the absence of a clear accompanying myocardial involvement and with a normal or near-normal ECG. From the electrocardiographic point of view, in the acute phase of pericarditis the ST-segment elevation is the most characteristic abnormality (Figure 4.48), which should be distinguished both from the ST-segment elevation of early repolarisation pattern (Figure 4.50) and from that seen in ACS (Table 7.1). In fact, computerised interpretation systems frequently confound the ST-segment elevation of the early repolarisation with that of a pericarditis (Willems et al.,

Table 7.1 Differential diagnosis between pericarditis, early repolarization, ACS and dissecting aneurysm.

		Pericarditis	Early repolarización	A C S	Dissecting aneurysm
M E D I C A L	1. Age	Any age	Any age. Often in young people with vagal overdrive /or sportsmen	Exceptional before the age of 30.	Adults and elderly
	2. Risk factors for isquemic heart disease	Sometimes	Sometimes	Often	Often. Very frequent in patients with hypertension
	3. Previous respiratory infections	Frequent. Sometimes fever.	No (occasional)	No (Occasional)	No (Occasional)
H I S T O R Y	4. Pain characteristics	Visceral pain often with: – Pain increase during respiration. *It may seem that pain increases with the exercise because the latter increases respiration frequency* – Typical irradiation towards the left shoulder – Sometimes recurrent	Can coexist with osteo-articular pain or pain of any other origin (see fig. 7.2 and fig. 7.3)	– Isquemic pain often with typical irradiation (see text) – During rest or light exercise – Can be present in any part of the thorax, and even any pain above the navel is suspicious	Intensive, visceral pain, mainly lo-cated in the back of the thorax. *If this occurs, it is always important to rule out a dissecting aneurysm or an MI of the lateral wall.*
	5. E C G	– ST elevation in the early phase. Often, but not always convex with respect to the isoelectric line; presented mainly in the precordial leads (figs. 4.48, 4.49) – Sometimes typical evolutive changes (fig. 4.48) – Often PR segment elevation in VR and depression in II (figs. 4.48, 4.49). – There is no change during an exercise stress test	– ST elevation, convex with respect to the isoelectric line. In general not always convex with respect to the isoelectric line. In general not >2–3 mm, mainly in precordial leads from V2–V3 to V4–V5. (fig. 4.50). Sometimes in the inferior wall. Often slurrings at the end of QRS – Elevation of PR segment not evident – The ST elevation disappears during a stress test (figs 7.2 and 7.3).	– ST elevation, which in its most typical form is concave with respect to the isoelectric line (see fig. 4.13). Sometimes, but not always is evident. – PR elevation in VR is not frequent. It can be present in MI of the atrium, but then there are clear signs of Q-wave MI.	– Not typical. In general is related to the associated diseases (HTA, previous isquemic heart disease). – Can give false ST elevation (see fig 7.4).
	6. Blood tests	Mild-moderate elevation of the troponin (perimyocarditis)	Within the normal range	Can be within the normal range (unstable angina) or elevated, very often with important increase.	In general, within the normal range
	7. Evolution	– In general, good clinical evolution – Sometimes evolutionary ECG changes, but not always typical (fig. 4.48) – Q-wave is missing	No change	Often evolution towards Q-wave infarction	Often bad evolution / prognosis

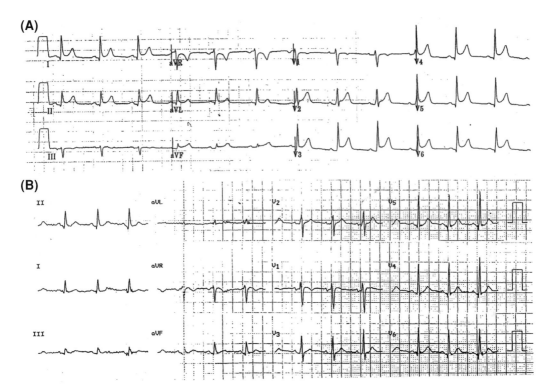

Figure 7.2 (A) A patient with thoracic pain and mild ST-segment elevation in many leads. ECG was considered by automatic interpretation as pericarditis. (B) The ST-segment elevation disappears with exercise, which favours the diagnosis of early repolarisation pattern. This is an example of misdiagnosis of automatic interpretation.

1991) (Figure 7.2). Additionally, in some cases pericarditis or ACS may occur in a patient with early repolarisation, which makes the diagnosis more difficult (Shu et al., 2005) (Figure 7.3). Nevertheless, even though the clinical features may be of much help (history of respiratory infection and chest pain with certain characteristics in pericarditis), the electrocardiogram presents some specific characteristics for the experienced cardiologist (e.g. presence of PR-segment elevation in VR due to atrial injury with, generally, PR-segment depression as a mirror image in lead II in pericarditis). In turn, in early

repolarisation, slurrings of the final part of the QRS complex are frequently present, and these are especially apparent in the mid-precordial leads. These slurrings can be well seen in Figure 7.3, but not in Figure 7.2. Also, the ECG response during an exercise stress test (abolishment of the ST-segment elevation in early repolarisation, and lack of change in pericarditis) is different and becomes definitive for the diagnosis in cases of doubt (Figure 7.3). Occasionally, ST-segment elevation concave with respect to the isoelectric baseline is recorded in pericarditis (Figures 4.48B and 4.49) with

---

The following may be of help in assessing the diagnosis of pericarditis versus an ACS:

1. Clinical history, including antecedents of respiratory infection
2. Pain characteristics, which are generally different in pericarditis from those of ischaemic pain

3. The presence of apparent atrial injury in the ECG (PR depression in II and elevation in VR; Figures 4.48 and 4.49), and the lack of evolving Q-wave MI
4. The evolution of the disease

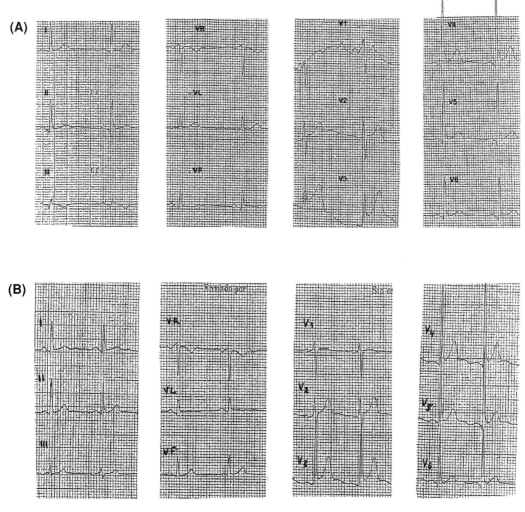

Figure 7.3 (A) The ECG corresponds to a patient presenting with thoracic pain. This ECG was considered to be suggestive of ACS with ST-segment elevation (see V2 and V3), and treatment with fibrinolytic agents was administered. Later, imaging and enzymatic tests were found to be negative. (B) The patient was discharged with the ECG presenting ST-segment elevation in V3 of 2 mm compared with the previous 5 mm. The whole clinical setting was thus considered as an atypical thoracic pain in a patient with an early repolarisation pattern. Nevertheless, properly performed history taking suggested the diagnosis of pericarditis (previous respiratory infection, fever, precordial pain, etc.) associated with an early repolarisation pattern. (C) The presence of early repolarisation was confirmed with an exercise test as the ST-segment elevation disappeared. This is a typical example of the incorrectly applied fibrinolytic treatment in a patient with thoracic pain and ST-segment elevation in ECG as a consequence of bad history taking and ECG interpretation.

myocardial compromise (perimyocarditis). Sometimes the ECG pattern of subepicardium ischaemia is quite difficult to distinguish from the negative T wave of IHD (Figure 3.29). In cases of doubt, the lack of evolution to evolving Q-wave MI is of much help. However, we have to remember that the troponin levels may increase in pericarditis (Bonnefoy, 2000). Therefore, troponin levels are not definitive for distinguishing without any doubt between pericarditis (perimyocarditis), in which they may be elevated, and ACS, in which they may be normal.

Occasionally, **acute myocarditis** may exhibit an ST-segment elevation, and rarely abnormal Q waves that are usually of a transient nature, generating an electrocardiographic pattern quite similar to that of an ACS. Characteristically, patients with an acute myocarditis that present an ECG similar to evolving Q-wave MI (Q wave and ST-segment elevation) exhibit low-voltage QRS complexes and sinus tachycardia that can help the differential diagnosis (Figure 5.43). The clinical history and the complementary tests help to clarify the case, although, as we have just mentioned, the troponin levels may rise in both situations and acute myocarditis can also present chest discomfort.

The acute aortic syndrome (dissecting aneurysm, aortic ulcer or intramural haematoma) usually presents with a very sharp and intense pain that is characteristically located predominantly at the back of the thorax. The prognosis is serious and adequate treatment should be performed immediately. However, these processes do not usually modify the ECG recording, which, frequently, is already abnormal. An ST-segment elevation in V1–V2 – the indirect (mirror) pattern of the left-ventricular enlargement that these patients frequently present in V5–V6 due to the frequent association with hypertension – is sometimes mistaken for the primary pattern of an ST-segment elevation due to an ACS. It is most important to consider this possibility, since this mistake could lead to the decision to employ fibrinolytic therapy. This might not only be unnecessary, but dangerous (Figure 7.4). In the mirror pattern, due to associated hypertension, the ST-segment elevation in V1–V2 is usually only of a few millimetres and convex with respect to the isoelectric baseline, as is clearly shown in Figure 7.4. On the other hand, in ACS the ST-segment elevation can be much more significant and, in general, concave. However, ST-segment elevation in an ACS may be convex with respect to the isoelectric baseline in the presence of a tall R wave, but when the morphology is 'rS', the convexity is not evident in ischemic cases as in some normal variants (Figure 3.1B) or in the mirror image of LVH seen in V1–V2 (Figures 7.4). The differential diagnosis is easier when 'Q' waves of necrosis are present. Rarely, the aortic dissection involves a coronary artery and then the case becomes clearly an 'atypical' ACS (Table 6.1, p. 266).

A pulmonary embolism usually causes dyspnoea rather than pain. Some of the following electrocardiographic changes usually appear in severe cases: ST-segment elevation, complete right bundle branch block (RBBB) (Figure 4.54), sinus tachycardia, negative T wave in the right precordial leads and/or the McGinn–White sign (SI QIII negative TIII) (Figure 7.5). McGinn–White pattern is transient and disappears when the situation is resolved. Sometimes, in elderly patients with poor sinus node function, sinus tachycardia may be misleadingly absent, even in the presence of a significant pulmonary embolism.

The most characteristic morphologies of ST-segment elevation in IHD and other situations are shown in Figure 4.13. The most important features that allow for differentiation of ACS from acute pericarditis, early repolarisation and dissecting aneurysm are given in Table 7.1.

Pain of doubtful origin

In these cases (at least 20% of all cases of chest pain arriving at the emergency department) a definitive diagnosis should be made as soon as possible and, especially, pain of an ischaemic origin (ACS) and other serious causes (dissecting aneurysm and pulmonary embolism) should be either confirmed or ruled out (Figure 7.1). It is also necessary to keep in mind other aetiologies, such as radicular, gastrointestinal and respiratory pain, and, principally, pericarditis and perimyocarditis. The possibilities of confusing perimyocarditis with an ACS are higher, since in perimyocarditis not only enzymatic elevation may exist, but also ST-segment elevation is sometimes evident. It is important to assess the presence of a recurrent pain, to analyse the pain characteristics and to perform another ECG. Whenever possible, ECG monitoring should be employed to check for dynamic changes in repolarisation. Enzymatic determinations may be repeated when the initial tests have not been conclusive. However, it is worth remembering that, as has already been stated, enzymatic levels usually rise in the acute pericarditis, although, in general, moderately and that the ECG does not evolve to a Q-wave myocardial infarction.

If necessary, other complementary tests should be carried out (chest X-ray, exercise stress test, echocardiography and other imaging techniques). When

(A)

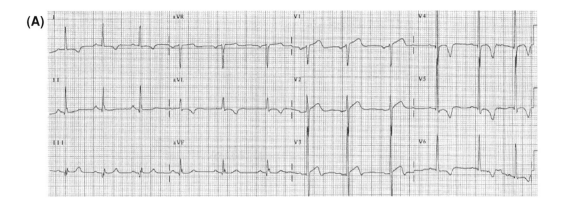

(B)

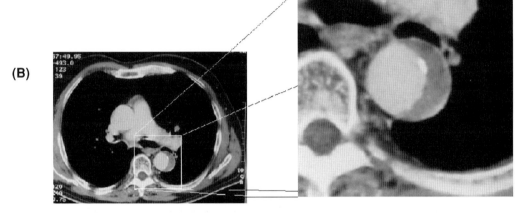

Figure 7.4 (A) A patient with thoracic pain due to a dissecting aortic aneurysm. An ST-segment elevation in V1–V3 can be explained by the mirror pattern of an evident LVE (V6) due to hypertension. This ST-segment elevation has been erroneously interpreted as due to an acute coronary syndrome. As a consequence, fibrinolytic treatment was administered, which was not only unnecessary but even harmful. (B) The CAT scan imaging shows the dissecting aneurysm of the aorta. This case demonstrates that before accepting a diagnosis of STE-ACS other diseases that may cause ST-segment elevation have to be ruled out.

the diagnosis of a dissecting aneurysm is suspected, a transoesophageal echocardiographic study and/or a computerised tomography (CT) scan should be done. If a pulmonary embolism is suspected, some blood test – D-dimer and ventilation/perfusion pulmonary scintigraphy or an angio-MRI – may be necessary. In cases of dubious precordial pain, an isotopic study or a stress echocardiogram will occasionally be needed, or even a coronary angiogram if possible, in order to confirm or to rule out an ischaemic origin. Recently, it has been reported (Hoffmann, 2006) that the non-invasive assessment of coronary arteries by coronary multidetector computed tomography may be, in case of relatively high prevalence of ACS, useful for early triage.

Some sophisticated techniques (CMTCE) or isotopic techniques are not available in the emergency department of majority of the centres. However, X-ray, exercise stress test, repeated determination of troponin levels and even an echocardiographic study can be performed in many of them. An exercise stress test should be carried out to clarify diagnostic doubts but only when a proper history and review of previous ECG recordings, if available, have ruled out that the patient is clinically unstable. The few serious problems that may arise during the practice of exercise test in these patients usually occur because these considerations have not been borne in mind (Ellestad, 2004). An example of the **usefulness of the exercise stress test in a**

(A)

(B)

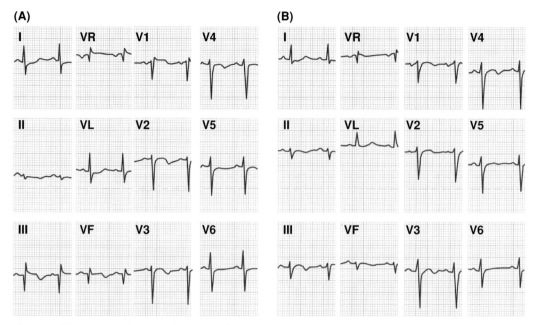

Figure 7.5 (A) A 58-year-old patient who presented a typical McGinn–White pattern (SI, QIII with negative TIII) in a course of pulmonary embolism. (B) The pattern disappeared during the follow-up (B).

patient with doubtful chest pain and a practically normal basal ECG is shown in Figures 4.62 and 4.64. After a few minutes of exercise, the ECG was abnormal. In the contrary, two cases of doubtful pain with ECG diagnosed as pericarditis by the automatic interpretation that normalised during the exercise stress test are shown in Figures 7.2 and 7.3. This result rules out the diagnosis of pericarditis and favours early repolarisation. With this approach the number of patients that are discharged with having a non-diagnosed ACS (accounting for 10% of the patients in some series) will decrease dramatically and hence the unnecessary admission of patients with non-ischaemic chest pain (more than 30% in some series) will also decrease.

In a small percentage of cases diagnosis is not clearly performed, and the patient's evolution sometimes provides the solution. When the clinical picture, the ECG recording, the enzymatic levels and the exercise stress test are not conclusive and the final diagnosis is an ACS, it is generally of low risk (Lee et al., 1985, 1993; Pastor Torres et al., 2002). The complication rate of an ACS with a normal baseline ECG that shows no changes during a chest pain episode is quite low. On the other hand,

cases with abnormal ECG presenting, in addition, changes during the anginal crisis have the highest rate of complications.

Pain of ischaemic origin: acute coronary syndrome

At least 40% of all cases of chest pain arriving at a hospital's emergency department (Figure 7.1) present an ACS (history taking, ECG, enzymes, complementary tests, etc.) that will either evolve or not towards an infarction (enzymes, ECG evolution, etc.).

In most cases the ACS is, from a pathophysiological point of view, the consequence of a coronary atherothrombosis, generally triggered by the rupture or erosion of a vulnerable plaque (a plaque with a large lipid content and thin and weak fibrous cap) (Figure 6.1A and Table 6.1; see Plate 1.4). When the plaque content is in contact with circulating blood, a coronary thrombosis occurs, with the resulting arterial occlusion (Braunwald, Zipes and Libby, 1998; Fuster and Topol, 1996). However, different ACSs, not due to coronary atherothrombosis, exist (Table 6.1). They are studied separately in the section '**Acute coronary syndrome not due to coronary** atherothrombosis' (p. 265). There are some patients with ischaemic chest pain suggestive of ACS that for several reasons does not seek attention in the emergency department. This means that we have to educate not only physicians but also the global population about the critical signs of heart attack and the importance to look for medical care very quickly.

The pain frequently has the typical ischaemic features (located in the precordium, oppressive, radiating to the jaw and/or arms, vegetative symptoms, etc.). However, in certain cases it may be atypical with respect to the localisation, irradiation and other characteristics. It may even be atypical increasing on movement, digital pressure, etc. These cases usually present a good prognosis (see later 'Prognosis of patients arriving at emergency department with chest pain' and p. 257). It should be considered that any exertional pain, not only of precordial location, but in any other upper part of the body, including the arms, has to be considered of ischaemic origin until the contrary has been demonstrated. Irradiation towards the arms and the jaw, especially, and the presence of vegetative signs support ischaemic origin.

Different clinical parameters exist that, independently of typical characteristics of the pain, favour its ischaemic origin. They are (1) age; (2) documented history of IHD and/or atherosclerotic artery disease, and/or evident risk factors (hypertension, diabetes and lipid disorders); (3) family history of IHD or sudden death. However, when these aspects are lacking, the ischaemic origin of the pain should not be ruled out. Occasionally, atypical ACS in a

young person, including a young woman, may occur (see 'ACS not due to coronary atherothrombosis', p. 265).

There are, as well, some cases with anginal pain that do not require urgent medical assistance in emergency department because the pain is stable (**classic exertional angina**), or their characteristics are frequently atypical and/or repetitive along the years (**X syndrome** or **myocardial bridging**, etc.). These cases (Tables 6.1-2) have been included in the section 'Clinical settings with anginal pain outside the ACS' (p. 297). However, in cases frequently coexisting with an underlying atherosclerotic disease, they may change their form of presentation or their duration, or may become repetitive, and give rise to a typical picture of an ACS. The cases of coronary spasm (p. 271), as the anginal pain occurred at rest, are considered an atypical ACS, because of transient nature of ST-segment elevation and because it is due to coronary spasm sometimes without evident atherothrombosis.

Prognosis of patients arriving at the emergency department with chest pain

(Braunwald et al., 2000; Diderholm et al., 2002; Lee et al., 1985, 1995; Morrow et al., 2000a,b; Pastor Torres et al., 2002; Ryan et al., 1999)

In chest pain of non-ischaemic origin, the prognosis is related to the aetiology of the pain. It can range from a benign prognosis (e.g. a musculoskeletal pain) to a poor or very poor prognosis (pneumonia, pulmonary embolism, dissecting aneurysm or other types of acute aortic syndrome).

Patients with chest pain of ischaemic origin correspond to the clinical picture of ACS. The ACS may be classified, according to the clinical, electrocardiographic and blood test characteristics, into three risk groups: high, intermediate and low. Further ahead, we will discussin detail the electrocardio-graphic markers found especially in these three groups (see section 'Risk stratification' p. 257). We will just recall here that patients presenting with an ACS, with atypical chest pain (increasing on movement or with digital pressure, etc.), normal or slightly abnormal ECG, and negative or not clearly positive enzymes, usually have a very good prognosis.

CHAPTER 8

Acute coronary syndrome: unstable angina and acute myocardial infarction

Pathophysiology and classification of ACS: the role of ECG

Majority of ACS occur due to coronary atherothrombosis, and thus they may be considered as classic or typical ACS. There are other causes that may in some occasions, usually rare, produce an ACS that we consider atypical (Table 6.1) (see 'ACS not due to coronary atherothrombosis' p. 265).

In the chronic phase of IHD the concept of Q- and non-Q-wave MI is still used and is valid to separate patients that usually present a larger infarction (Q-wave infarction) than the others with usually less extensive infarction (non-Q-wave MI), as has been demonstrated by CMR (Moon et al., 2004). However, in acute phase of IHD, the best classification after the results of TIM11B trial (Bertrand and Spencer, 2006) is ACS with or without ST-segment elevation, because it was demonstrated that fibrinolytic therapy is clearly beneficial in patients with ACS and ST-segment elevation (STE-ACS),* and no clear benefit was found in patients without ST-segment elevation (NSTE-ACS). Angiographic findings have demonstrated that these differences in outcome are due to the status of the infarct-related artery that present acute coronary occlusion in more than 80% of cases in STE-ACS and only in 10–25% in NSTE-ACS. The group of NSTE-ACS includes patients with unstable angina (UA) and NSTEMI that present similar physiopathology but patients

with non-NSTEMI have a worst outcome. Other differences between stable angina, STE-ACS and NSTE-ACS are shown in Figure 8.1 and Table 8.2. This figure shows that patients with NSTE-ACS present white thrombi (platelet-rich thrombi) as compared with STE-ACS that present red thrombi. The difference between the two groups is also important regarding the degree of occlusion, as we have already mentioned. Patients with STE-ACS usually present total occlusion of the infarct-related artery due to thrombosis that if persists, evolves to a Q-wave MI. Meanwhile, in patients with NSTE-ACS the obstruction is not usually complete and localised but presents active lesions with irregular borders and superimposed thrombus in a lesion that frequently presents a ruptured or eroded plaque, and usually if infarct occurs, is of non-Q-wave type.

In patients with STE-ACS, early achievement of an open infarct-related artery (**the open artery theory**) is associated with an improved outcome. However, if occlusion persists for more than 30 minutes, usually Q-wave-type MI develops. Fibrinolytic therapy interrupts this cascade of events by lysing the coronary thrombus and clearly improving survival. On the other hand, among patients presenting NSTE-ACS the coronary artery is usually patent, although the presence of ulcerated/ruptured plaque with non-occlusion thrombus makes necessary to prevent the progression to complete occlusion (**theory of passivation of disrupted plaque**).

From ECG point of view, we have to mention that patients with **new onset persistent ST-segment elevation (>30 min) belong to the group STE-ACS**, which indicates transmural ischaemia due to epicardial coronary occlusion by a thrombus that evolves

---

* In English literature, it is usually named STEMI (ST elevation myocardial infarction), but we consider the name STE-ACS better because currently with quick reperfusion treatment some of these cases present aborted MI.

	Stable angina	Non-ST elevation ACS	ST elevation ACS evolving to Q-wave MI
Angiographic thrombus	0–1%	40–75%	>90%
Morphology	Smooth	Ulcerated	Occluded
Acute coronary occlusion	0–1%	10–25%	>90%
Angioscopy	No clot	'White Clot'	'Red Clot'

Figure 8.1 Angiographic findings in chronic stable angina and all the spectrum of ACS. (Modified from Cannon, 2003.)

to Q-wave MI and needs immediate reperfusion therapy. When there are transient episodes of ST-segment elevation and ST-segment depression there is no clear decision, and usually these cases are ultimately classified as NSTE-ACS. When only ST-segment elevation is present but the crises are very transient, these cases usually correspond to non-typical ACS as is variant angina (coronary spasm). Therefore, in all patients with suspected ACS it is very useful to perform ST-segment monitoring in order to detect or rule out ST-segment changes during chest pain or to detect silent ischaemia.

The ECG patterns found in patients with NSTE-ACS (Table 8.1) (usually non-occlusive thrombosis) **include cases with ST-segment depression (horizontal or downsloping)** greater than 0.5 m in at least two adjacent leads for some authors (Holper et al., 2001) or ≥1 mm for others (McConhay, 1971) (p. 111). Also included are the cases of **flat or negative T wave**, which are usually not very deep and more often in leads with predominant R waves. It should also be appreciated that a **completely normal, near-normal or unchanged ECG** in patients presenting with suspicious symptoms are also included in NSTE-ACS, but the presence of completely normal ECG recorded during an episode of significant chest pain should direct attention to other possible causes for the presenting symptom.

In both groups of ACS, the ECG pattern may be different according to the following factors: (a) duration, severity and extension of ischaemia; (b) presence of collateral flow; (c) variation of coro-

nary anatomy; and (d) presence of confounding factors.

From the electrocardiographic point of view in the presence of ACS, first it is necessary to assess whether the QRS complex is narrow or wide. More than 80% of ACS present narrow QRS. The diagnosis and prognostic implications of both types are different. Patients with hemiblocks are included in ACS with narrow QRS because repolarisation is not modified by hemiblocks. However, those with complete bundle branch block, Wolff–Parkinson–White syndrome, or pacemaker are not included and will be studied later on (see 'ACS with wide QRS and/or LVH') (p. 247).

In first part we have discussed the criteria for diagnosis and location of ST-segment elevation (pattern of subepicardium injury) and ST-segment depression or negative T wave (pattern of subendocardial injury and subepicardial ischaemia). Now we will discuss the clinical evolution, prognostic implications and risk stratification of these patterns.

Typical and atypical pattern of STE-ACS and NSTE-ACS (Table 8.1, and Figures 8.2 and 8.3)

In clinical practice patients with ACS and narrow QRS may be classified in two groups: **ACS with persistent ST-segment elevation (typical and atypical patterns)** and **ACS without ST-segment elevation that also includes cases of normal, near-normal (pseudonormal) or unchanged ECG.** We will briefly comment on the clinical characteristics and prognostic implications of these two types of clinical ECG syndromes.

Table 8.1 ECG patterns of ACS seen in emergency services at admission

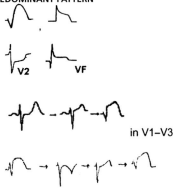

A. ECG PATTERNS IN STE-ACS AS THE MOST PREDOMINANT PATTERN

1. **Typical** = ST elevation in frontal or horizontal planes with mirror image of ST depression in other leads

2. **Atypical:**

–   Equivalent = ST depression in V1-V3 with smaller ST elevation in II, III, VF / V5–V6 (pattern C fig 8.3) or even without ST elevation in these leads

–   Patterns without ST elevation during some period of the evolving process
    –   **Hyperacute phase.** Tall T wave with rectified or even small ST depression (pattern A fig 8.3) (pattern A fig 8.3)
    –   **Deep negative T wave in V1-V4-5 (reperfusion pattern)** (pattern B figs 8.3, and fig 8.9). May evolve to an STE-ACS

B. ECG PATTERNS IN NON STE-ACS

1) **ST depression as the most predominant pattern**

–   **In ≥7 leads (circumferential involvement)**
Corresponds to 3-vessel disease or critical LMT subocclusion or equivalent (LAD + CX). If T wave is negative in V4-V6 usually is LMT

–   **In less than 7 leads (regional involvement)**
May be 2–3 vessel disease but usually with 1 culprit artery. More frequently in leads with dominant R wave. Cases of worst prognosis present ST depression in V4–V6 and in FP leads, with negative T wave in V4–V6.

2) **Flat or negative T wave as the most predominant pattern** The negativity of T wave usually is <2-3 mm (fig 3.23). Sometimes a negative U wave may be seen.

3. **Normal ECG, nearly normal or unchanged during ACS**

C. ECG PATTERNS IN PRESENCE OF CONFOUNDING FACTORS = LVH, LBBB, PM, WPW

(a) Patients with persistent STE-ACS present an ST-segment elevation as a new or presumably new and most characteristic electrocardiographic change of this syndrome and correspond to group of patients that demonstrated that fibrinolytic treatment is beneficial (type A; Figure 8.2 and Table 8.1). The treatment has to be very urgent. If possible, it is always the best option, especially after 3 hours of pain, to perform a primary percutaneous coronary intervention (PCI). The following ECG patterns are included:

(1) **Typical cases with ST-segment elevation (Table 8.1A(1)):** The arterial occlusion is complete or nearly complete, and the ventricular wall is globally and homogeneously severely compromised, and usually collateral circulation is

not very developed. The ischaemia occurs first predominantly in the subendocardium, but it soon becomes transmural and homogeneous (Figure 3.7, and Tables 2.1 and 4.1).

(2) **Atypical ECG patterns (see Table 8.1A(2), Figure 8.3):**

(i) **ST-segment depression in leads with non-dominant R wave, especially V1–V3** corresponds to a mirror pattern of the ST-segment elevation, recorded in leads of the back and represents injury mainly located in lateral and inferobasal wall due to left circumflex coronary artery (LCX) occlusion (Table 8.1). Under these circumstances, **ST-segment depression in V1–V3 as a mirror pattern** is seen as the main

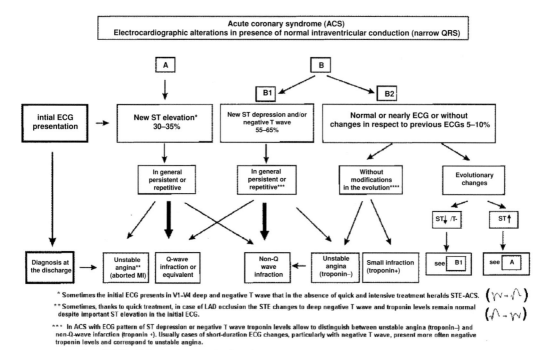

Figure 8.2 Acute coronary syndromes: ECG abnormalities at admission and diagnosis at discharge.

electrocardiographic change, but often (not always) **small ST-segment elevation is recorded in inferior or lateral leads** (Figure 4.47). Also, it has been reported that posterior (back) leads increase the detection of ischaemia in this area (Khaw et al., 1999). It is very important to perform the correct diagnosis because the therapeutic approach in this case has to be urgent revascularisation (primary PCI or thrombolytic therapy as a reasonable alternative – Antman et al. (2004)) (Figure 8.3C).

(ii) In early phase of STE-ACS there is a brief initial period in which often, in case of left anterior descending coronary artery (LAD) occlusion, a tall and symmetric T wave corresponding to subendocardium ischaemia is recorded in **V1–V2**. The first ECG taken to the patient may present this atypical pattern (Figures 8.4 and 8.6). It is very important to not consider this pattern as a nor-

mal variant. It is necessary to perform urgent treatment when the dynamic changes start (Figure 8.3A).

(iii) The presence of deep negative T wave in V1–V4–V5, as the most striking ECG finding in the course of an ACS, is the expression that critical stenosis exists in LAD (Wellens syndrome) (De Zwane, Bär and Wellens, 1982) (see p. 42). Also, a similar pattern may be seen in STE-ACS after reperfusion (fibrinolysis or PCI), as it is a good sign of opened artery (see p. 220).

On the other hand, to know where is the site of occlusion (see Table 4.1) in STE-ACS is important, to decide the need and the urgency to perform a primary PCI. As a consequence of reperfusion treatment (fibrinolytic or PCI) it has been shown that the area at risk during the acute phase is larger than the final infarcted area.

(b) Patients with NSTE-ACS correspond to the cases that have not demonstrated that fibrinolytic

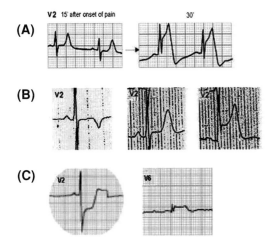

Figure 8.3 Atypical patterns of STE-ACS. (A) Tall and positive T wave in V1–V2. Hyperacute phase of LAD occlusion. (B) Deep and negative T wave in V1–V4–V5. Impending STE-ACS or reperfusion pattern after treatment. New occlusion may appear. (C) ST-segment depression in V1–V2 clearly greater than ST-segment elevation in inferior/lateral leads due to LCX occlusion.

treatment is beneficial. The following ECG patterns may be found (Figure 8.1B and Table 8.1):

(1) **ST-segment depression** (Table 8.1B(1)): The culprit artery, in these cases of NSTE-ACS, is not completely occluded and a transmural though not homogenous involvement usually exists, with subendocardium predominance.

This also occurs in some cases when the artery is completely occluded but much collateral circulation is present, or when the thrombus has been rechannelled.

(i) **Cases with ST-segment depression are sometimes very striking in many leads** (generally seven or more) with or without dominant R wave, presenting along with ST-segment elevation in VR (Table 8.1B(1)). The T wave in V3–V5 may be negative (usually left main trunk (LMT) subocclusion) or positive. Both cases present a **circumferential involvement** (p. 114). It is compulsory to start medical treatment and perform coronariography as a coronary angiography emergency.

(ii) **Cases with ST-segment depression:** In a few leads **(generally from two to six)** (Table 8.1B(1)) more frequently in leads **with dominant R wave** (**regional involvement**) the need of emergent coronary angiography depends on the clinical situation.

(2) **Flattened or negative T wave** (Table 8.1B(2)): Usually, it is not necessarily an emergent coronariography. This morphology is usually seen in leads (generally from two to six) with or without dominant R wave.

(3) **Normal or unmodified ECG** (Table 8.1B(3)): In approximately 10% of the cases, the

---

(1) **The distinction between an ACS with or without ST-segment elevation is of critical importance in order to determine the need for urgent fibrinolytic therapy. This therapeutic approach is beneficial in the ACS with ST-segment elevation, but not in the ACS without ST-segment elevation.**

(2) **The differences between ACS with or without ST-segment elevation are shown in Table 8.2.**

(3) From the electrocardiographic point of view an ST-segment depression or a negative T wave will be recorded, **depending on the area (with or without subendocardial predominance) of the ventricular wall that is affected** (see Table 8.1 and Figure 3.9).

(4) **The pattern of negative T wave recorded in patients with IHD probably is not due to 'active' ischaemia.**

a. In case of very negative T wave in V1–V4–V5 (LAD occlusion), it is probably a **reperfusion pattern (pattern induced by ischaemia but not due to 'active ischaemia').** However, if this pattern is present in the absence of reperfusion treatment, most probably, it represents that an STE-ACS has partially spontaneously reperfused, but usually an important proximal LAD occlusion existed (p. XX).

b. **Flat or negative T wave** is probably explained as a postischaemic changes (reperfusion pattern).

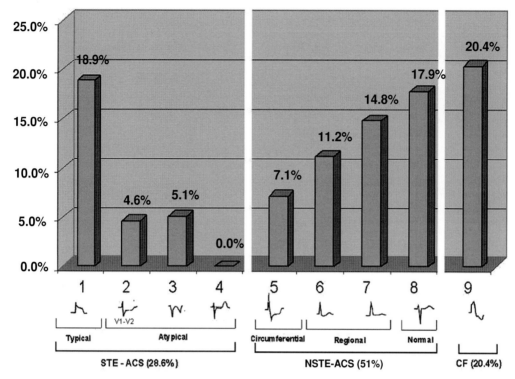

Figure 8.4 Incidence of different patterns of STE-ACS and NSTE-ACS in our hospital (pilot study of 200 consecutive cases of ACS). There is no case of hyperacute phase (tall and peaked T wave – no 4) because the patients arrive at emergency room at least after 30 minutes from the onset of pain (see Figure 8.3(A) and Table 8.1). CF, confounding factors. (see p. 242).

ECG is normal or nearly normal, or unchanged with respect to previous ECG recordings usually the prognosis is better. However, it has to be considered that some cases of apparently normal ECG may correspond to atypical patterns of STE-ACS (see Figure 8.2 and Table 8.1).

All these situations will be dealt with now, with a special focus on the clinical evolution and the coronary angiogram correlation in each case, and with emphasis on the prognostic implications and risk stratification.

Incidence of STE-ACS and NSTE-ACS

The incidence of NSTE-ACS has increased in the recent years. Large data (Roe et al., 2005; Scholte et al., 2006) have reported that currently STE-ACSs are present in 30–50% of cases and NSTE-ACS in 50–70% (see Table 8.2). Figure 8.4 shows the incidence of different ECG patterns of ACS at ar-

rival to our emergency department (see footnote). The in-hospital mortality of these ECG patterns is shown in p. 221 and 234.

Patients with ACS and ST-segment elevation (STE-ACS): from the aborted infarction to the Q-wave infarction

In Chapter 1 the mechanisms of ST-segment elevation were discussed, along with the criteria of the ST-segment deviations that allow for the diagnosis, differential diagnosis and location of first STE-ACS. Now, the following will mainly be discussed: (1) the evolving electrocardiographic patterns of STE-ACS; (2) the risk and prognosis stratification of STE-ACS at entrance; (3) the ECG data indicative of a poor prognosis during evolution; (4) the ECG changes developing during the thrombolytic therapy; (5) the possibility to know through the ECG changes

Table 8.2 Comparative study of ACS with and without ST segment elevation

	STE-ACS ST elevation or equivalent ($\downarrow$ ST V_1-V_3)	NSTE-ACS Without ST elevation ($\downarrow$ ST and/or negative T-wave or normal ECG)
Occurrence (Roe 2005, Scholte 2006)	30%–50%	50%–70%
Type of occlusion and thrombus	– Usually complete occlusion – Red	– Non-complete occlusion – White
Level of the previous ventricular ischemia	In general, small	In general evident, especially in the subendocardial area
Type and location of the ischemia due to ACS	– Usually transmural and homogeneous – Located in anteroseptal ($\uparrow$ ST V_{1-2} a V_3) I or VL) or inferolateral zone ($\uparrow$ ST II, III, and sometimes I, VL, V_6 and/or $\downarrow$ ST V_1–V_3. – See atypical patterns (fig 8.3)	– Often not easy to locate – When ST depression is in $\geq$7 leads with elevation in VR, the injury is very extensive (circumferential) and predominantly subendocardial – non-complete occlusion of the main trunk (LMT) or proximal occlusion of LAD + LCX (equivalent) – The ischemia is regional when the ST depression is only present in a few leads ($\leq$6) – Flat or negative T wave is due to delay of repolarization that has no subendocardial predominance.
Diagnostic criteria (present at least, in two leads	– $\uparrow$ST $\geq$2 mm PH – ST $\geq$1 mm PF – $\downarrow$ST $\geq$1 mm V_1-V_3 (mirror image)	**ST segment depression:** – ($\downarrow$ ST $\geq$ 0.5 mm in at least 2 consecutive leads (see p. 111). **Negative T wave:** – Usually not very deep (<2-3mm). May be present in HP and/or FP. – When is very negative and present in V_1 to V_{4-5} usually is an atypical pattern of STE-ACS (see fig 8.3)
Mirror image	– In general, yes. – Sometimes more prominent than the direct image: V_1- V_3 in some cases of lateral MI.	– In general, no. – ST elevation in VR and sometimes in V_1 in case of non-complete occlusion of the left main trunk or equivalent and in 3 vessel disease.
Type of ECG evolution	Usually Q-wave infarction. Sometimes limited infarction or even aborted by the treatment (see fig 8.2)	Non Q-wave infarction or unstable angina
Clinical setting: prognostics	In case of a clear Q-wave infarction the importance of the ventricular area at risk depends on the location of the occlusion. – Fewer coronary arteries are involved. – Variable prognostic. In general good if treatment is started early	– Often more ventricular mass involved. – More coronary arteries involved – Prognosis may be worst in case of very extensive infarction (LMT or equivalent)
Fibrinolytic treatment vs. PCI	If possible, urgent PCI is preferable specially after 3 hs of anginal pain.	– In principle, no fibrinolytic treatment – At least in high-risk patients, PCI is advisable

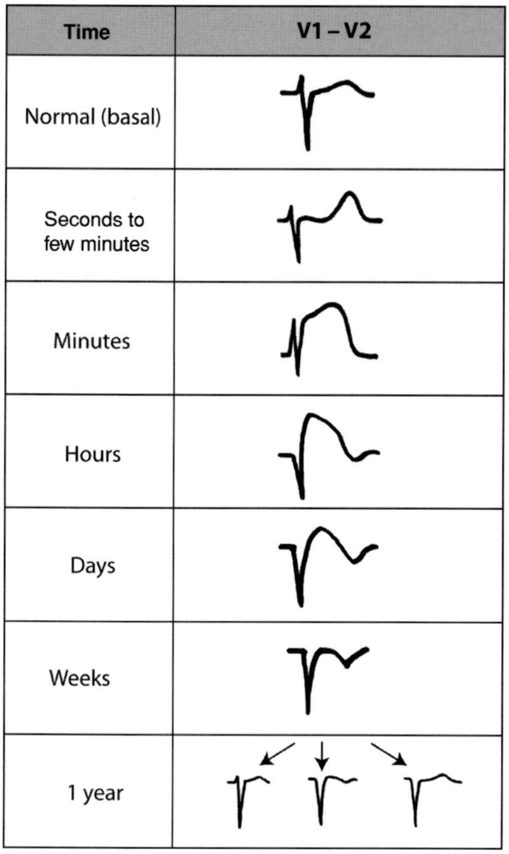

Time	V1 – V2
Normal (basal)	
Seconds to few minutes	
Minutes	
Hours	
Days	
Weeks	
1 year	

Figure 8.5 A flow chart drawing of the ECG changes in case of Q-wave anterior MI (records in V1–V2) from the very onset (rectified ST and positive T wave) till the different evolution patterns that may be present along a year in case where no treatment has been administered.

which is the culprit artery in the presence of multi-vessel disease.

Evolving electrocardiographic patterns in the STE-ACS (Figures 8.2 and 8.5)

The typical pattern of evolving STE-ACS represents the presence of persistent (≥30 min) ST-segment elevation[†] and expresses the successive phenomena that occur during a complete occlusion of an epicardial artery; CMR has demonstrated (Mahrhold et al., 2005) that the 'wavefront' of ischaemia and consequent infarction begin in the subendocardium and grow towards the epicardium over the next

hours. During this period the ischaemic area is very soon transmural (ST) and the infarcted area within the ischaemic area increases continuously towards a transmural infarction (Figure 8.6). This is a clear demonstration 'in vivo' of the previous experimental work, some of them already 50 years old (Lengyel et al., 1957), that after a coronary occlusion first predominant subendocardial ischaemia arises and then the ischaemia becomes more severe and transmural (ST elevation) (see 'Experimental point of view' and Figure 3.4, p. 32). However, according to our knowledge, it is the first demonstration in human beings that the MI starts from the subendocardium to subepicardium, becoming often transmural but has never been exclusively subepicardium.

In this group of STE-ACS are included the ECG patterns described earlier: (1) typical pattern of ST-segment elevation, and (2) atypical patterns (peaked and tall T wave in V1–V2; negative T wave in V1–V4 and ST-segment depression in

---

[†] Transient ST elevation lasting a few minutes corresponds to atypical ACS especially due to coronary spasm (variant or Prinzmetal angina) (p. 272). Sometimes ACS due to atherothrombosis may present transient ST shifts in the form of ups and downs. These cases usually finalise as clinically NSTE-ACS.

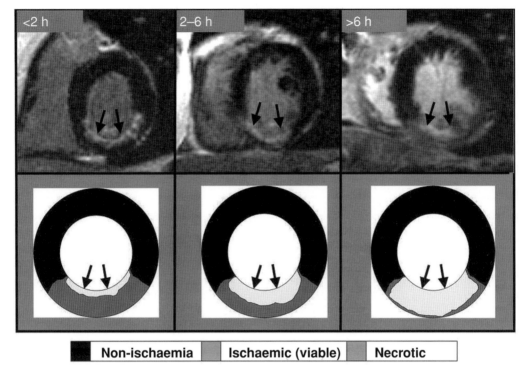

Non-ischaemia   Ischaemic (viable)   Necrotic

Figure 8.6 The typical pattern of ischaemic heart disease can be explained by the pathophysiology of ischaemia studied with CE-CMR. Little or no cellular necrosis is found until about 15 minutes after occlusion. After 15 minutes, a 'wavefront' of necrosis begins subendocardial and grows towards the epicardium over the next few hours. During this period the infarcted region within the ischaemic zone increases continuously towards a transmural infarction. (Adapted form Mahrholdt et al., Eur Heart J, 2005.)

V1–V3 > ST-segment elevation in inferior lateral leads) (see Figure 8.3 and Table 8.1A).

Now we will discuss the evolving electrocardiographic patterns that can appear throughout the occlusion of an epicardial coronary artery and its prognostic implications (Figures 3.18, 3.19 and 8.5).

(a) **Subendocardial ischaemia (symmetric and peaked T wave and usually taller)**

This pattern is not always seen. Surely, if we have the opportunity of recording the ECG during the **hyperacute phase of the coronary occlusion**, it could be more frequently recorded as in case of the experimental coronary occlusion (Figure 3.3) and in more than half the cases of coronary spasm (Prinzmetal angina) (Figure 10.5; Bayés de Luna et al., 1985). In the hyperacute phase of STE-ACS, a usually tall and peaked T wave with QTc prolongation indicative of subendocardium ischaemia, preceded by a rectified ST segment or even slightly depressed ST segment, can be seen especially in V1–V3

(Figure 8.7A). If the base is wide (Figure 3.8A,C), it is the expression of an intermediate situation between the typical pattern of subendocardium ischaemia and the pattern of subepicardium injury (Figure 3.8A and 8.8).

(b) **Subepicardial injury (ST-segment elevation)**

This pattern, which ECG expression starts during the first part of repolarisation (see Figure 4.5 and p. 61), is characterised by ST-segment elevation in some leads of variable magnitude and morphological features with usually mirror patterns showing ST-segment depression in opposite leads. In some atypical cases the mirror images of ST-segment depression are more predominant than the direct pattern of ST-segment elevation. This occurs especially in some cases of LCX occlusion (Figure 4.47). In cases of severe ischaemia (grade 3) (see 'To identify the grade (intensity) of ischaemia through the ST/T morphology') (p. 224) the ST-segment elevation is accompanied by a change in the QRS

V2

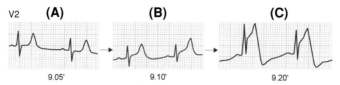

(A)   **(B)**   **(C)**

9.05'   9.10'   9.20'

Figure 8.7 A 45-year-old patient with an acute precordial pain who presents a tall T and peaked T wave that follows a rectified ST segment in right precordial leads as the only ECG sign suggestive of ischaemia (A). Some minutes later ST-segment elevation appears (B) and very soon becomes very evident, accompanied by R-wave increase and S-wave decrease (C). The ECG pattern recorded in (C) presents ratio J point/R wave >0.5 which corresponds to more severe ischaemia (grade C or 3 of Birnbaum–Sclarovsky) (see p. XX). This patient presents ventricular fibrillation some minutes after the ECG only presents peaked T wave (A). This is a clear evidence of the importance to make a good interpretation of ECG at entrance, especially in a patient with acute chest pain.

complex morphology, which is 'swept' upwards by the ST-segment elevation (Figures 8.7 and 8.9). This occurs because the injury pattern is recorded during systole (see p. 61), starting as of the final portion of the QRS complex, and decreases while the ST segment is recorded. In this case there is a delay in the intramyocardial conduction of the stimulus in the area involved by a severe and hyperacute ischaemia, generally before the appearance of infarction Q wave. Therefore, in severe cases **the ST-segment changes appear along with changes in the final portion of the QRS complex**. They consist, in leads with rS morphology, in an increase of R-wave voltage and, frequently, abolishment of the S wave when the ST segment is upwardly deviated. According to Birnbaum et al. (1993, 1996b) (see 'To define the grade (intensity) of ischaemia through ST/T morphology') (p. 224) if the ratio J point/R wave is less than 0.50, the ischaemia is type B or grade 2, and if the ratio is greater than 0.50, it is type C or grade 3. Even in grade 3 of ischaemia the S wave may disap-

pear (Figures 8.7 and 8.9). To a lesser degree, the opposite occurs in leads with ST-segment depression that S wave may increase. These QRS abnormalities are generally transient and are only found in cases with severe ischaemia, but do not necessarily imply the existence of an intraventricular block (e.g. hemiblock).

A new onset ST-segment elevation, evident (≥ 1 mm in the inferior wall and ≥ 2 mm in the precordial leads), persistent or repetitive, is explained by a coronary occlusion due to thrombosis occurring on a ruptured or eroded plaque, and it will most probably evolve towards a Q-wave myocardial infarction (Table 2.1-A1). Therefore, this ST-segment elevation may be considered typical of an **evolving Q-wave myocardial infarction** (Wagner et al., 2000). However, on certain occasions, when reperfusion therapy has been initiated early on and/or the patient is suffering from a transient thrombotic occlusion, the ST-segment elevation may be transient, though it is quite important at the beginning. At

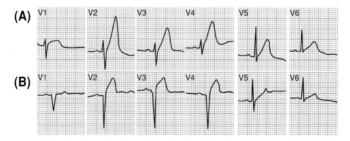

(A) V1   V2   V3   V4   V5   V6

(B) V1   V2   V3   V4   V5   V6

Figure 8.8 (A) A 48-year-old patient in an acute phase of anterior infarction (less than 1 h from the pain onset). Observe a tall, wide and not quite symmetric T wave without clear ST-segment elevation in V2–V4, which may be explained by intermediate situation between typical ECG pattern of subendocardial ischaemia and the pattern of subepicardial ischaemia. Slight ST-segment elevation may be noted in V1 lead. (B) Few hours later appeared typical pattern of subepicardial injury (ST-segment elevation) with QS of necrosis in V2–V4.

(A) **(B)** **(C)** **(D)**

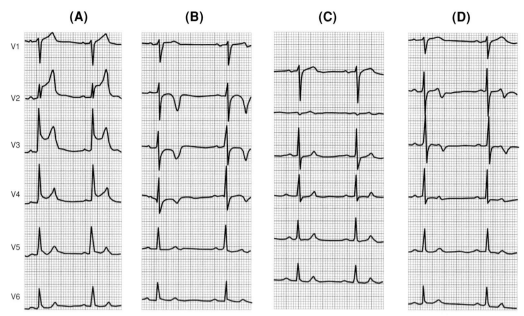

Figure 8.9 (A) A patient with ACS with ST-segment elevation with the pattern found in cases of severe transmural ischaemia (increase in R, disappearance of S wave, ratio J point/R wave >0.5). Troponin levels were normal. (B) The ECG after primary PCI of proximal LAD presents a deep negative T wave from V2–V4, suggestive of opened artery (reperfusion pattern).
(C) Some hours after PCI the patient presented precordial pain with pseudonormalisation of ECG as a sign of reocclusion. (V2 lead presents artefacts.) (D) After having controlled the pain, a new PCI demonstrates intrastent thrombosis and a new stent was inserted, and again non-prominent negative T waves were recorded. The ECG was normalised after a few days. The troponine levels were not elevated during the whole clinical setting. Therefore, it is a clear case of aborted myocardial infarction. Some years before, this ECG would certainly evolve into extensive Q-wave infarction (see Figures 8.5 and 3.18).

other times the ECG may show minor ST-segment elevation or perhaps, just in case of basal negative T wave, a pseudonormalisation pattern may appear without ST-segment elevation (Figure 3.21), though the ST may be clearly elevated in another crisis. Under these circumstances, the patient might not suffer irreversible myocardial damage (troponin is negative) neither evolve towards a Q-wave infarction. Therefore, with the therapies currently available, the STE-ACS may be of short duration and evolve towards a non-Q-wave infarction or unstable angina (**aborted infarction**) depending on troponin levels (Figures 8.1 and 8.2).

The term **aborted infarction** (Dowdy et al., 2004; Lamfers et al., 2003) refers to clinical situation that presents the following features:
(1) ACS with evident ST-segment elevation suggesting a transmural ischaemia (Figure 8.7)
(2) Absence of enzyme elevation or, an increase of less than double the normal values

(3) The summation of the ST-segment elevation and depression decreases to a value lower than 50% in less than 2 hours of reperfusion therapy

The number of aborted infarctions has been shown to be much higher (18%) when fibrinolytic therapy is begun in the pre-hospital setting than when it is begun after admission (4.5%). Moreover, more aborted infarctions occur when the ST-segment elevation, though evident, is not so striking. The same occurs in patients with a prior history of angina because they present more collateral circulation. Therefore, when reperfusion therapy is begun early, the ST-segment elevation pattern lasts for less time and the condition may end in a non-Q-wave infarction or even in an aborted infarction (UA) (Figures 8.2 and 8.9). Recently, it has been suggested that Tako–Tsubo syndrome may be an aborted MI with spontaneous thrombus autolysis (Ibañez et al., 2006) (see 'Transient left ventricle apical ballooning') (p. 267).

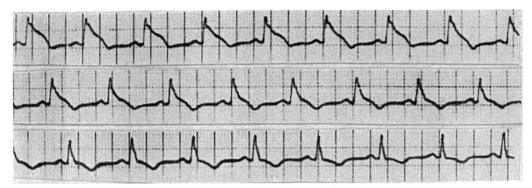

Figure 8.10 Patient with crises of Prinzmetal angina, who presented during these crises typical of subepicardial injury pattern. During the remission of pain (Holter method recording) the injury pattern disappeared within a few seconds.

In case of proximal LAD occlusion the ST-segment elevation in precordial leads after successful revascularisation is followed by **negative and deep T wave** in the same leads, with usually little or no ST-segment elevation or more frequently mild ST-segment depression. This is currently considered an **expression of reperfusion and opened artery**. However, sometimes the same ECG may be seen in case of proximal LAD subocclusion probably with spontaneous partial reperfusion that is necessary to treat quickly to avoid the presentation of an STE-ACS (De Zwan, Bär and Wellens, 1982). The same may also happen in patients presenting this ECG pattern after revascularisation (reperfusion pattern), if spontaneous rethrombosis or new intrastent thrombosis appears. In this situation the ECG will present an ST-segment elevation or a pseudonormalisation of T wave, which may be confused with an improvement of the clinical situation but really represent an important complication (Figure 8.9).

Therefore the presence of negative and deep T wave in precordial leads, especially in V1–V4, is usually the expression of evolutive phase of STE-ACS that occurs when the LAD occlusion is opened (reperfusion ECG sign). However, in some cases may herald, especially if the angina pain is recurrent, a new occlusion with the appearance of pseudonormal T wave and occasionally a new ST-segment elevation (Figures 8.3B and 8.9).

In cases with coronary spasm, ST-segment elevation lasts from seconds to a few minutes (Figure 8.10, p. 271). Often the ST-segment elevation is very striking presenting in rare cases, even

an ST/TR alternance (Figure 8.11). The duration of classical STE-ACS is much longer, though this is greatly related to the onset of reperfusion therapy (see 'ECG changes induced by fibrinolytic therapy') (p. 228).

(c) **Infarction Q wave and negative T wave pattern of subepicardial ischaemia**

This is the electrocardiographic pattern that is recorded when the ACS with ST-segment elevation evolves towards a transmural infarction with homogenous involvement of the full wall. First, the Q wave of infarction develops and then, after a few hours, the negative T wave is observed (see Figures 8.15, 3.18 and 3.19). It has been shown **in the fibrinolytic era** that **at 9 hours of the onset of an ACS with ST-segment elevation, the changes occurring in the QRS complex (Q wave) have already been completed** and the QRS morphology is already stable. Therefore, at that time it has been possible to estimate not only the exact location of the infarction, but also the infarct size, on the basis of the presence of an infarction Q wave (Bar et al., 1996; Hindman et al., 1985).

On rare occasions, the pathological Q wave that develops during an ACS may be transient. The pathological Q wave recorded at the initial phase of the infarction indicates the presence of tissue unable to be activated electrically. More than likely, this will end up being an infarcted tissue (Q wave of necrosis). However, certain possibilities of recovery exist. Should this happen, R wave will again be recorded. This sometimes occurs in coronary spasm and in aborted MI. However, one should remember that transient 'q' waves are also seen at times in

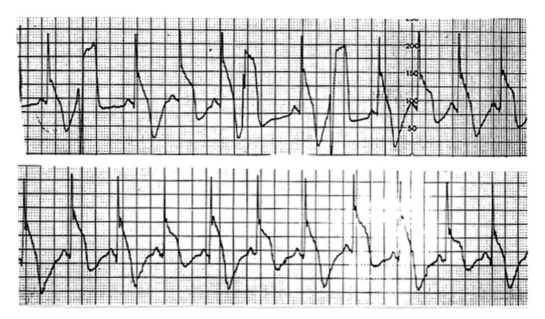

Figure 8.11 Holter recording of a patient with a severe crisis of Prinzmetal angina. Observe the presence of clear ST-segment and TQ alternance together with some PVC.

myocarditis (Figure 5.43) or these develop due to other causes (Table 5.5, p. 175).

What is more frequently seen in the subacute phase is that patterns of ST-segment elevation that begin to return to the baseline coexist with the development of an infarction Q wave and a negative T wave (Figure 8.5). The evolution and approximate duration of the different morphologies in case that treatment was not administered observed throughout the first year following a Q-wave MI are shown in this figure. The appearance of negative and often deep T wave is related with the changes that Q-wave MI has induced in the repolarisation process and does not represent the existence of 'active' ischaemia. On the contrary, the disappearance of ST-segment elevation and the appearance of negative T wave are a sign of good evolution after MI. As a matter of fact the lack of appearance of negative T wave is a marker of bad outcome and possible mechanical complications (see Figures 8.27 and 'ECG in mechanical complications of an ACS evolving to MI') (p. 244).

The disappearance of the infarction Q wave may be the result of an improvement of the disease (Figure 8.5). Generally, this is due to the presence of collateral vessels. The involved area may recover its ability to generate measurable vectors. However, it may also be explained by a new infarction that has developed in the opposite area and by the appearance of ventricular block usually LBBB. In the first case, the ECG improvement will be progressive (Figure 8.12), whereas it will occur more rapidly in the latter two cases (Figures 5.38 and 5.39).

In mid-1990s the **Anderson–Wilkins score** was introduced (Wilkins et al., 1995). This score is provided as a continuous scale from 4.0 (hyperacute T wave) to 1.0 (subacute) on the basis of the comparative hyperacute T waves versus abnormal Q waves in each of the leads with ST-segment elevation. Although it is an interesting approach to study the ischaemia/infarction (ischaemic acuteness) for quantifying the timing of an MI to guide decisions regarding reperfusion therapy, it is too complex for manual clinical application. Furthermore, additional studies are needed to validate these scores using non-ECG reference standards (Wagner, Pahlm and Selvester, 2006).

ST-segment elevation on admission: prognosis and risk stratification

The electrocardiographic abnormalities described above are observed in different leads, in accordance

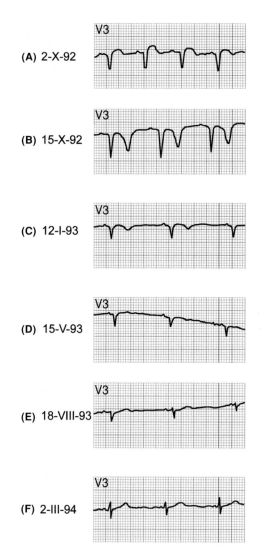

(A) 2-X-92

(B) 15-X-92

(C) 12-I-93

(D) 15-V-93

(E) 18-VIII-93

(F) 2-III-94

Figure 8.12 Patient with extensive anterior infarction. ECG normalisation with Q wave disappearing and positivation of T wave during 18-month follow-up.

ST-segment elevation related with prognosis and risk stratification.

Despite substantial progress in the diagnosis and treatment of STE-ACS and the evidence that PCI is the preferred method of reperfusion if it can be performed in a timely manner, the implementation of this knowledge in clinical practice has been variable (Henry et al., 2006). To improve that it is necessary to develop a coordinate system of care that has to start taking ECG to all patients with acute chest pain and improving the diagnostic accuracy of all health care professionals involved in emergency services.

In order to correctly stratify the risk in a patient having an STE-ACS, the characteristics of these changes in the admission ECG could be studied in the following manner to know the burden of ischaemia:

(a) **Assess the elevation and depression of ST in different leads**, which allows one to localise the coronary occlusion site and the area at risk.

(b) **Sum up in millimetres the ST-segment elevations and depressions**, which helps to quantify, approximately, the area at risk.

(c) **Assess the morphology of the ST-segment elevation**, which allows one **to know better the severity of ischaemia.**

(d) **Check the dynamic changes of ECG from the pre-hospital phase to the catheterisation laboratory**, which gives an idea about the evolutive phase.

All these four aspects have their own prognostic implications, but also are complementary amongst themselves and with the clinical and enzymatic risk markers (age, history of infarction, risk factors and level of enzymes; risk score) (Morrow et al., 2000a,b) (p. 257). We will now discuss these in detail.

with the occluded coronary artery and, consequently, the involved myocardial area. In the first part the correlation in the acute phase (ST-segment elevation) between the abnormal ECG, the involved myocardial area and the occluded artery was discussed (Table 4.1) (see p. 70), and later on the correlation in the chronic phase between the infarcted area and the presence of an infarction Q wave in different leads was also commented Figure 5.9) (p. 140). We will now describe the importance of these changes and other aspects of

Correlation between the ST-segment changes, the occlusion site and the area at risk

We have already discussed (p. 101) the algorithms that give key information about how different ST-segment changes are related to the occlusion of different coronary arteries and locations (see Table 4.1, p. 70, and Figures 4.43 and 4.45). **The correlation between the ST-segment elevations and depressions in the different leads has already been** stated, which is key information to know what the area at risk of infarction is and to identify the culprit artery and the occlusion site. This area could be identified by determining the segments involved (Figures 1.8, 1.9 and 1.14, and Table 4.1). In Figures 4.43 and 4.45 the SE, SP and PV of different criteria used in these algorithms are presented.

Regarding the prognosis, we can confirm that the STE-ACS involving the anteroseptal zone (LAD occlusion) has globally worst prognosis than STE-ACS of inferolateral zone (Elsman et al., 2006; see 'Anteroseptal versus inferolateral MI') (p. 282). On the other hand, the ACS of anteroseptal zone with the poorest prognosis is that with a larger extension, generally secondary to the occlusion of the **LAD proximal to the take-off of D1 and S1. Under these circumstances in presence of ST-segment elevation in precordials, the following ECG criteria are related with proximal occlusion of LAD:**

1. A clear ST-segment depression in II, III, VF and V6, and ST-segment elevation in VR and V1 and ST-segment depression in V6: LAD occlusion proximal to D1 and S1. These cases present usually clear evidence of lower ejection fraction and haemodynamic impairment. Other authors (Sclarovsky, 1999) used other criteria (ST↑ > 1 mm in VL) to locate the occlusion proximal to D1. According to our experience this criteria has lower specificity. Table 8.3 shows that the presence of ST ↓ III + ↓VF>0.5 mm and Σ ST **deviations in VR + V1–V6 ≥ 0** represent a group of patients with a higher incidence of proximal occlusion of LAD, worst haemodynamic status, more important grade of ischaemia and more clinical complications (MACE) compared with the rest of the patients. However, during their stay in the hospital the two groups presented similar incidence of death. Further follow-up of these patients is in process and will give us the real importance of these findings.

2. New bundle branch block: We have already explained that the presence of intermittent RBBB is higher in the group of patients with very proximal LAD occlusion (Figure 4.66). The prognosis is worst, especially if the ST-segment elevation resolution is slowed and the QRS is very wide (Wong et al., 2006a, b). In case of new LBBB, which occurs very

Table 8.3 ACS due to LAD occlusion: Two groups of risk

	GROUP A	GROUP A	
	ST↓III + ↓ VF > 0,5 and Σ ST deviations in VR + V1–V6 ≥ 0 n = 65	Rest of the patients n = 35	p
Age	56,4 ± 14,3	57 ± 15,6	ns
EF	47 ± 12	56,3 ± 11	0,001
Killip index	1,76 ± 1	1,37 ± 0,6	0,040
Killip ≥ III	24,2%	5,7%	0,026
Grade C of ischaemia	54,7%	21,4%	0,005
Proximal to S1	48%	3%	0,000
Proximal to D1	83%	8,6%	0,000
Distal to D1	17%	91,4%	0,000
MACE (major cardiac events)	57,1%	17,1%	0,000

rarely, we only have a worse prognosis of the cases with evident ST-segment deviations (Sgarbossa et al., 1996 b).

On the other hand, the STE-ACS involving the inferolateral zone, presenting with the poorest prognosis, is that with the largest extension, with evidence of significant involvement of the inferior and lateral walls and the RV. Those cases with the highest risk present the following ECG criteria:

1. RCA occlusion proximal to the RV marginal branches: manifested by the presence of an isoelectric or elevated ST segment in V1–V2 (Figure 4.31)

2. Presence of a very dominant RCA: ST-segment elevation in V5–V6 ≥2 mm (Nikus et al., 2005) (Figure 4.36)

3. Evidence of very predominant LCX: Evident ST-segment depression in V1–V3 and/or elevation in III > II and/or ST-segment depression in VL and very evident ST-segment elevation in V5–V6 (Figure 4.42)

4. Development of an Mobitz-type AV block

5. The combination of ST-segment elevation in the inferior wall and depression in V4–V6, because it represents involvement of two or three vessels

Quantification of the burden of ischaemia by the summation of the ST-segment deviations

In order to quantify the area at risk and burden of ischaemia, both ST-segment elevations and depressions should be assessed. The latter are not the expression of subendocardium injury, but the real expression of subepicardium (transmural) injury in a distant area. Therefore, in LAD occlusion, an ST-segment depression detected in II, III and VF, more significant compared with an ST-segment elevation in the same leads, represents more ischaemia (compare Figures 4.21 and 4.23).

In patients with an STE-ACS, **the TIMI group has reported a risk score** in which one of the parameters to be assessed is ST-segment deviation (Morrow et al., 2000a,b). This will be further discussed in the next sections (see 'Risk stratification') (p. 257).

On the basis of the **information derived from the GUSTO trial**, Hathaway (1998a,b) reported a nomogram, for the quantification of involved area and to stratify the 30-day mortality risk, on the basis of the ST-segment abnormalities (elevation or depression) at the time of hospital admission (between 1 and 4 h from the onset of pain). Also, electrocardiographic (QRS complex width) and clinical (age, risk factors, Killip class, etc.) data were included (Table 8.4). From a practical point of view, **an ST-segment deviation (upward or downward deviation) above 15 mm is supposed to indicate the existence of a large area of myocardium at risk** (see 'Risk stratification') (p. 257).

However, some limitations may occur, e.g. in the case of an infarction due to occlusion of a dominant RCA proximal to the RV branches. In spite of the large area involved, the ST segment is frequently isodiphasic in the right precordial leads, since the RV involvement counteracted the ST-segment depression that is usually seen in the large infarctions due to the right coronary artery occlusion. For that reason, the injury vector is directed more rightwards (Figure 4.30) and masks the ST-segment depression in V1. Therefore, an RCA occlusion before the RV marginal branches may present, even with the same dominance, globally fewer ST-segment changes (Figure 4.31) than an RCA occlusion after the take-off of these branches (Figure 4.34).

The prognosis has been shown to be worse (higher possibilities of developing a primary ventricular fibrillation (VF)) **when the summation of ST-segment elevation in the three most compromised leads is more than 8 mm** (Fiol et al., 1993). This finding, along with the presence of hypotension, is a marker of the poorest prognosis, especially in cases with inferior infarction.

Lastly, at the same location of occlusion in two arteries relatively of the same size, the sum of ST-segment elevations will be higher when the degree of occlusion is more important, because this represents a higher amount of ischaemia.

In the late 1980s **the Aldrich score** was introduced (Aldrich et al., 1988) for estimation of the extent of myocardium at risk for infarction in the absence of successful reperfusion therapy. It is based on the slope of the relationship between the amount of ST segment in the presenting ECG and the Selvester score of the pre-discharge ECG and is expressed as percentage of LV infarcted. This score is obtained using a mathematical formula. Although it is an interesting approach to know the extent of ischaemia/infarction, it needs to be validated using non-ECG reference standards and is too complex for manual clinical application (Wagner et al., 2006a).

To define the grade (intensity) of ischaemia through the ST/T morphology

Three ST/T morphologies that can have prognostic implications have been described (Figure 8.13; Birnbaum et al., 1993). In cases with slight ECG changes such as tall and wide stable T wave (not the evolving transient pattern seen in hyperacute phase – Figure 8.7) (type A or grade 1), the prognosis is better than that when exists a convex ST segment elevation with respect to the isoelectric baseline (type B or grade 2) or, especially, when it is concave with distortion of the final portion of the QRS complex (type C or grade 3). This means decrease or disappearance of S wave in leads with a usual rS morphology (V1–V3) with R/S ratio ≥50% in two adjacent leads. In the latter case, the coronary occlusion is probably proximal, and not much collateral circulation exists. The type C morphology expresses the involvement of the Purkinje fibres, which are more resistant to ischaemia than are the myocytes. Therefore, it probably suggests larger area of acute ischaemia, higher mortality, less myocardial salvage by fibrinolytic

Table 8.4 Nomogram for estimating 30-day mortality from initial clinical and electrocardiographic variables (Hathaway et al. JAMA 1998).

Systolic Blood Pressure		Pulse		Sum of Absolute St-Segment Deviation		QRS Duration, milliseconds			
mm Hg	Points	bpm	Points	mm	Points	Nonanterlor MI	Points	Anterior MI	Points
1. Find Points for Each Risk Marker									
40	46	40	0	0	0	60	22	60	16
50	40	60	0	10	7	80	23	80	21
60	34	80	6	20	15	100	25	100	26
70	28	100	11	30	19	120	26	120	34
80	23	120	17	40	19	140	27	140	36
90	17	140	23	50	19	160	29	160	41
100	11	160	29	60	19	180	30	180	47
110	6	180	34	70	19	200	32	200	52
120	0	200	40	80	18				
130	0								
140	0								
150	0								
160	0								

Age		Height				Killip		ECG	
y	Points	cm	Points	Diabetes	Points	class	Points	Prior MI	Points
20	0	140	30	No	0	I	0	Yes	10
30	13	150	27	Yes	6	II	8		
40	25	160	23			III	18	No	
50	38	170	19			IV	30	Inferior MI	0
60	50	180	15					Noninferior MI	10
70	62	190	11	Prior					
80	75	200	8	CABG	Points				
90	87	210	4	No	0				
100	100	220	0	Yes	10				

2. Sum Points for All Risk Markets

Systolic Blood pressure	———
Pulse	———
Sum of Absolute ST-Segment Deviation	———
QRS Duration	———
Age	———
Height	———
Diabetes	———
Prior CABG	———
Killip class	———
ECG prior MI	———
Total	

3. Look up Risk Corresponding to Point Total

Total Points	Probability of 30-Day Mortality
61	0.001
87	0.005
98	0.01
117	0.03
122	0.04
125	0.05
129	0.06
131	0.07
134	0.08
136	0.09
138	0.10
151	0.20
167	0.40
180	0.60
196	0.80

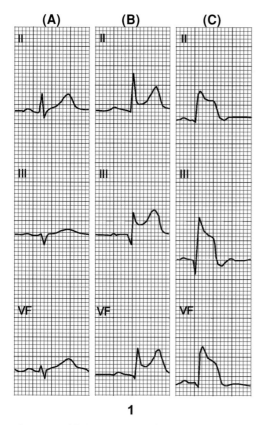

1

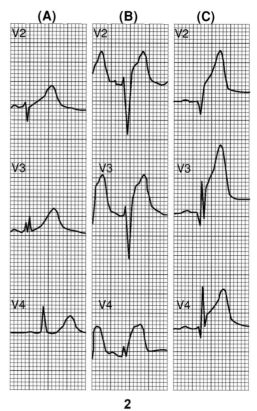

2

Figure 8.13 (1) The three types of repolarisation abnormalities that may be seen in an acute phase of myocardial infarction involving the inferolateral zone: (A) tall and/or wide T waves in inferior leads; (B) abnormal ST-segment elevation, with no changes of the final part of QRS; (C) important ST-segment elevation and distortion of the final part of QRS. (2) The three types of repolarisation abnormalities that may be seen in an acute phase of myocardial infarction involving the anteroseptal zone wall: (A) tall and/or wide T waves especially seen in right precordial leads; (B) abnormal ST-segment elevation, with no changes of the final part of QRS; (C) important ST-segment elevation and distortion of the final part of QRS.

treatment and more rapid progression of infarction over time.

Type C patterns may appear shortly after severe acute ischaemia. Therefore occasionally it has been seen in Prinzmetal angina. These electrocardiographic findings are especially of great importance if the chest-pain duration is similar in the different groups when the patients arrive at the hospital. Evidently, when a patient arrives at the emergency room after 6 hours of chest pain with a near-normal ECG recording (type A), the prognosis is better than the lack of ECG changes after just 15 minutes from the onset of pain. Therefore, it is very important to check if the A (or I) pattern is transient and soon becomes B or C pattern, or if it is

persistent. In the latter case either the ischaemic area is well protected by collateral circulation or the occlusion is not very important (Sagie et al., 1989). In both situations the grade of ischaemia is much lower than that in B (or II) pattern or especially in C (or III) pattern. In the latter the grade of ischaemia is very important due to complete occlusion of an area that does not present collateral circulation (unprotected area).

It is important to emphasise that the most dangerous complications occur in patients with a C (III) pattern. These include severe bradycardia and AV block, usually in case of LCX or RCA occlusion, and VF leading to sudden death.

STE-ACS: global prognostic value of the ST-segment changes on admission (Birnbaum et al., 1993; Elsman et al., 2006; Hathaway, 1998a,b; Morrow et al., 2000a,b)

The ST-segment deviation that is frequently recorded in opposite leads allows for assuring not only which artery is occluded, but the occlusion site as well. The cases at higher risk are those caused by a proximal LAD occlusion, by a very dominant RCA occlusion (especially when the obstruction is proximal to the RV branches) or by a very dominant LCX occlusion.

• Additionally, the sum in millimetres of the ST-segment elevations and depressions is also useful in assessing the size of the myocardial area at risk. Figures above 15 mm along with other electrocardiographic and clinical data allow for establishing a risk score when the patient is first assessed, which is useful for prognosis stratification (see 'Risk stratification') (p. 257).

• The ST-segment morphology on admission is also useful. Cases with the poorest prognosis are those presenting with a concave ST segment with regard to the isoelectric baseline, with distortion of the final portion of the QRS complex.

• Because of its great value in risk stratification, ST/T changes are part of the most frequently used risk scores (TIMI risk score) (see 'Risk stratification') (p. 257).

• The in-hospital prognosis of both STE-ACS and NSTE-ACS has improved very much in the era of new antithrombolytic and antiplatelet drugs and primary PCI.

The dynamic changes of the ST-segment elevation from the pre-hospital phase to the catheterisation laboratory

Continuous ST-segment monitoring performed in the pre-hospital phase in STE-ACS shows that the ST-segment elevation may present in 29% of the cases spontaneous ST resolution, and this is a marker of good prognosis (Bjorklund et al., 2005). On the other hand two-thirds of the patients who present ST-segment elevation on arrival at the interventional hospital achieve complete ST-segment resolution after PCI and these patients have much better prognosis compared to the group of patients that presents an increase of ST-segment elevation during PCI. This increase in ST-segment elevation is expected to be associated with impaired microvascular integrity indicative of poor patient outcome.

Although both strategies of reperfusion, fibrinolysis and PCI improve very much the prognosis of STE-ACS, there are evidences (Sejersten, 2004, 2006) that PCI compared with fibrinolysis shows a 40% relative decrease in the composite end point of death, reinfarction and stroke at 30 days and that quantitative value of the sum of ST-segment elevation on the admission ECG is useful for predicting outcomes after PCI or fibrinolysis, correlating the magnitude of Σ ST-segment elevation with increased mortality at 30 days. **However, if** the patients are treated in the first 3 hours after the onset of symptoms, the outcome is similar with both approaches (fibrinolysis vs primary PCI). This means that a great effort has to be made to start the treatment in the ambulance (pre-hospital fibrinolysis) because it is much more feasible in the majority of the world even in developed countries than to perform very quickly a primary PCI. Nevertheless, in the case that the patient has already arrived at emergency unit, it is compulsory to shorten as much as possible the door-to-balloon time for PCI, because this results in a better outcome for the patient (Brodie et al., 2006).

Electrocardiographic data of short- and long-term bad prognosis during the evolution of STE-ACS

The ECG recording does provide much useful information for assessing the prognosis and global risk over time of a patient suffering STE-ACS (Patel et al., 2001; Piccolo et al., 2001). During the evolution of a patient who has been admitted to the hospital, the electrocardiographic changes depicting the poorest prognosis at short and long term are the following:

(a) **Persistent sinus tachycardia** or development of rapid supraventricular or ventricular arrhythmias.

(b) Persistent ST-segment elevation or evidence of transient changes in its magnitude. This indicates the presence of an evolving infarct and implies that when the patient has received thrombolytic agents, reperfusion has not been efficient (see 'ECG changes induced by fibrinolytic therapy') (see below). **The persistence of the ST-segment elevation with no development of negative T wave** after a week is a marker of poor prognosis and of the potential for subsequent cardiac rupture (see 'ECG in mechanical complications of an ACS evolving to MI') (p. 244).

(c) Classically, **the occurrence of VF** during the evolution of an acute infarction with ST-segment elevation has been thought not to influence the prognosis. However, it has been demonstrated to be a marker of poor prognosis in the presence of an anterior infarction (Schwartz et al., 1985).

(d) The presence of wide QRS is a sign of worst prognosis. This especially includes the **development of complete bundle branch block**, especially RBBB in anterior infarctions (Figure 4.66) **or advanced AV block** in inferolateral infarctions (Figure 8.36) (Lie et al., 1975). **In patients receiving thrombolytic agents, the development of LBBB is much rarer** because the left bundle receives double perfusion (p. 249). Currently, it is considered that LBBBs that do not present ST/T changes described by Sgarbossa et al. do not represent a very bad prognosis, especially when these are of transient nature.

(e) Several studies have been reported that revealed an evident **decrease in QT-segment dispersion in patients undergoing a primary PCI** restoring a normal flow (TIMI III). However, patients presenting VF during the evolution of an infarction have not been shown to present a more significant QT-interval dispersion on arrival at the hospital (Fiol et al., 1995). Currently, it is not considered that QT dispersion plays an important role in the prognosis after MI.

(f) In general, **the evidence of STE-ACS of the anteroseptal zone is a strong determinant of lower EF and a worst prognosis than STE-ACS of inferolateral zone**, even at similar amount of myocardial necrosis detected by enzymatic level (Elsman et al., 2006).

(g) The **evidence of an extensive Q-wave infarction also implies a poor prognosis**. These data may be derived from the ECG when a large number of involved leads are found (ST-segment abnormalities – elevations and depressions evolving to Q-wave MI). Furthermore, the presence of high QRS score estimated in the first ECG after hospital admission is an independent predictor of incomplete ST recovery and 30-day complications in STE-ACS treated with primary PCI (Uyarel, 2006).

(h) The presence of Q wave during an ACS usually indicates myocardial necrosis. However, extensive ischaemia and large myocardial area at risk can in fact result in **transient Q wave** due to electrical inexcitability in the zone under the electrode. Therefore, the presence of Q wave not always implies irreversible damage. Reperfusion therapy has not to be ruled out simply because Q wave is present (Wellens, 2006).

(i) In patients with normal intraventricular conduction, 30-day mortality was higher among those with than those without initial Q wave, accompanying ST-segment elevation in the infarct leads (Wong et al., 2006a). This is consistent with the finding that patients presenting with Q wave at admission have worse epicardial recanalisation, tissue reperfusion and less salvage myocardial area than patients without Q wave at admission (Wong et al., 1999, 2002a,b).

(j) Recently, Petrina, Goodman and Eagle (2006), making a review of the literature of the admission ECG in patients presenting with acute myocardial infarction, have identified **the ECG changes that better predict the prognosis**. These include ST-segment deviations, arrhythmias, QRS duration and others. A summary of the independent risk factors for short- and long-term mortality is depicted in Figure 8.14. In general this review is in agreement with what we have explained in the previous items.

Electrocardiographic changes induced by fibrinolytic therapy (Figures 8.15–8.17) (Corbalan et al., 1999; Zehender et al., 1991)

The most typical electrocardiographic changes are the following:

(a) Rapid resolution of the ST-segment elevation is a very sensitive sign of reperfusion, especially in the anterior infarction, though is not very specific. The GISSI trial has demonstrated that a higher than 50% reduction of ST-segment elevation during the first 4 hours is a marker of good prognosis (Mauri et al., 1994) (Figures 8.15 and 8.16). Furthermore,

(A)

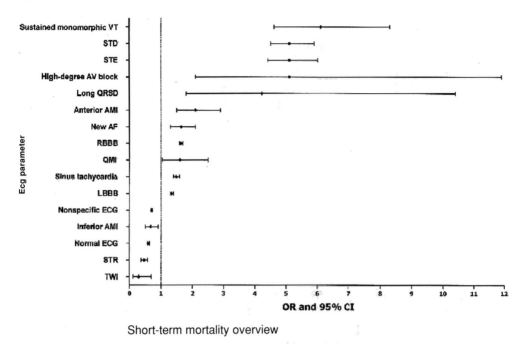

Short-term mortality overview

(B)

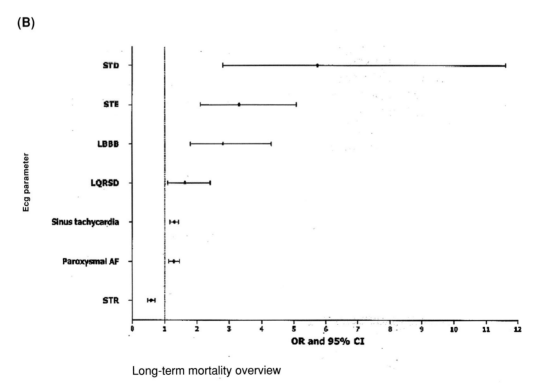

Long-term mortality overview

Figure 8.14 Short-term (A) and long-term (B) mortality of different parameters found in admission ECG. (Taken from Petrina, 2006.) STR, ST resolution; TWI, T-wave inversion; STD, ST depression; STE, ST elevation; QRSD, QRS deviation.

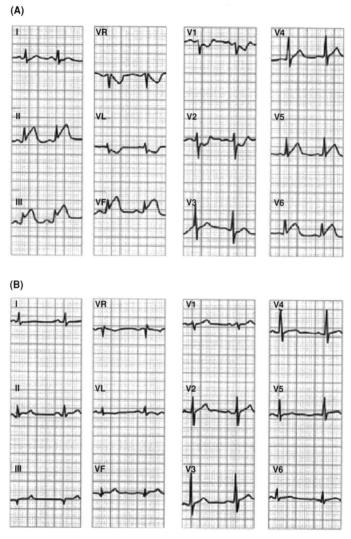

Figure 8.15 A 48-year-old patient with an acute inferior myocardial infarction due to RCA occlusion after the RV branches with an evident alteration of ST segment (ST↓ in I, ST↑ in III > II and ST↓ in V1–V2). The fibrinolytic treatment was started at 3 hours from the pain onset (A). At 4 hours (B) the ST segment was quite normal and there were no definite criteria of MI.

it is considered that when the summing up of the ST-segment elevations decreases by more than 50% in 2 hours, the infarction may be aborted (Lamfers et al., 2003) (p. 219). It has recently been reported that when the ST segment exhibits a slight deviation (≤1 mm in inferior infarctions or ≤2 mm in anterior infarctions) at 90 minute following fibrinolysis, it is likely that the artery is patent (reperfusion) (Cooper et al., 2002). It has also been demonstrated that the decrease (more than 75% in inferior infarc-

tions and more than 50% in anterior infarctions) of the ST-segment elevation in a few hours is a sign that suggests effective reperfusion. The correct interpretation of this information could avoid the practice of urgent coronary angiography.

(b) The early development (within the first 12 h following fibrinolysis) of a negative and usually deep T wave in the leads in which an ST-segment elevation was initially appreciated in patients with an anterior infarction (LAD occlusion) is a specific

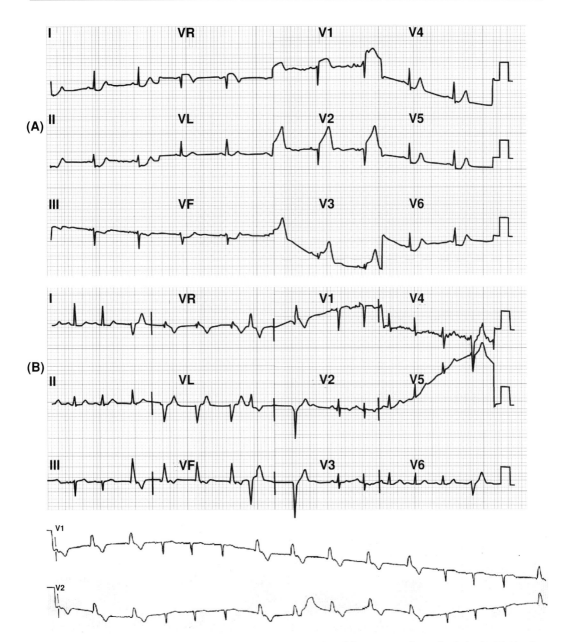

Figure 8.16 (A) The ECG of a patient with an acute myocardial infarction due to LAD occlusion proximal to D1 and S1 (ST-segment elevation from V1 to V4 and in VR, and ST-segment depression in II, III, VF (II > III), V4 and V5–V6). The injury vector is slightly directed to the right (see Figures 4.18 and 4.19) and this explains the isoelectric ST in VL and a mild ST-segment depression in lead I. (B) After 3 hours from fibrinolytic treatment ST segment is practically normal and accelerated idioventricular rhythm appears. In lead III a sinus complex, a fusion complex and a premature ventricular complex are shown. Lower part displays salvos of accelerated idioventricular rhythm in V1–V2 leads.

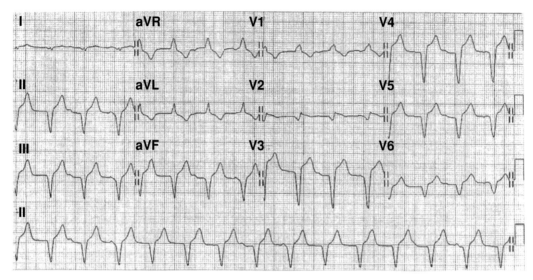

Figure 8.17 Twelve-lead ECG recordings showing AIVR during reperfusion of the LAD in a patient with an acute myocardial infarction. The morphology of AIVR suggests that it arises in mid-apical area of inferior wall (vector of depolarisation addressed upwards and backwards).

marker of reperfusion and good prognosis (**Doevendans et al., 1995**). This corresponds to one of the atypical patterns of STE-ACS that we have previously discussed (see 'Evolving ECG patterns in STE-ACS' p. 216, Figures 8.2 and 8.5 and Table 8.1). The reperfusion with primary PCI may also induce negative and deep T wave, especially in cases of LAD proximal occlusion (Figure 8.3). For more explanation about PCI and ECG changes, see 'Percutaneous coronary interventions'. When an isoelectric ST segment with negative T wave is seen in the ECG, blood flow through the LAD is much better (TIMI III in 65% of the cases) compared with cases with an ST-segment elevation and positive T wave (TIMI III in just 7% of the cases). Additionally, the EF is much better (57%) in the first group as compared with the second group (41%) (Matetzky et al., 1994). It should also be highlighted that the persistence of ST-segment elevation with no negative T wave after several days is a marker of poor prognosis and of risk of cardiac rupture (Figures 8.27 and 8.29).

(c) **The presence of Q wave in the admittance ECG** and **lower ST-segment resolution** despite early infarct artery patency are **markers of worse tissue reperfusion and epicardial recanalisation** (Wong et al., 1999, 2002a, 2006b).

(d) **Efficient reperfusion of the right coronary artery is highly specifically associated with sinus bradycardia and, sometimes, AV block** (Zehender et al., 1991).

(e) **The twofold increase in PVC, the development of accelerated idioventricular rhythm** (AIVR) and **runs of non-sustained ventricular tachycardia** (NSVT <30 s) **are supportive of successful reperfusion** (**reperfusion arrhythmias**) (Wellens, Gorgels and Doevendans, 2003; Figures 8.16 and 8.17). According to some authors, an AIVR preceded by an increase in PVCs is a specific sign of reperfusion (>80%), with a high positive predictive value (PPV) (Figure 8.17). The location of AIVR may be deduced from ECG morphology during AIVR and may help to assess what the occluded artery is (Wellens, Gorgels and Doevendans, 2003). The specificity of the AIVR increases when it occurs repeatedly (>30 episodes per hour) or when it lasts over 3 hours, or when it coincides with the abolishment of the ST-segment upward deviation. The positive predictive value of AIVR is higher than that of NSVT (Zehender et al., 1991). On the contrary, monomorphic sustained ventricular tachycardia is not a sign of reperfusion (Fiol et al., 2002).

(f) Recently, **vectocardiographic dynamic monitoring of the QRS-T loop** has been described as a non-invasive technique that provides a higher positive predictive value for the detection of reperfusion (Dellborg et al., 1991). However, this technique has not been widely used.

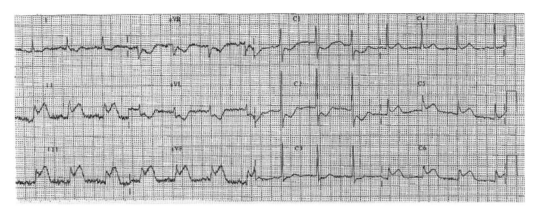

Figure 8.18 ECG in STE-ACS with very dominant RCA occlusion distal to RV branches and diffuse but not critical LAD occlusion. ST-segment depression in I points towards RCA occlusion. The ST-segment elevation in III > II and ST-segment depression V1–V3 or ST-segment elevation II–III–aVF ratio <1 also favours RCA involvement. The ST-segment elevation in V5–V6 suggests that the RCA is large enough to reach the low-inferolateral wall (superdominance). Accurate interpretation of ECG assures that the culprit artery is RCA and therefore a PCI was performed in this artery.

(g) Additionally, **score criteria for the prediction of ventricular function** following thrombolytic therapy have been reported (Pahlm et al., 1998).

STE-ACS in patients with multivessel occlusion: which is the culprit artery

In the first part (see 'ST-segment changes in patients with active ischaemia due to multivessel disease' and p. 105) we have described the ECG characteristics that may suggest the implication of more than one vessel in the genesis of STE-ACS. Usually, in these cases, the area at risk is higher and the outcome is worst. However, in spite that in some cases it seems clear that more than one vessel actively participates in the ischaemia that induce the ACS, usually even in the presence of multivessel disease there is one culprit artery responsible for ACS.

Now we will discuss the importance of the catheterisation laboratory in a patient with multivessel disease, which is the culprit artery responsible of the ACS. In clinical practice, when an STE-ACS occurs, a critical occlusion has developed usually in only one culprit artery. In most cases, due to the fact that multivessel disease is often present, what is most important is that in the catheterisation laboratory, in a patient with STE-ACS and multivessel disease, the interventionist cardiologist may, thanks to the correct and quick interpretation of the ECG, take the correct decision on which coronary artery the PCI has to be performed in. With the coronary angiograhic results at hand the ECG gives an important information that helps in defining which is the culprit artery in cases of multivessel disease. Unfortunately, this information is largely underused in clinical decision making (Nikus et al., 2004, 2005). Figure 8.18 shows an example of the relevance of these correlations. Therefore, a closer collaboration between clinicians, experts in ECG and interventionists should be emphasised, and this may be possible nowadays with modern technology that gives us an expert opinion on the ECG interpretation at any distance, even in seconds (Leibrandt et al., 2000). The possibility to transmit ECGs directly to a consulting centre with web-browsing capabilities may also be an alternative approach to take the best decision to immediately start revascularisation procedure in the appropriate culprit artery.

Patients with ACS and non-ST-segment elevation (NSTE-ACS): from unstable angina to non-Q-wave infarction

First of all we have to consider that small or even relatively significant negative T waves or ST-segment depression may be seen in several clinical situations, outside IHD and even in the absence of an apparent explanation (Table 3.2 and Figure 4.65).

The electrophysiological mechanisms of ST-segment depression and negative T wave that allow for the diagnosis of NSTE-ACS have already been explained in Figure 3.9 (see 'Electrophysiological mechanism of ECG pattern of injury') (p. 32). The importance of ST-segment depression and T-wave morphologies will now be commented on, from prognosis and risk stratification standpoint. We also included in this section the case of ACS with normal, near-to-normal or unchanged ECG.

Most of the patients included in this group of ACS (ST-segment depression/negative T wave) will present unstable angina or will evolve towards a non-Q-wave infarction. Just a few (10–20%) will end up developing a Q-wave infarction (Figure 8.2). This corresponds to pattern B (Table 8.1B(1–3)).

There are some groups of patients (already discussed on p. 210) that presenting with ECG features of non-ST elevation are not included in this section because they are seen in the clinical context of STE-ACS. Therefore, they are considered atypical ECG patterns of STE-ACS (see Table 8.1A(2)). We have already commented on some aspects of them in the previous pages (see 'Typical and atypical patterns of STE-ACS and NSTE-ACS') (p. 210).

After the consensus of ESC/ACC was reported (Alpert et al., 2000), the differential diagnosis between UA and non-Q-wave infarction has been especially based on the rise of troponines. Nevertheless, it should be borne in mind that a small number of patients with ST-segment depression may end up with a Q wave infarction (Figure 8.2).

On the other hand, the most important differences between the ACS with ST-segment depression/negative T wave and those presenting with ST-segment elevation or an equivalent are shown in Table 8.2.

The ST/T morphology on admission: prognosis and risk stratification

The presence of different ECG patterns plays a decisive role in the risk stratification of patients with NSTE-ACS. Table 8.1 shows the different ECG patterns found in STE-ACS and NSTE-ACS. We will just highlight here that in case of NSTE-ACS the prognosis is worse when the patient evolves towards a non-Q-wave infarction and even more so when it ends up as a Q-wave infarction. **Factors, such as age, the presence of refractory angina and previous infarctions, ejection fraction, enzymatic level,** etc., **also influence the prognosis**. All these will be explained later (see Risk stratification ACS p. 257) (Antman et al., 2000; Holmvang et al., 1999; Holper et al., 2001; Hyde et al., 1999; Lee et al., 1993). Regarding the ECG, it is important from prognostic point of view the cases in which the ECG changes of ST/T give us the clues to detect occlusion of LMT/three-vessel diseases (see 'Location criteria' p. 113). It is also important to recognise that the presence of confounding factors (found in nearly 25% of the cases) as LBBB, ventricular enlargement or pacing also represents a poor prognosis (Holmvang, 2003). Let us explain all these aspects in more detail.

ST-segment depression (Figures 8.19–8.22)

• **Circumferential subendocardium involvement**: ST-segment depression, sometimes very evident and present in many leads, (7 or more) with or without dominant R wave (Table 8.1, and Figures 4.59 and 8.19).

In these cases there is an extensive predominant subendocardial ischaemia (**circumferential subendocardial ischaemia**). The ST-segment depression is evident and, sometimes, striking. It is found in seven or more leads, some with a dominant R wave and others with rS morphology (presence of ST-segment depression in two planes). The precordial leads V4–V5 are those presenting a more significant ST-segment depression (often ≥5 mm) and appear often concomitantly without positive T wave in these leads (Figures 4.59 and 8.19). An ST-segment elevation is seen in VR and, sometimes, in V1 and III, but the ST-segment elevation is always greater in VR than in V1 (Yamaji et al., 2001). The ST-segment depression in V2–V3 is not accompanied by ST-segment elevation in inferior leads (except sometimes III), so it should not be confounded with inferolateral infarction due to LCX occlusion (Table 8.1B(2) and Figure 4.9).

This typical electrocardiographic finding corresponds to a **left main incomplete occlusion** and is present in patients with a prior large subendocardium ischaemia (Sclarovsky's circumferential involvement; Figure 5.51) and when collateral circulation is present. **Similar ECGs** with sometimes somewhat less ST-segment depression, and

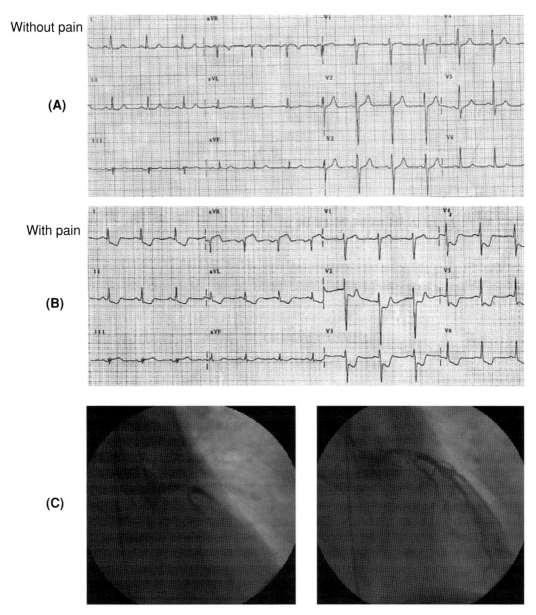

Figure 8.19 (A) ECG without pain is practically normal. (B) ECG shows during pain ST-segment depression and inverted T waves in more than eight leads, maximally in leads V4–V5 where there is not a positive T wave and ST-segment elevation in lead aVR (circumferential subendocardial involvement). (C) Coronary angiography shows tight stenosis in the left main coronary artery before and after primary PCI.

more often **with positive final T wave in V4–V5**, are seen in patients that may present with **multivessel disease, usually very tight occlusion of proximal LAD + LCX** (Figures 4.60 and 4.61), but also in case of LMT incomplete occlusion.

The baseline ECG of patients with important occlusion of the left main coronary artery or three-vessel disease frequently is relatively normal. The important ST-segment deviations appear with spontaneous angina (Figures 5.51, 4.61 and 8.18) or during exercise testing (Figure 8.23). Only few

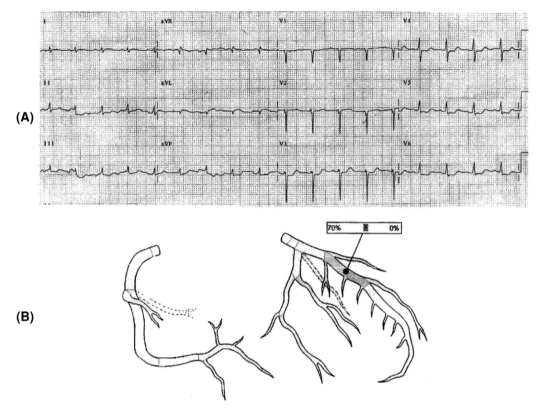

Figure 8.20 (A) ECG shows ST-segment depression especially in precordial leads (V3–V6) with positive T wave very evident in leads V3–V5 (regional subendocardial involvement). There is no ST-segment elevation in VR.

(B) Drawing of coronary angiography that shows tight stenosis of the mid-left anterior descending coronary artery.

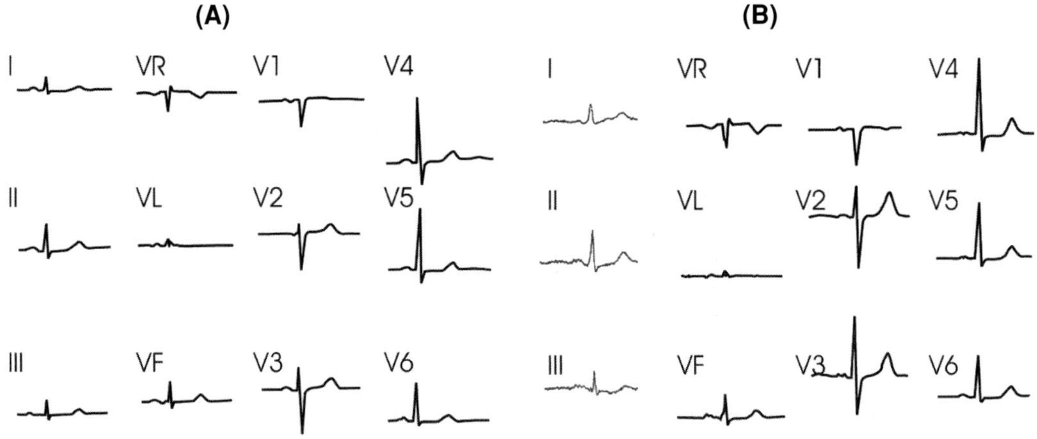

Figure 8.21 The ECG recorded during ACS (B) represents subtle changes of the repolarisation (more positive T wave in V2–V4, somewhat more evident ST-segment depression in inferior leads and V6) as compared to previous ECGs (A). These features suggest inferolateral involvement, as it was

confirmed by coronary angiography. Note the importance of using in these cases an ECG machine that allows us to record amplified ECG in order to detect easily small changes (0.5 mm) of ST-segment deviation (see Figure 4.3).

(A)

(B)

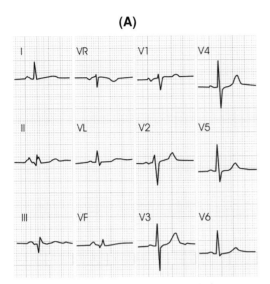

Figure 8.22 (A) ECG of 62-year-old patient with multivessel chronic coronary artery disease. (B) During an NSTE-ACS MI an ST-segment depression in V1–V2 and low-voltage R wave in V6 with flattened T wave, compared to pattern displayed in previous ECG (A), was observed. This patient presented an ACS due to OM occlusion.

patients present at rest ST-segment elevation in aVR or evident ST-segment depression in several leads. Sometimes these patients present RBBB or LBBB. This group of NSTE-ACS **represents the worst prognosis** and in our experience the highest mortality of all ECG patterns (Figure 8.4). These cases needs urgent treatment and an emergent coronariography to confirm the diagnosis and decide the need of revascularisation, which usually is surgical. Because of this it is recommended to not start with clopidogrel treatment.

• **Regional subendocardium involvement: ST-segment depression in less than seven leads (Table 8.1, and Figures 3.3 and 4.64)**

By the pathophysiological point of view ST-segment depression in only some leads (<7 leads) during ACS represents regional area of predominant subendocardium ischaemia. The ST-segment depression is frequently smaller than that in circumferential involvement. The following new or dynamic repolarisation abnormalities have to be at least present: **ST-segment depression horizontal or downsloping, between 0.5 and 1 mm, with a normal or flattened T wave** (Holper et al., 2001). At least, two leads with ST-segment depression is the minimum requirement for a diagnosis of ACS (Table 8.2), and to **give exact value to these small electrocardiographic abnormalities**

they must develop during exercise testing or ACS or disappear when the syndrome resolves (Figures 4.62–4.64).

The specificity of the ST-segment and its prognostic value are based on the number of leads showing those changes and significance of the ST-segment depression. The specificity is very high when the ST horizontal or downsloping depression is greater than 1 mm (McConahay, McCallister and Smith, 1971). The prognosis is worse in patients with evident ST-segment depression, especially if this change is found in four or more leads, and when despite the implementation of therapy, dynamic ECG changes exist (Akkerhuis et al., 2001). The Gusto IIB trial demonstrates that **the cases of worst prognosis are those with ST-segment depression in precordial leads with dominant R wave (V4–V6) and in some leads of FP, with negative T wave in V4–V6** (Birnbaum and Atar, 2006). Similar results have been published by others (Barrabes et al., 2000). On the contrary, the presence of ST-segment depression in the precordial leads with positive T wave was associated to a single-vessel disease (Sclarowsky et al., 1988). Furthermore, it should be highlighted that mild ST-segment depression (0.5–1.0 mm) during spontaneous angina or exercise testing with angina in leads with dominant R wave (I, VL and V4–V6) may be seen in case of

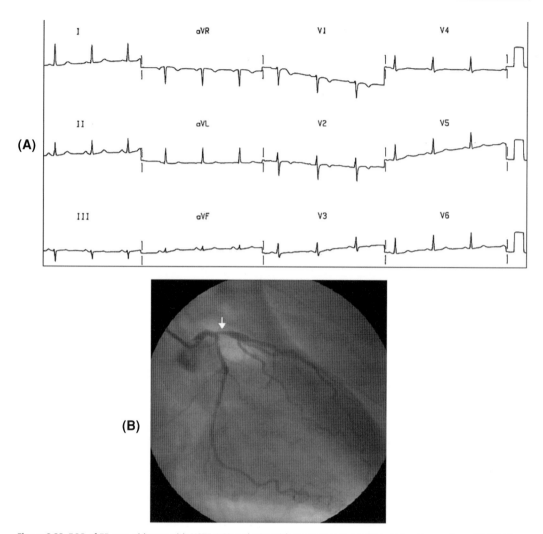

Figure 8.23 ECG of 55-year-old man with NSTE-ACS and ECG with symmetric and mild negative T wave from V1–V3. The coronariography shows important LAD proximal occlusion.

severe two- and three-vessel diseases (Figure 4.62). Therefore, as has already been stated (Figure 4.3), the recording of an amplified ECG (1 mV = 4 cm) is important for measuring slight ST-segment depressions.

This ACS with regional involvement is usually secondary to an incomplete coronary artery occlusion in patients frequently presenting with prior predominantly regional subendocardial ischaemia and single- or multivessel disease, but one culprit artery. Any coronary artery may be the culprit one and the occlusion often is not proximal (Table 8.2).

The correlation between the leads exhibiting this type of NSTE-ACS depression and the culprit artery is not as good as in case of NSTE-ACS with circumferential involvement (LMT) (Table 8.1) or in cases of STE-ACS (see Table 4.1). However, the careful assessment of subtle ST-segment or T-wave changes may give important information about the affected area and the culprit vessel in these patients with NSTE-ACS (Figures 8.21 and 8.22).

The ST-segment depression in precordial leads, especially V1–V2 to V4–V5, followed by an evident positive T wave in V3–V5, corresponds usually to proximal LAD incomplete occlusion in a patient with previous subendocardial ischaemia (Nikus, Eskola and Virtanen, 2004). When the ST-segment depression is present, especially in V4–V6, more often incomplete occlusion in the mid-late LAD is present (Figure 8.20). However, in both cases there is often multivessel disease, although usually the culprit artery is the LAD. The cases of proximal LAD occlusion are at risk for large MI and urgent PCI has to be performed, but not as emergency as is the case of involvement of LMT. As the injury pattern starts at the end of QRS and appears early in the ST segment, it is logical that if not very severe it may finish before the end of repolarisation, and this makes possible the appearance of final positive T wave. Negative T wave appears in the second part of repolarisation, and due to that sometimes presents a ± morphology in V1–V3 (Figure 3.21).

The ST-segment depression, even slightly, has generally been shown to imply a worse prognosis than the T wave changes because represent clearly "active" ischaemia. Patients with ST-segment depression or bundle branch block have been described to have a fivefold higher risk (15%) than those exhibiting just a flattened or slightly negative T wave (3%) (Collinson et al., 2000). However, in our experience with the current intensive treatment of NSTE-ACS including primary PCI, there is no difference of in-hospital mortality in case of NSTE-ACS due to regional involvement between ST-segment depression and the presence of flattened and mild negative T wave.

The invasive treatment of regional NSTE-ACS is now under revision. For some authors (Diderholm et al., 2002; Gomez-Hospital and Cequier, 2004) in cases with even slight ST-segment depression, the best approach seems to be to perform a **coronary angiography and revascularisation**. With this approach morbidity and mortality have been greatly

reduced (from 18 to 12% per year). However, despite of increasing acceptance of this approach, a recent publication (De Winter et al., 2005) demonstrates that the non-invasive strategy may give even better results. **We consider that the final decision has to be taken at individual level on the basis of presence of symptoms and global clinical evaluation of each patient.**

Flattened or negative T wave

Sometimes in patients with NSTE-ACS the only abnormality is a new flattened or negative T wave with no apparent ST-segment depression (see Table 8.1, and Figures 3.23 and 8.23).

The presence of negative or flattened T wave may be explained by delay in repolarization probably in all the wall but without subendocardial predominance that is more consequence of postischaemic changes than to the presence of "active" ischaemia. However, sometimes in spite of benign appearance of small T-wave negativity the coronary stenosis may be tight (Figures 3.26 and 8.23). The location of these small changes of T wave may be usually in leads with prominent R wave (Figure 3.23), but occasionally are present in leads with rS morphology (V1–V2) (Figures 3.26 and 8.23).

Also, **a positive T wave, which has evidently increased its positivity** with respect to the baseline T wave, may be considered abnormal (Jacobsen et al., 2001). Furthermore, the presence of a **negative U wave, or a positive U wave when the T wave is negative** in leads with a dominant R wave, is considered abnormal (Figures 3.24 and 3.26).

We have to remember that in case of reperfused LAD proximal occlusion may be seen in the ECG as a deep negative T wave (Figure 8.9). In these cases with new chest pain the ECG usually pseudonormalises and rarely even presents ST-segment

---

NSTE-ACS: prognostic implications (Antman et al., 2000; Boden, 2001; Braunwald et al., 2000; Diderholm et al., 2002; Erhardt et al., 2002)

- Overall, patients with ST-segment depression on arrival at the hospital have a worse prognosis than patients with negative T wave. Also, in general, they more frequently have two- or three-vessel diseases and many more complications than those presenting with a small negative T wave.

- Also, patients with higher millimetres of ST-segment depression (score >3 mm) in the different ECG leads have the worst prognosis. In these patients an early invasive strategy may reduce the risk up to 50% of death or MI (Holmvang et al., 1999).

- The recording of ST-segment monitoring is very important to access changes during the follow-up with and without pain.
- The presence of confounding factors that are relatively frequently found in NSTE-ACS represents by themselves poorest prognosis.
- The differentiation between an unstable angina and a non-Q-wave infarction is mainly based on the presence or not of increased enzyme levels (troponine).
- Patients with UA usually refer fewer pain crises and their ECGsare less abnormal (flattened or negative, but not deep T wave) with normal levels of troponins.
- Patients with non-Q-wave infarction generally refer more frequent crises of longer duration, and their ECG recordings exhibit more frequently ST-segment depression than negative T waves. Usually cases with deep negative T wave in precordials (V1–V4–V5) correspond to proximal non-complete LAD occlusion and are included in the group of atypical patterns of STE-ACS (reperfusion pattern) (Figure 8.3).
- The presence of evident ST-segment depression in seven or more leads with ST-segment elevation in VR and sometimes V1 (circumferential involvement) (Yamaji et al., 2001) suggests LMT involvement and represents a pattern of very bad prognosis (Figures 5.51 and 8.19). The T wave in V4–V5 may be negative or positive but more often is negative.
- When there is tight occlusion of proximal LAD and LCX (LMT equivalent) with or without non-critical involvement of LMT, the ST-segment depression may or may not be huge, but usually the T wave is positive in V3–V5 (Figures 4.60 and 4.61).
- The cases with ST-segment depression in less than seven leads with worst prognosis present ST-segment depression in V4–V6 and in some leads of FP and negative T wave in V4–V6 (Birnbaum, 2007).
- The cases of NSTE-ACS with only mild flat or negative T wave are of better prognosis. However, when these small changes are present in V1–V3, we recommend coronary angiography because sometimes there is a tight proximal LAD occlusion in a patient without at this moment probably "active" myocardial ischaemia.

elevation. This pattern corresponds to an atypical pattern of STE-ACS.

Global mortality and morbidity (refractory angina and/or new infarction) in patients with flat or negative T wave are low. **Patients with a less –than 1 mm of negativity or flattened T wave in leads with a dominant R wave**, and, even more, those presenting with a normal ECG, have a low risk of a large infarction or death, even though they may suffer from multivessel disease but without proximal stenosis. Due generally to their good prognosis, medical therapy is usually advised, which includes the new drugs, IIb/IIIa inhibitors, unless the patient's age, the clinical presentation and the enzyme level increase recommend the practice of a coronary angiography to decide the convenience to perform PCI. However, some patients with mild T changes in V1–V3 (Figures 3.26 and 8.23) may present critical non-distal subocclusion of LAD in the absence of "active" subendocardial ischaemia because in its presence probably an ST depression would be recorded. In these cases of negative T wave in V1-V2 may be convenient to perform coronariography.

Patients with NSTE-ACS with normal ECG, or without evident changes with respect to previous ECG recordings (Figure 8.24 and Table 8.1B 3).

The patients with ACS that have been included in this group exhibit minimal or doubtful ST-segment/T-wave changes ($\leq$0.5 mm). The T waves are somewhat flattened but are not very different from those found in prior ECG recordings. We would like to stress the importance to perform an exercise test in case of normal or nearly normal ECG with dubious previous precordial pain, or without pain but important presence of risk factors, because sometimes an ST-segment depression as a sign of probably 'active' ischaemia with or without angina appears (Figure 4.64).

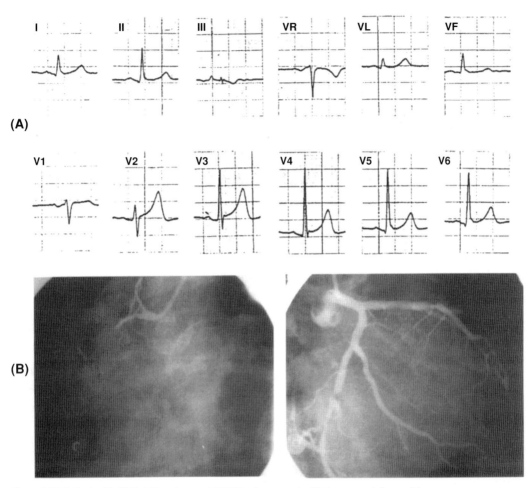

Figure 8.24 Patient with NSTE-ACS and normal ECG (A) who present with three-vessel disease (B).

The ECG may be normal even in presence of two- and three-vessel diseases or LMT subocclusion when pain is absent. Around 10% of patients who end up with an ACS (MI or UA) present a normal or unchanged ECG in the emergency department. However, **in the presence of significant and, especially, repetitive chest pain, it is highly improbable that a completely normal ECG corresponds to an ACS. This is especially true when the ECG shows no changes with respect to previous ECGs recorded in the absence of chest pain.** In any case, if **ACS is finally shown to be present, it is generally of good prognosis.** It should be pointed out that we are referring to ACS with a narrow QRS complex. In the presence of a wide QRS complex, the approach is different, since an **ACS with a wide QRS complex always has a worse prognosis. This is true even when apparent changes are not present in the ECG,** since these are sometimes masked.

Because of the high sensitivity of the new infarction markers (troponins), the number of patients with ACS who present chest pain and elevated enzyme levels, but without electrocardiographic changes, has been increasing (ESC/ACC; Alpert et al., 2000). Therefore, there is no doubt that more infarcts than before may be diagnosed, although it is also evident that the prognosis of these infarctions, named *necrosettes*, micronecroses or enzymatic infarctions, is much better than that of the typical non-Q-wave infarction.

Occasionally, the first change observed in an anteroseptal infarction, even extensive, is the increase in the T-wave amplitude in the right precordial leads, due to the acute subendocardium ischaemia in a heart without much prior ischaemia. **This T-wave morphology may be interpreted as pseudonormal**, and it should be readily recognised and differentiated from the normal T wave. In this case the recording of evolutionary ECG is mandatory (Figure 8.7).

Management: The following aspects should be borne in mind in a patient presenting at the hospital with **suspicion of ischaemic chest pain and a normal or near-normal ECG**:

(a) Frequently, **the ECG exhibits evolutionary patterns of ST-segment elevation or depression**. Consequently, the repetition of the ECG during the first hours or better still, if possible, ST-segment monitoring is required to assess whether transient ST-segment elevations or depressions exist.

(b) Whenever possible, **a comparison with previous ECGs should be made** (Figure 3.26).

(c) Two further enzyme-level determinations (troponins) (at 6 and 12 h of admission) should also be performed.

(d) When especially in coronary patients the pain is suggestive of ischaemia and troponins are slightly positive, but the ECG remains normal, the existence of a '***necrosette***' (enzymatic infarction) **is confirmed**. In some cases, the ECG remains normal, even with clear evidence of enzyme-level increase. It usually corresponds to **a distal occlusion, generally in the LCX. When troponins are negative and the evolution demonstrates the presence of an ACS, a diagnosis of UA is made**, which usually represents a good prognosis.

(e) In cases of doubt, an exercise stress test should be performed, if possible in the same emergency department (Figures 4.62 and 4.64). One should be convinced that the patient is haemodynamically stable and not presenting an evolving ACS and that the baseline ECG is normal or near normal. When, in spite of all, diagnostic doubts persist, imaging techniques should be performed, whenever possible, to assess the presence of ischaemia (exercise stress echocardiogram or scintigraphy) and to know the coronary anatomy non-invasively (Hecht, 2000). When the tests performed are evidently positive and the patient continues referring chest pain, the performance of an urgent coronary angiography is advisable, and a PCI should be done, if possible.

When reasonable doubts persist with regard to the pain's origin and the complementary tests performed are negative, including the imaging techniques and the coronary angiography, other causes of chest pain should be reassessed (Figure 7.1). If patients with all the tests performed sequentially over several hours being negative and finally diagnosed as ACS, it is usually of low risk (see above).

In hospital mortality of different ECG patterns at arrival

The in-hospital mortality of different ECG patterns of Figure 8.4 is the following: The global in-hospital mortality of STE-ACS was 6.5% and of NSTE-ACS 2.02%. Characteristically, the highest mortality in the group of STE-ACS corresponds to the atypical C pattern on admission (11%) (ST-segment depression in V1–V3 > ST-segment elevation in inferior lateral leads; Figure 8.3 and Fig. 2.10 pattern 2). This probably is related with the number of mechanical complications that these patients present (cardiac rupture, etc.) (see p. 243). In the group of NSTE-ACS the highest mortality corresponds to the group of LMT involvement (14%). In our study the ECG pattern with confounding factors does not represent worst outcome, as was classically considered. This concept however has to be reconsidered after the Wong's paper (2005) (see p. 249). Globally, these results are very similar to results obtained in the Euro Heart Survey (Mandelzweig et al., 2006), which presents an in-hospital mortality for STE-ACS of 7% and for NSTE-ACS 2–4%. On the contrary, compared with a series of cases of our own hospital before 24-hour PCI was implemented and all the new antithrombotic and antiplatelet drugs were used, the current in-hospital mortality is much better (globally 11.6% vs 4.6%).

Recurrent ACS

This term means repeated episodes of ACS either with or without ST-segment elevation usually evolving to MI, in patients who are chronologically and anatomically unrelated to each other. Now the recurrence of ACS with clear change of

ST segment occurs less with all the new medications. However, it is not an infrequent event that usually appears after 2–3 years after the index MI and often in a different location. Roth et al. (2006) have demonstrated that most patients (76%) who were admitted two times due to a recurrent ACS have new episode of the same type STE-ACS (44%) or NSTE-ACS (32%). Rest of the patients (24%) presented both STE-ACS and NSTE-ACS. These episodes were also noted in patients with two recurrences, thus supporting the validity of the results. Therefore, most patients with recurrent episodes will have STE-ACS or NSTE-ACS, but not the two types suggesting that some patients present factors that predispose to repeat episodes of STE-ACS, such as thrombus formation, complete coronary occlusion, low flow, high-grade stenosis, spasm, some coagulation factors, etc., or NSTE-ACS, such as inhibition of thrombus progression, small rapidly healing lesion, high natural lysis, etc. (Davies, 1996).

Other electrocardiographic abnormalities in patients with an ACS

P wave and PR segment

The deviations of PR interval are especially seen in pericarditis (Figures 1.106 and 1.107) and atrial involvement in case of myocardial infarction (Figures 2.60 and 2.61). The diagnosis of atrial infarction is based especially on the presence of PR-segment deviations (elevation or depression in different leads) associated with reciprocal changes in other leads (specially ST-segment elevation in VR and ST-segment depression in II) and any atrial arrhythmias (Liu, Greenspan and Piccirillo, 1961). Recently, it has been demonstrated (Jim et al., 2006) that PR-segment depressions ≥ 1.2 mm in patients with inferior STE-ACS (ST-segment elevation in II, III and VF) are a marker of high risk of AV block, supraventricular arrhythmias, cardiac rupture and in-hospital mortality (p. 246).

The morphology of P wave may change especially in V1 in case of left ventricular failure (see Figure 13.3).

Changes of QRS complex

ACS with ST-segment elevation and severe ischaemia often present changes in the final portion of the QRS complex (see Figures 8.7 and 8.13). Also severe ischemia may induce QRS widening with or without classic patterns of intraventricular block (see p. 247 and 287). The importance from a prognostic point of view of some of these changes is discussed in p. 224 and 247 (Birnbaum et al., 1993).

QT interval

During the acute phase of ischaemia, a lengthening of the transmembrane action potential (TAP) is recorded in the area of ischaemia (p. 39). The presence of a long QTc interval at the time of admission of a patient with ACS has been shown to be a marker of poor prognosis (Flugelman et al., 1987). Additionally, patients with non-Q-wave infarction, in comparison with those with UA, have overall longer QTc intervals (Rukshin et al., 2002). However, this is not useful when applied to an individual patient. Therefore the troponin levels remain as the best way to distinguish whether an ACS with no ST-segment elevation has evolved to a non-Q-wave infarction or has remained as a UA. One should also recall that discrepancies exist with regard to the prognostic value of QT-interval dispersion in STE-ACS (Fiol et al., 1995).

U wave

A normal U wave is always positive in the presence of a positive T wave and, under normal conditions, it is negative only in VR. In patients with different clinical settings of IHD, U-wave abnormalities may be recorded, generally as a negative U wave, while the T wave may be negative, positive or flattened (Figures 3.24–3.26). The U wave may be positive when the T wave is negative (T-U discordance) (Reinig, Harizi and Spodick, 2005).

In all these situations, the U wave is pathological, and when it is recorded in patients with coronary heart disease (CHD), it is highly probable that the LAD is involved. Also, it should be highlighted that a negative U wave may be the only electrocardiographic sign of ischaemia, it sometimes precedes ST-segment changes and, among other things, it may increase the sensitivity of the exercise stress test (Correale et al., 2004).

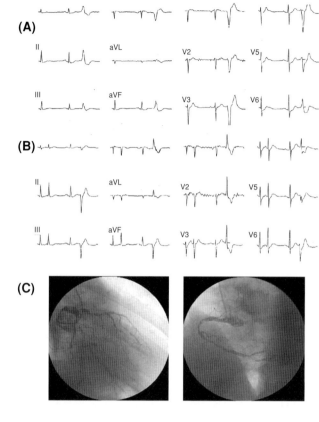

Figure 8.25 Exercise test of a patient with doubtful precordial pain and frequent (A) ventricular and (B) supraventricular premature beats. Observe that ST-segment depression was little evident in sinus rhythm complexes, while it was very significant in premature complexes (see V3 and V4 in (B) and V5 and V6 in (A)). (C) The patient presented severe three-vessel disease.

Arrhythmias

All the different issues of ACS-related arrhythmias will be commented on in the next sections (see 'Arrhythmias and intraventricular conduction blocks'). We will just state here that frequently, both during the exercise stress test and in the resting ECG in a chronic patient, or during an ACS (Figures 1.105, 8.25 and 8.26), **the repolarisation abnormalities may be more visible in the premature ventricular complexes (PVCs) than in normal ones and sometimes even are seen in PVC only** (Figure 8.25). Additionally, the ST-segment depression in the PVCs in the exercise stress test has been described as possibly being more useful than the ST-segment depression in normal complexes for predicting myocardial ischaemia. The ST-segment depression in the PVCs higher than 10% of the R-wave amplitude in V4–V–V6 has a 95% sensitivity and a 67% specificity for predicting ischaemia (Rasouli and Ellestad, 2001) (Figures 8.25 and 8.26). However, in spite of that, there frequently exist cases of repolarisation abnormalities in the PVC of healthy patients, and therefore the specificity of the test is not so high. It is, however, useful in doubtful cases (Figures 8.25 and 8.26).

Furthermore, the meticulous study of the QRS complex or the T-wave morphology of the PVC allows for suspicion of an old infarction (qR morphology, with a wide q wave or slurred QS complex, with a sometimes symmetric T wave).

ECG in mechanical complications of an ACS evolving to myocardial infarction (Figures 8.27–8.29)

The most important mechanical complications of ACS evolving to MI occur in transmural infarctions, usually Q-wave infarction. They consist in **cardiac rupture, which may occur in the free wall, the interventricular septum or the papillary muscles and the ventricular aneurisms.**

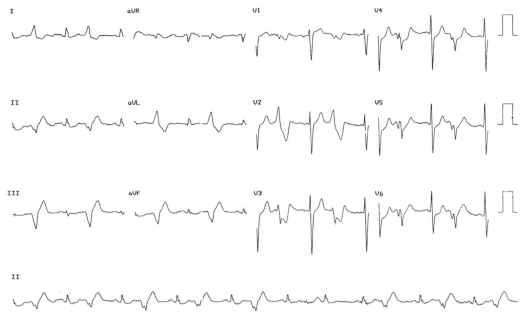

Figure 8.26 Other example of exercise test in a patient with ischaemic heart disease that demonstrated the presence of significant ST-segment changes in premature beats (see V3–V4) that were not so evident in normal sinus complexes.

Cardiac ruptures are much less frequent with the currently available therapies. However, they may still be found in 2–3% of Q-wave infarctions and are still an important cause of mortality in the acute phase (Figueras et al., 1995). Additionally, cardiac rupture may occur without prodromal signs in patients with evolving Q-wave or equivalent infarction, sometimes small and for that their occurrence is even more dramatic. Therefore, it is extremely important to assess correctly the subtle premonitory data, such as some electrocardiographic details. Contrary to what occurs in primary VF, which may be virtually always resolved in the coronary care unit, cardiac rupture requires urgent surgical treatment. The mortality rate is only below that of cardiogenic shock secondary to a massive infarction. Fortunately, also the latter is much less frequent with the currently available therapies.

Free-wall rupture is the most frequent and may be acute, followed by sudden death secondary to electromechanical dissociation, or subacute with recurrent chest pain and haemorrhage within the pericardial sac, with or without cardiac tampon-

ade and cardiogenic shock (Figure 8.29A; see Plate 2.2). Sometimes it is presented as pseudoaneurysm (López-Sendón et al., 1992). A pseudoaneurysm is a cavity formed by a free-wall rupture that has been self-limited by the formation of pericardial adherence and organised fibrin. A cavity is also present in an authentic ventricular aneurysm, but in this case it is secondary to the dilation of a non-ruptured ventricular wall, so myocardial fibres are present throughout the entire extension of the cavity.

From an electrocardiographic standpoint, during the evolution of a Q-wave acute myocardial infarction, some ECG changes may be recorded that herald cardiac rupture. In the free-wall rupture, frequently, the persistence of an ST-segment elevation may be detected. This is usually accompanied by the lack of T-wave negativisation throughout the acute phase. Therefore, the persisting ST-segment elevation, sign of regional pericarditis, is an indirect risk marker of cardiac rupture (Figure 8.27; Reeder and Gersh, 2000). The persistence of ST-segment elevation is seen more frequently in the inferior and, especially, in the lateral wall MI, than in the anterior wall MI (Figure 8.28A). The k

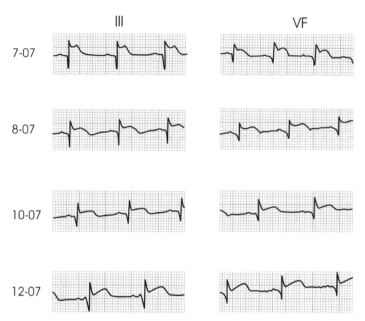

Figure 8.27 The ECG recordings (lead III and VF) performed during 1 week of evolution of STE-ACS. ST-segment elevation persists without appearance of negative T wave. This is a risk marker of cardiac rupture, as happened in this case.

ST-segment elevation is, generally, more persistent than significant, and though the ECG is clearly abnormal, a striking ST-segment elevation is not usually seen (Figure 8.28A) (Oliva, Hammill and Edwards, 1993). Consequently, the degree of ST-segment elevation during the acute phase of evolving MI does not correlate with the risk of rupture. Coronary artery disease is not usually very extensive (one- or two-vessel disease) in cases with free-wall cardiac rupture. Generally, the RCA and the LCX are more frequently involved than the LAD, and collateral circulation is not too developed, which favours the occurrence of transmural MI (Q wave or equivalent) with homogeneous involvement of the entire wall. When a free-wall cardiac rupture is suspected, it should be confirmed with imaging techniques, thereafter proceeding to an urgent surgical procedure. In patients with an evolving inferior acute MI the presence of PR-segment depression ≥1.2 mm in II, III and VF is associated with a higher risk of in-hospital mortality and free-wall cardiac rupture and/or atrial rupture compared with cases without PR-segment deviations (Jim et al., 2006) (see 'P wave and PR segment') (p. 243).

Septal rupture usually occurs, in turn, in larger infarctions, especially due to a proximal LAD oc-

clusion. It is also accompanied by recurrent pain and, in this case, a systolic murmur may be heard, suggestive of a ventricular septal defect; frequently, the patient presents cardiogenic shock if surgery is not urgently carried out. Sometimes rupture of the lower part of the septum occurs in patients with inferior MI (Figure 8.28). Septal rupture may sometimes be associated with free-wall rupture. The ECG may also show the persistence of ST-segment elevation. Higher incidence compared to control Q-wave infarctions exists of RBBB with or without added superoanterior hemiblock (SAH), advanced AV block and atrial fibrillation.

Finally, **papillary muscle rupture or dysfunction causes acute mitral regurgitation** (generally, the development of an intense systolic murmur), frequently with acute pulmonary oedema. Urgent surgery is also required. The posteromedial papillary muscle is more frequently involved (Figure 8.29B), since its perfusion is derived only from the posterior descending artery (RCA or LCX), while the anterolateral papillary muscle has double perfusion (LAD and LCX). As in free-wall cardiac rupture, they are usually small infarctions with, generally, few collateral vessels and single-vessel disease. However, in this case, contrary to free-wall cardiac

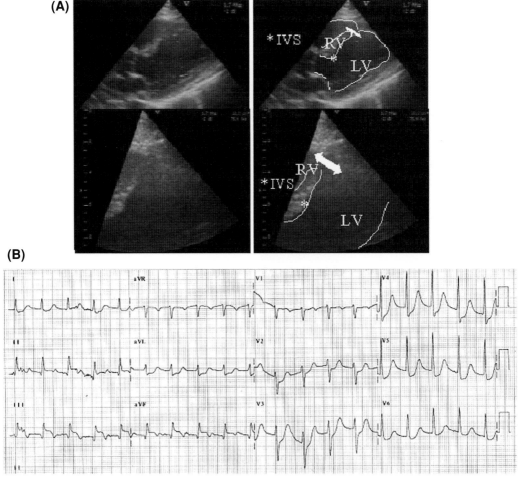

Figure 8.28 Echocardiogram showing rupture of lower part of septum (see arrow) in (A), in a patient with previous extensive non-Q-wave MI during the course of new inferior MI due to LCX occlusion (B).

rupture, the infarct is frequently of the non-Q-wave type (>50% of the cases).

With regard to **ventricular aneurysms**, their presence has classically been suggested by the persistence of ST-segment elevation. In chronic patients, the sensitivity of this sign is poor. Just 10% of the patients in the post-infarction setting with ventricular aneurysm exhibit a higher than 0.1 mV ST-segment elevation (East and Oran, 1952). Also, it has been described that some changes of mid-late part of QRS including rsR' in left surface leads (Sherif, 1970) and other morphologies (fractioned QRS) are very specific of ventricular aneurysm (Reddy et al., 2006) (see 'Usefulness and limitations of ECG in chronic IHD') (Figure 13.2) (p. 304).

ACS with wide QRS complex and other confounding factors: complete bundle branch block, Wolff–Parkinson–White syndrome, pacemaker or LVH pattern

These account for around 10–20% of ACSs. The electrocardiographic diagnosis of an ACS in the presence of complete LBBB, Wolff–Parkinson–White syndrome or pacemaker is more difficult than in cases with a narrow QRS complex. RBBB does not interfere with the diagnosis (Figure 4.66). In case of LBBB in the **acute phase**, ST-segment often presents deviations (Figure 4.67) (Sgarbossa et al., 1996a,b), and in presence of LVH or pacemaker also,

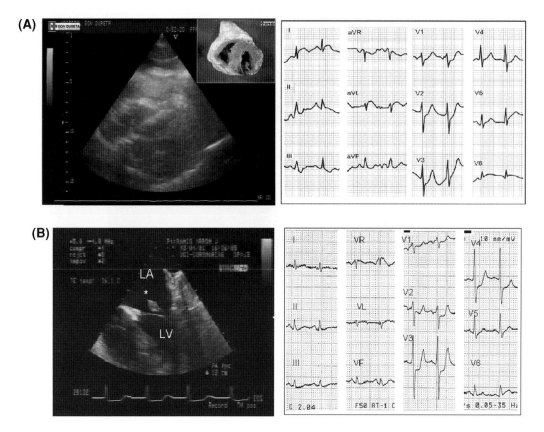

Figure 8.29 (A) Rupture of inferior wall in a patient after 7 days of inferior MI due to LCX occlusion. See the echocardiography with great haematic pericardial effusion and the pathological aspect of the rupture. In spite of that, the ECG shows relatively small ECG changes (mild ST-segment elevation in I and VL and mirror image of ST-segment depression in V1–V3 that remains after a week of MI). (B) Rupture of posteromedial papillary muscle (see asterisk in the echocardiography) in a patient with inferolateral MI due to LCX occlusion. The ECG shows ST-segment depression in V1–V4 as a mirror image of inferolateral injury without ST-segment elevation in inferior leads, just mild ST-segment elevation in lateral leads (I, VL and V6). This figure can be seen in colour, Plate 6.

frequently, ST-segment deviations compared with previous ECG are visible (Figure 4.68). Diagnostic criteria have also been described for the **chronic phase** (Figures 5.48–5.52; Table 5.6). **All these diagnostic aspects have been discussed at length in the first part** (see sections 'ECG pattern of ischaemia in patients with ventricular hypertrophy and/or wide QRS' (p. 54), 'ECG pattern of injury in patients with ventricular hypertrophy and/or wide QRS' (p. 120) and 'diagnosis of the infarction Q wave') in the presence of intraventricular conduction disturbances (p. 170). Hemiblocks are not included since the QRS complex is not widened and, consequently, repolarisation abnormalities are seen as in normal conditions, if present. However, recently it has been

reported that the association of SAH represents a marker of worst outcome (Biagini et al., 2005) (p. 255). **Some prognostic and clinical considerations of ACS with wide QRS and other confounding factors will now be addressed.**

Prognostic and clinical considerations

With regard to prognosis, it has been considered for a long time that the mere **presence of a wide QRS complex is a poor prognostic sign**. Therefore, contrary to what occurs in cases with narrow QRS complexes, in which a normal or near-normal ECG is a sign of good prognosis it was thought that in the presence of a wide QRS complex, especially in the presence of a LBBB or pacemaker, no good

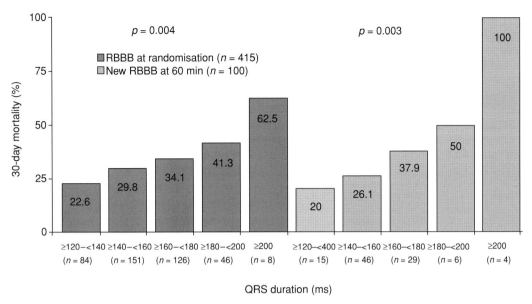

Figure 8.30 Increasing 30-day mortality with increasing QRS duration in patients with RBBB at randomisation and new accompanying anterior STE-AMI.

prognostic value is obtained by the absence of evident signs of ischaemia (Q wave or evident repolarisation changes).

In the pre-fibrinolytic era, RBBB appeared frequently during the course of anteroseptal infarction in case of very proximal occlusion of LAD because the right bundle is perfused by first septal branch (Figure 4.66) (see p. 223). The patient was at high risk for sudden death, usually not secondary to a bradyarrhythmia, but to VF. To prevent sudden death, 6 weeks was the minimum period of in-hospital time advised (Lie et al., 1975). **In the reperfusion era** the risk of mortality of patients with STE-ACS evolving to anterior MI that present RBBB is still very high. The ECG changes are very useful for risk stratification. In the HERO-2 trial (Wong et al., 2006a) the 30-day mortality was similar in patients with RBBB at randomisation or new RBBB at 60 minutes after streptokinase treatment had begun. However, an increasing QRS duration was associated in a multivariable analysis with increasing 30-day mortality in both RBBB groups (at randomisation and new RBBB at 60 min) (see Figure 8.30). Also for both groups of RBBB (presenting at randomisation and at 60 min) 30-day mortality was lower if ST-segment elevation had been resolved by ≥50% at 60 minutes. The group

of patients at lowest risk (14%) are the few number of patients (2%) that the RBBB resolved to normal intraventricular conduction after 60 minutes and do not present ST-segment elevation. On the contrary, the group of patients with higher mortality (≥50%) are the cases with widest QRS complex especially if the RBBB is a new appearance at 60 minutes after streptokinase began.

The presence of complete LBBB is itself considered indication for fibrinolytic therapy. Additionally, the rare cases of **LBBB**, which develop during the acute phase, usually were indicative of a two-vessel disease, large infarction and a worse prognosis. This is explained because left bundle has double perfusion (LAD + LCX). However, this concept has to be reconsidered after the paper of Wong et al. (2005). According to Wong et al., patients with ACS evolving to MI that present presumed new LBBB have heterogeneous outcome dependent on the type of ST-sement changes. The patients with ST-segment deviations of the type described by Sgarbossa et al. (1996a,b) (see 'ECG pattern of injury in patients with ventricular hypertrophy and/or wide QRS', p. 123) had a higher 30-day mortality rate than those without these ST-segment changes. In fact this latter subgroup of LBBB patients had a lower 30-day mortality rate

> **The ACSs with bundle branch block are considered to have a worse prognosis.**
>
> This is especially true
> (a) when the bundle branch block has developed during the ACS
> (b) when the duration of QRS is very wide
> (c) it ST-segment elevation resolution is delayed
> (d) if the ST deviations are very striking

than the patients with STE-ACS and narrow QRS. This surprising lower risk may be related to differences in clinical characteristics (age, comorbidities, etc.), smaller MI and/or ACS of the NSTE type. In our experience patients with confounding factors (BBB and/or LVH with strain) at arrival represent 20% of all cases of ACS and do not present worst prognosis (p. 242).

As it happens with **all types of arrhythmias the incidence in the acute MI phase, of RBBBs and LBBBs, has decreased very much since the introduction of reperfusion therapy**, because this treatment improves intraventricular conduction system perfusion. Furthermore, the prognosis is better, as in general the ventricular function is also more preserved (Roth et al., 1993).

Finally, the development of a **bifascicular block** (RBBB plus SAH, or RBBB plus inferoposterior hemiblock (IPH)) during the acute myocardial infarction usually is considered a poor prognosis, since this is indicative of a large infarction and the involvement of, at least, two territories (LAD and RCA or LCX). However, on the basis of HERO-2 trial, no data (Wong et al., 2006a) have been found showing that there was no difference in 30-day mortality.

In an ACS with bundle branch block, it is convenient to know whether the bundle block was already present or if it was caused by the ACS. In case of RBBB the presence of qR pattern in V1 makes probably that the pattern is new and caused by the MI (Wellens, Gorgels and Doevendans, 2003).

Arrhythmias and intraventricular blocks in ACS

Ventricular arrhythmias: risk of sudden death (Figures 8.31–8.33)

Acute ischaemia frequently triggers ventricular arrhythmias that may lead to sudden death. From an experimental point of view, ventricular arrhythmias have been shown to develop following ligature of a coronary artery in two phases. The first one occurs after a few seconds, probably induced by a re-entry mechanism, and the second one after a few hours, which is most likely explained by post-potentials (Janse, 1982).

From experimental and clinical points of view, severe ventricular arrhythmias, runs of ventricular tachycardia and, occasionally, ventricular fibrillation appear in relation to most severe degrees of ischaemia. This is especially true in case of long-lasting ischaemia and hearts with poor ventricular function (Bayés de Luna et al., 1985; Janse, 1982). Those cases with the most severe ischaemia, such as after the ligature of an epicardial coronary artery or, in the clinical setting, a coronary spasm with total occlusion of a large epicardial vessel (Prinzmetal angina), are accompanied by significant ST-segment elevation even with subepicardium injury pattern with morphology of a TAP (Figure 8.45). In the most extreme cases, T-wave or ST-segment alternance is observed (Figure 8.11). In general, severe ventricular arrhythmias, in the clinical setting, if present do not appear immediately, but do so after a few minutes.

The incidence of **PVCs** in the course of ACS is high. As it happens in cases of coronary spasm (Bayés de Luna et al., 1985; Figure 8.46B), they have been shown to be related to the magnitude of the ST-segment elevation and to the duration of the spasm. PVCs in the course of an ACS are considered hazardous when they are frequent, especially if they occur in runs of non-sustained VT, or if they are associated with poor ventricular function and significant ischaemia (Figure 8.31A). In turn, an R/T phenomenon that was described by Lown et al. (1967) as a marker of a very poor prognosis in the course of an ACS is not currently, in post-thrombolytic era, considered to have same significance (Chiladakis et al., 2000). However, a primary VF may develop in acute phase of

(A)

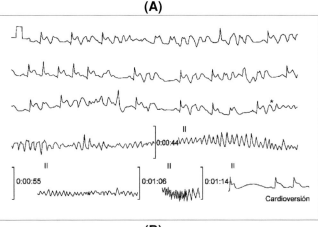

(B)

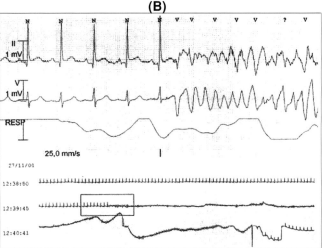

Figure 8.31 (A) A patient with an acute myocardial infarction with evident ST-segment elevation and frequent, polymorphic, repetitive, PVC that triggers VF (asterisk) that was resolved with cardioversion. (B) Primary ventricular fibrillation in a patient with acute MI. VF appears suddenly, without previous PVC and without evident ST-segment elevation. However, the underlying sinus rhythm is fast, which can often be present in cases of primary ventricular fibrillation and express the sympathetic overdrive that is usually present in acute phase of MI (see p. 252). The electric cardioversion resolved the problem.

MI without important ST-segment elevation but with basal rapid sinus rhythm and with isolated PVCs with R/T phenomenon (Figure 8.31B). Additionally, PVCs may detect ischaemia (ST-segment depression) more evidently than sinus complexes (Figures 8.25 and 8.26) (Rasouli and Ellestad, 2001).

An **accelerated ventricular rhythm**, which is defined as a ventricular rhythm with a rate higher than the escape ventricular rhythm rate and lower than the ventricular tachycardia rate (between 25–40 bpm and 90–110 bpm), usually occurs in runs that cease spontaneously and is well tolerated. It sometimes occurs during reperfusion (see p. 228; Figures 8.16 and 8.17) and generally does not require a specific treatment.

A **monomorphic sustained ventricular tachycardia** does not occur frequently in ACS, especially in patients without prior infarctions. However, it has been shown to have worse prognosis in 1-year follow-up period than that of patients with primary VF (Newby et al., 1998). It is partly related to prior infarction scar, which explains its lower incidence following a first myocardial infarction (Fiol, 2001; Mont et al., 1996). Rarely, it may appear during the course of a significant and sustained coronary spasm.

A **polymorphic ventricular tachycardia** usually exhibits characteristics that mimic the **torsades de pointes ventricular tachycardia with normal QT interval**. It frequently degenerates into VF. Fortunately, it is infrequent and usually appears in

(A)

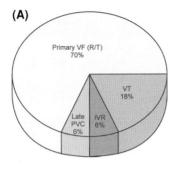

(B)

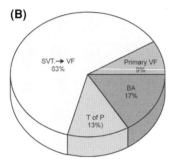

Figure 8.32 Final arrhythmias in case of sudden death in different clinical situations. (A) In the acute phase of an ischaemic heart disease (Adgey et al., 1982). In the majority of cases final arrhythmia was primary ventricular fibrillation and only in few cases it was sustained ventricular tachycardia, which developed in fibrillation. (B) In ambulatory patients the most frequent final arrhythmia was sustained VT leading to VF (Bayés de Luna, Coumel and Leclercq, 1989).

large infarctions with poor ventricular function. It is probably secondary to prolonged ischaemia (poor reperfusion), and thus urgent revascularisation is advised.

Pre-hospital mortality in acute myocardial infarction is approximately 20–30% (Braunwald, Zipes and Libby, 1998; Fiol, 2001). More than half of these deaths occur within the first hour and are generally caused by sudden death due to primary VF. This is generally triggered by a PVC with R/T phenomenon in the setting of autonomic nervous system (ANS) dysfunction (sinus tachycardia) (Figure 8.32A; Adgey et al., 1982). In the thrombolytic era, this phenomenon has already been mentioned to be less frequent (Chiladakis et al., 2000). Furthermore, in ambulatory patients, primary VF only explains 10% of all sudden death cases, with sustained ventricular tachycardia leading to VF be-

ing the most frequent cause of sudden death (Figures 8.32B and 8.33; Bayés de Luna, Camacho and Guindo, 1989; Bayés de Luna, Coumel and Leclercq, 1989).

Once the patient has been admitted to the hospital, the mortality rate is lower (5–10%) and is caused by cardiogenic shock because though VF may occur, it may be resolved with cardioversion. Fiol et al. (1993) have demonstrated that once the patient is in the hospital, VF occurs particularly in the presence of (a) summation of the ST-segment elevation in the three leads, with the most prominent ST-segment elevation higher than 10 mm; (b) systolic blood pressure lower than 110 mm Hg; (c) inferior and/or lateral infarction. According to other authors, a long QT interval and the presence of sustained ventricular tachycardia on admission are markers of poor prognosis (Flugelman et al., 1987). In a small number of cases of acute MI, sudden death is due to a bradyarrhythmia, often secondary to electromechanical dissociation (Figure 8.34).

The incidence of primary VF (Figures 8.30 and 8.31) in patients admitted to the coronary care unit has decreased significantly (2–3%) due to the new therapies employed, though it is still higher in more compromised patients (Killip 1: <1%; Killip 3 and 4: >4%) (Fiol, 2001). In patients with an ACS, only the VF that occurs in the course of an anterior infarction has subsequent negative prognostic implications (Schwartz et al., 1985). Evidently, VF requires treatment with electric cardioversion and all measures required to treat cardiorespiratory arrest (Fiol, 2001). The most important is to adopt the measures necessary to avoid it, since it occurs outside the coronary care unit; the possibilities of survival are very low.

Supraventricular arrhythmias

Sinus tachycardia in patients with ACS is a sign of poor prognosis. A clear increase in sinus heart rate (from a mean rate of 80 bpm to almost 100 bpm) was demonstrated by Adgey et al. (1982) prior to VF in patients developing primary VF while on their way to the hospital during the hyperacute phase of an acute myocardial infarction. Sinus tachycardia is a manifestation of ANS imbalance and is seen in large infarctions and, characteristically, in the presence of heart failure, risk of cardiogenic shock and risk of cardiac rupture. It can also be the expression of extracardiac complications, such as a pulmonary

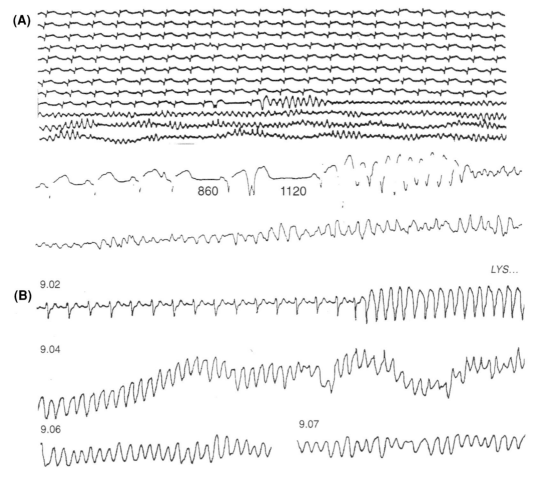

Figure 8.33 (A) Ambulatory recording of a patient with ST elevation due to acute coronary syndrome an R on T PVC triggering VF. (B) Ambulatory recording of a patient that presented VF triggered by sustained VT, which appears without previous PVC in presence of basal sinus tachycardia.

embolism, anaemia, fever, etc. In the absence of any evident contraindication, sinus tachycardia should be corrected with beta-blocker agents. Sinus tachycardia that persists over the follow-up (subacute phase) is a sign of subsequent poor prognosis (Crimm et al., 1984). In acute phase of MI, VF usually appears in presence of basal sinus tachycardia with or without ambient PVC (Figure 8.31). In post-MI patients, sustained VT triggers VF, usually also in presence of sinus tachycardia (Figure 8.33).

Premature atrial complexes are benign. However, when frequent, they can be premonitory of atrial flutter and, especially, of atrial fibrillation.

Atrial flutter rarely occurs. When the heart rate is rapid, i.e. above 150 bpm, it is usually poorly tolerated. It requires immediate medical assistance

and, in the presence of haemodynamic impairment, electrical cardioversion is mandatory.

Atrial fibrillation is a relatively frequent supraventricular arrhythmia (10–12% of cases) (Figure 4.16; Sugiura et al., 1985), as other supraventricular arrhythmias are typically related to atrial involvement (Liu, Greenspan and Piccirillo, 1961; Zimerman, 1968) and/or pericarditis. Atrial fibrillation occurs usually in the most extensive ACSs. However, in patients with ACS due to RCA occlusion, it may be explained by vagal overdrive and may be accompanied by AV block. Age, presence of abnormal P wave (Agarwal, 2003), chronic obstructive pulmonary disease (COPD) and heart failure are triggering factors. The incidence of atrial fibrillation has decreased in the post-thrombolytic era.

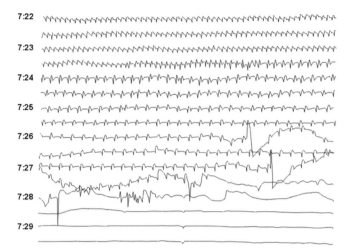

7:22
7:23
7:24
7:25
7:26
7:27
7:28
7:29

Figure 8.34 Patient of 68 years of age who suffered sudden death 10 days after an acute infarction. A progressive depression of the automatism (with the appearance of a slow escape rhythm) is shown in the Holter ECG recording, until cardiac arrest occurs, due to an electromechanical dissociation caused by cardiac rupture.

Atrial fibrillation usually is self-limited; thus, electric cardioversion is advised only when the heart rate is rapid and causes haemodynamic impairment. The P-wave late potentials technique may identify candidates for atrial fibrillation in ACS (Rosiak, Bolinska and Ruta, 2002).

Other supraventricular arrhythmias, such as **supraventricular paroxysmal tachycardia or atrial tachycardia secondary to an ectopic focus**, are much less frequent.

Bradyarrhythmias and intraventricular conduction abnormalities

Sinus bradyarrhythmia is frequent in patients with acute inferior MI, especially during the first hours, because the sinus node is perfused by RCA or LCX (see p. 18). It is found in 30% of cases (Pantridge, Webb and Adgey, 1981). It is most frequently secondary to depression of automatism than to sinoatrial block. Indications for the administration of atropine and pacemaker implantation have been defined by the ACC/AHA guidelines for the treatment of patients with an acute myocardial infarction (1999). **Advanced SA block** suggests a proximal occlusion of RCA or LCX and is often accompanied by an atrial infarction and corresponds usually to a large MI. Pacing is indicated in case of low cardiac output or bradycardia-related ventricular arrhythmias.

The **progressive depression of sinus node automatism** and the occurrence of a progressively slower escape rhythm that leads to cardiac arrest (Figure 8.34) are usually detected in patients with electromechanical dissociation (Bayés de Luna, Coumel and Leclercq, 1989).

The prevalence of different types of **AV blocks** has also decreased in the fibrinolytic era. A complete AV block is currently recorded in approximately 3–4% of all cases, while it previously occurred in nearly 10% (Harpaz et al., 1999). In patients with acute inferior MI, the incidence of AV block was significantly higher in the pre-fibrinolytic era (Melgarejo et al., 1997). **The first-degree AV block** has few clinical implications, but sometimes may evolve towards advanced AV block that is usually of infrahisian level if bundle branch block or anterior infarction is present. The **second-degree AV block of Wenckebach type** is more frequent in the inferior MI (RCA), since it is due to AV node ischaemia and/or a significant vagal overdrive. Atropine should be administered to accurately identify its origin. AV blocks due to vagal overdrive disappear following the administration of intravenous atropine, while those of ischaemic origin persist. Also, the latter usually presents fast heart rate, while the former does not. An AV block of Wenckebach type is usually transient and is of suprahisian level. The prognosis is usually good, with pacemaker implantation not being necessary, although administration of atropine is required. The **second-degree AV block of the Mobitz type** is less frequent and is more associated with anterior infarction than with inferior infarction. It occurs paroxysmally and may disappear or progress to advanced AV block. It is usually generated at the infrahisian level and implies a worse prognosis. Pacemaker implantation is frequently required, at

(A)

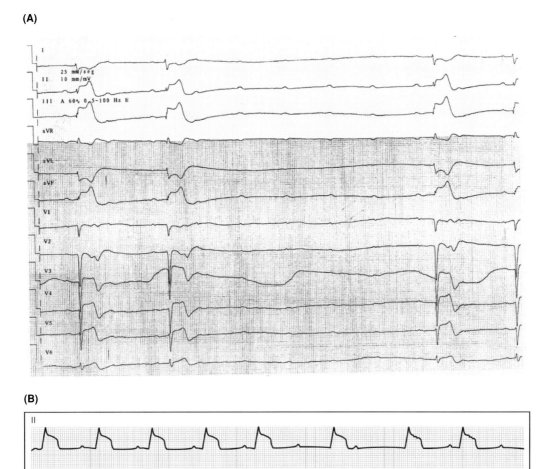

(B)

Figure 8.35 (A) Patient with STE-ACS due to proximal occlusion of dominant RCA (ST↓ in I, ST ↑ III > II, ST isodiphasic in V1 and ST ↑ in V6). The patient presented 2×1 AV block and suddenly advanced AV block. (B) Patient with STE-ACS due to RCA occlusion. Different degrees of AV block may be seen in continuous recording of lead II.

least temporarily. The **third-degree (complete) AV block** has a different significance according to the location of the MI, inferior or anteroseptal (Melgarejo et al., 1997). **When it occurs associated with inferior MI**, it usually evolves from a first-degree block, the QRS complex is narrow and the block is of suprahisian level. Thus, the prognosis is relatively good, though the mortality rate is higher than that in cases with no advanced AV block, especially if fibrinolytic therapy has not been administered (Mavric et al., 1990). When haemodynamic impairment develops (Figure 8.35A), a temporary pacemaker is mandatory. **The advanced AV block presenting in an anteroseptal infarction** is usually accompanied by an infrahisian escape rhythm with a wide QRS complex, and the insertion of a temporary pace-

maker is mandatory. In these cases, the infarction is large and the prognosis is poor. Sometimes in the same record there is evidence of different types of AV blocks (Figure 8.35B).

The presence of an **SAH associated with an ACS** was considered to not have many clinical implications. However, the development of an SAH in the course of an inferior infarction (RCA or LCX) represents the involvement of at least two vessels, since LAD perfuses the superoanterior division. Recently, Biagini et al. (2005) reported that the presence of previous SAH implies worst prognosis. Patients with suspected IHD and LAH referred for stress test presented an increased risk for cardiac death. This risk is persistent after adjustment for major clinical data and abnormalities

(A)

(B)

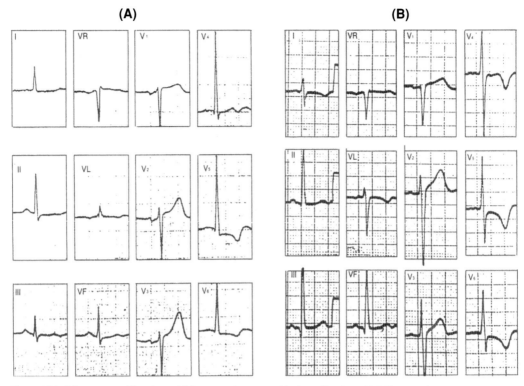

Figure 8.36   (A) A 55-year-old patient with hypertension and heart failure. (B) One month later, during an ACS, the patient presents a very evident change in the ECG – the ÂQRS changes rightwards, lead VF changes from Rs to qR, with time of intrinsicoid deflection of 0.06 seg and in lead V6 qR changed to Rs. These changes may be explained by the association of IPH. Also, there are more ST/T changes.

on the stress echocardiogram. Therefore, the presence of associated SAH should not be considered a benign abnormality in this group of patients. These results, which are in line with what we have already said about the development of SAH in patients with inferior MI, imply the involvement of at least two-vessel disease. The appearance of **IPH** during ACS is observed less frequently. In this case there is clear rightward change of ÂQRS (Figure 8.36).

The occurrence of an **RBBB or LBBB** has already been mentioned to have an evident prognostic sig-

nificance (see p. 248). We have already mentioned that RBBB at randomisation, but especially of new appearance, has worst prognosis especially when the QRS is very wide (Figure 8.30). Furthermore, the LBBB that appears during ACS has worst prognosis, although it has been described that this is also true for cases with ST-segment deviations described by Sgarbossa et al. (1996b) (see p. 120). Cases of RBBB with or without associated left SAH occur in presence of very proximal LAD occlusion (before S1 and D1). The acquired forms of bundle branch block, with very wide QRS complex and with slowed

Acquired RBBB presents QR or qR morphology in V1 (Figures 4.66), whereas pre-existing RBBB that is more frequent in elderly patients usually shows an rsR' morphology in V1.

Acquired LBBB occurs rarely (Figure 4.67)

because the left bundle has double perfusion, but when it occurs it represents by itself a worst prognosis, especially if significant ST-segment deviations are present.

ST-segment elevation resolution, present the worst prognostic implications, because they are associated to a large MI.

Risk stratification in ACS: role of ECG (Antman et al., 2000; Bertrand et al., 2003; Hathaway et al., 1998a,b; Morrow et al., 2000a,b)

During the **initial assessment of a patient with an ACS**, **risk stratification** is of critical importance in **deciding patients who will require urgent or invasive treatment** (fibrinolysis, PCI or surgical revascularisation), since risk is higher in this case.

In clinical practice we used for risk stratification clinical, electrocardiographic, enzymatic variables and also imaging techniques and coronary angiography. In each case the parameters may be used isolated or clustered in a score. The scores of risk may be formed only by clinical parameters or may be a mixture of clinical and other non-clinical parameters. The most useful data are the following:

(a) Clinical: Age, gender, heart rate, blood pressure, diabetes, history of previous infarction, time from the onset of symptoms, type of symptoms (dyspnoea, pain, etc.), physical examination, presence of rales, third cardiac sound, pulmonary and renal function, other comorbidities, etc.

(b) Electrocardiographic: Rhythm and heart rate, type and location of ST-segment deviations – elevation versus depression – ST-segment morphology; number of leads involved and summation of ST-segment deviations, most probable occlusion site according to the involved leads; QRS morphology; QRS score; presence of arrhythmias and conduction disturbances, location of area at risk, the Aldrich score, the Anderson–Wilkins score (see p. 221 and 224), etc. (Elsman et al., 2006; Johanson et al., 2003; Uyarel, 2006).

(c) Enzymatic: Repeated determination of enzymes, currently especially of troponin levels.

(d) Imaging techniques: Echocardiography, scintigraphy, MRI (EF, number and localisation of involved segments, type of perfusion or contractile impairment).

(e) Coronary angiography: Number of vessels involved and location of stenosis; type of plaque. Currently, it may be performed with non-invasive imaging techniques (coronary multidetector computer

tomography), although in the ACS, coronary angiogram is advisable because if necessary a PCI may be readily performed.

The importance of the ECG in ACS is highlighted in this book**, since it is of **critical importance for the classification** (ACS with or without ST-segment elevation) **and for therapeutic decision making** (thrombolysis, urgent PCI or bypass surgery).

Using risk scores

Risk scores use combination of different variables. They have a higher predictive value than does each variable alone, **so they stratify the risk in clinical practice in a reproducible and easily applied way. This stratification may be made on the patient's admission to the coronary care unit, or during the follow-up.** The use of risk scores, although important from the prognostic point of view, has to be considered carefully because it has been demonstrated that according to the different parameters used with similar enzymatic levels, the risk stratification may be very different (Jacobs et al., 1999; Singh et al., 2002). It is not the purpose of this book to make a critical review of the scores used in ACS, but especially to emphasise the importance that the ECG has as a marker of prognosis. So, we will mention only the most important with special emphasis in the most commonly used. For more information about the limitation of risk scores, consult Cannon (2003) and Singh et al. (2002).

Selected scores have been proposed for stratifying risk after MI. These scores have been derived either from clinical trials (TIMI, PURSUIT, GUSTO, etc.) or from registries and cohort studies (PREDICT, CCP, etc.). The majority of them divide the ACS into two groups with and without ST-segment elevation (STE-MI or STE-ACS vs NSTE-MI or NSTE-ACS). This classification is very useful for a better approach of treatment. The GUSTO score includes QRS duration and ECG (Hathaway et al., 1998a,b) prior MI (Table 8.4), and the PREDICT score uses other ECG parameters (ECG severity score) that include ST, Q wave and branch block criteria (Jacobs et al., 1999; Table 8.5).

In **STE-ACS the TIMI risk score is most commonly used** (Morrow et al., 2000a,b). This score is formed by seven variables that may be easily obtained, including history taking, ECG changes,

Table 8.5 PREDICT score components, definitions, and risk computation.

Patient Name: _____

Medical Record Number: _____ Date: _____

Clinical Descriptor	Minnesota Heart Survey Definition	Preliminary Assessment	Predict Points
Shock			
Normal	None of the conditions below		0
Moderate	Any one of the following:		2
	first observable SBP 61–99 or first blood pressure unobrainable or		
	first recorded heart rate 100–119 beats/min		
Severe	At least 2 of the above or		4
	first observable SBP <60 mmHg or first recorded beart rate ≥120 beart/min		
Clinical History			
a) myocardial infarction, b) stroke, c) angina >8 weeks before admission d) coronary artery bypass grafts, e) cardiac arrest, f) hypertension			
Normal	None of the above		0
Mild	1 or 2 of above		1
Moderate	3 or more of the above		2
Age			
	35–59 years old		0
	60–69 years old		1
	70–74 years old		3
ECG Severity Score	Preliminary Assessment – circle all that apply		
Q-wave Infarction	Major: Q duration ≥ 0.03 sec, Q/R amplitude ≥ 1/3: MN codes 1.1.1–1.1.7		
	Anterolateral (leads I, aVL, V6)	2	
	Anterior (leads VI-V5)	2	
	Minor: 0.02 sec ≤ Q duration <0.03 sec, Q/R amplitude ≥ 1/3: MN codes 1.2.1–1.2.7		
	Anterolateral (leades I, aVL, V6)	1	
	Anterior (leads V1-V5)	1	
Non Q-wave infarction	Major: ST segment depression ≥1.0 mm, horizontal or downward sloping:		
	MN codes 4.1.1-4.1.2		
	Anterolateral (leads I, aVL, V6)	2	
	Anterior (leads V1–V5)	2	
	Poterior/inferior (leads II, III, AVF)	2	
	Minor: 0.5 mm ≤ ST segment depression <1.0 mm, horizontal or downward sloping:		
	MN code 4.2		
	Anterolateral (leads I, aVL, V6)	1	
	Anterior (leads V1–V5)	1	
	Posterior/inferior (leads II, III, AVF)	1	
	Summarize Q/ST itmes for use in PREDICT point computation Q/ST Score		
	Add scores to got Q/ST score (enter 0–15) ——		
	Circle any bundle branch block (BBB) for use in PREDICT point Computation		
	Right BBB: MN code 7.2.1 RBBB		
	Left BBB: MN code 7.1.1 LBBB		
	Intraventricular: MN code 7.4 IVB		
	PREDICT point computation		
No BBBor infarction	Q/ST score = 0 and no BBB		0
Mild	(Q/ST score = 1.4 and no BBB) or (Q/ST score = 0 and RBBB)		1
Moderate	(Q/ST score ≥ 5 or LBBB		2
Severe	IVB or (RBBB and Major Q finding)		3

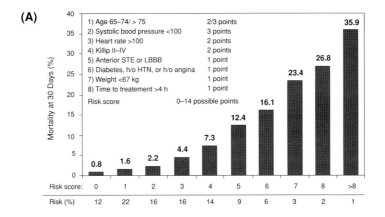

(A)

1) Age 65–74/ > 75   2/3 points
2) Systolic bood pressure <100   3 points
3) Heart rate >100   2 points
4) Killip II–IV   2 points
5) Anterior STE or LBBB   1 point
6) Diabetes, h/o HTN, or h/o angina   1 point
7) Weight <67 kg   1 point
8) Time to treatement >4 h   1 point

Risk score   0–14 possible points

Risk score:	0	1	2	3	4	5	6	7	8	>8
Mortality (%)	0.8	1.6	2.2	4.4	7.3	12.4	16.1	23.4	26.8	35.9
Risk (%)	12	22	16	16	14	9	6	3	2	1

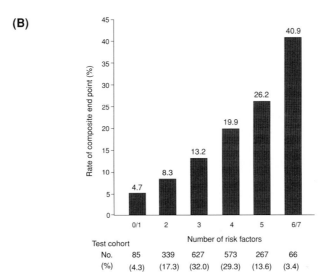

(B)

Number of risk factors	0/1	2	3	4	5	6/7
Rate of composite end point (%)	4.7	8.3	13.2	19.9	26.2	40.9
Test cohort No.	85	339	627	573	267	66
(%)	(4.3)	(17.3)	(32.0)	(29.3)	(13.6)	(3.4)

Figure 8.37 (A) TIMI risk score for STE-ACS for predicting 30-day mortality (Morrow et al., 2000a,b). (B) Rates of all-case mortality, myocardial infarction and severe recurrent ischaemia prompting urgent revascularisation through 14 days after randomisation were calculated for various patient subgroups based on the number of risk factors present in the test cohort (the unfractioned heparin group in the thrombolysis in MI (TIMI) 118 trial; $n = 1957$). Event rates increased significantly as the TIMI risk score increased ($p < 0.001$ by x^2 for trend) (Antman et al., 2000).

ST-segment elevation, etc. (see Figure 8.37). The results of this score significantly correlate with prognosis. For example, patients presenting with lower scores (0/1 points) have 14-day combined event rate of 4.7% (death/ischaemic events). In those with a higher score (6/7 points) there is an almost nine-fold increase in event rate (41%). The advantage of this score is that it has already been widely validated and may be rapidly assessed (Antman et al., 2000; Holper et al., 2001; Morrow et al., 2000a,b). The score reported by Hathaway et al. (1998a,b), on the basis of GUSTO trial, for estimating 30-day mortality from initial, clinical and ECG variables reported that summation of ST-segment elevation and depression, greater than 15 mm, represents higher risk mortality (Table 8.4).

Also in **NSTE-ACS** the TIMI risk score is the most used score (Antman et al., 2000) because it is easy to assess and combines the same variables used for cases with ST-segment elevation. Its use provides prognostic information at the short and long term (14 days and 6 months) of patients with NSTE-ACS

(UA and non-Q-wave MI). In addition to its prognostic information, the patients with higher scores will have a higher risk of events over time and, thus, will benefit the most from antithrombotic treatment (low-weight heparins, IIb/IIIa GP inhibitors and clopidogrel) and early revascularisation (PCI or surgery).

One community-based MI cohort (Singh et al., 2002) the PREDICT cohort was superior to that of the TIMI scores across time, largely because PREDICT include morbidity lacking from the TIMI score.

Also, the inclusion of EF and different biomarkers added significant prognostic information over TIMI and PREDICT scores. Recently, other markers, such as CRP, and different interleukins have been added to the risk assessment (Anguera et al., 2002; Zairis et al., 2002), as well as BNP (Bassan et al., 2005) and PAPP (Heeschen et al., 2004). Even the value of multiple biomarkers added to the value of quantitative ST-segment depression has been recently published (Westerhout et al., 2006).

However, it is convenient to use a simple score that may be widely accepted for everybody and give enough information for good stratification. In this sense, a **risk index based only on clinical parameters** (age, blood pressure and heart rate)[‡] (Morrow et al., 2000a,b) **was established first in patients with STE-ACS** and is predictive of mortality. Recently, Wiviott et al. (2006) have demonstrated that this single risk index (TRI) provides important information about in-hospital mortality **in both STE-ACS and NSTE-ACS**, with some differences between three groups (STE-ACS with reperfusion, STE-ACS without reperfusion and NSTE-ACS (Figure 8.38)). This risk index provides clinicians important information for risk stratification and confirms that with simple clinical and ECG parameters derived from bedside diagnosis are possible to obtain important information for initial triage and treatment.

According to what has just been discussed, patients with ACS may be classified into different risk groups.

[‡] Risk index $= \dfrac{\text{Heart rate} \times (\text{age}/10)^2}{\text{Systolic blood pressure}}$ (see Figure 8.38)

Risk groups: the role of the ECG

ACS with or without ST-segment elevation may be classified, according to its **clinical, electrocardiographic and enzymatic characteristics**, into three large risk groups: high, intermediate and low (Antman et al., 2000; Bertrand et al., 2003; Braunwald et al., 2000; Diderholm et al., 2002; Jernberg, 2002; Lee et al., 1995; Morrow et al., 2000a,b; Ryan et al., 1999).

In this book we will emphasise the most important electrocardiographic, clinical and enzymatic abnormalities that define a more favourable or less favourable prognosis. Naturally, **risk scores have their main role in the overall risk assessment.**

High-risk ACS

This term is applied to ACS evolving towards a large (Q-wave or non-Q-wave) myocardial infarction. Currently, the 30-day mortality rate is greater than 20–30%.

The following characteristics are considered as of high risk:

A. Clinical

Advanced age, heart rate, systolic blood pressure, diabetes mellitus, recurrent or persistent pain. **The prognosis is worse** in diabetics and elderly patients, especially in presence of renal failure, sinus tachycardia and evident haemodynamic impairment (hypotension, pulmonary oedema, etc.) (grade 3–4 of Killip classification) (Wiviott et al., 2006).

B. ECG changes

The markers of poor prognosis are the following:

(1) **Repolarisation changes (ST/T)**

(a) **STE-ACS: dynamic and persistent ST-segment changes (ST-segment elevation $\geq$2 mm in several precordial leads or $\geq$1 mm in the inferior leads)**

–The higher the **number of leads with ST-segment elevation** and the **greater their importance, the higher the risk of a large infarction will be, and therefore the higher the risk of ventricular arrhythmias and haemodynamic complications.**

–In patients who present within 3 hours of symptoms onset, **terminal QRS distortion** in two or more adjacent

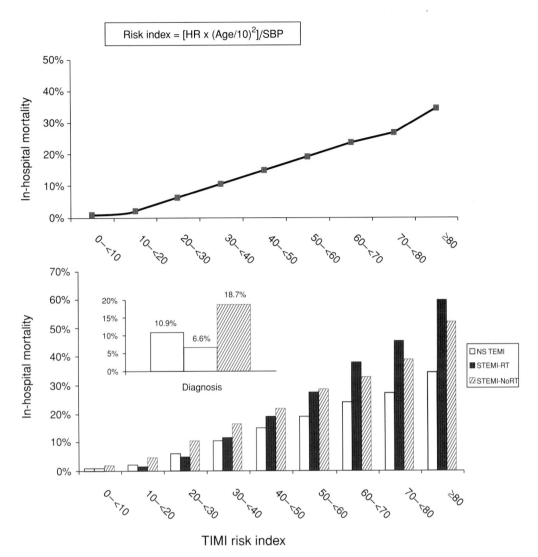

Figure 8.38 (A) Relationship between Thrombolysis in Myocardial Infarction (TIMI) risk index and mortality in non-ST-segment myocardial infarction (NSTE-ACS). (B) Relationship between TIMI risk index and mortality in three groups of ACS (STEMI, NSTEMI and STEMI without reperfusion therapy). Inset graph shows mortality in full group by diagnosis. HR, heart rate; RT, reperfusion therapy; SBP, systolic blood pressure (Wiviott et al., 2006).

leads (no S wave in leads with rS pattern) (V1–V3) and/or J/R ratio $\geq$0.50 in any lead represents higher mortality and infarct size, less myocardial salvage by fibrinolytic treatment and more benefit from PCI than from thrombolysis (Sejersten, 2004).

–Recurrent ST-segment elevation, especially with pain, detected with continuous multilead ST-segment monitoring (Akkerhuis et al., 2001).
–According to the ST-segment elevation in the precordial or inferior leads and the presence of mirror patterns, the ECG allows for location of the coronary

artery occlusion. It helps to identify cases requiring an urgent coronary angiogram (proximal RCA, very dominant RC and LCX and proximal LAD).

–Persistence of ST-segment elevation over days, without negativisation of the T wave. **This sign suggests the risk of cardiac rupture**.

–According to the **initial morphology** of the **ST-segment elevation, the prognosis may be better or worse** (**Figure 8.13**).

–The most dangerous situation for the development of **VF** is the existence of **ST-segment alternance during ischaemia**.

(b) NSTE-ACS: evident ST-segment depression in many leads (≥ 7) especially if the ST-segment depression is very important with ST-segment elevation in VR and V1 and without positive T wave in V4–V5. In one study Westerhout et al. (2006) developed for knowing 30-day and 1-year risk for NSTE-MI, ST-segment depression was the strongest contributor predicting mortality, even more than troponin and the others biomarkers. Patients with ≥ 2 mm ST-segment depression were 2.4 times more likely to die in the first year compared with those without ST-segment depression ($p < 0.001$).

–**Any case presenting with dynamic ST-segment deviations**

In all these situations, the therapeutic approach (emergent coronary angiogram, if possible) should be decided upon with the clinical history and the ECG.

(2) Bundle branch block

–Especially when it is **of new onset**. As has been already stated (p. 223), the development of **complete RBBB** is characteristic of a LAD occlusion, proximal to the first septal branch (Figure 4.66). The prognosis is even worse in case of a bifascicular block. The prognosis is worst in cases of RBBB with wide QRS especially if the BB is of new appearance.

The presence of **LBBB** is in itself a marker of poor prognosis. When it develops during an ACS, which occurs rarely, it implies the involvement of both the RCA and the LAD, since it is usually perfused by both, or it may indicate that one of them is very dominant and perfuses part of the opposed wall. The prognosis is especially worst when the LBBB presents ST-segment changes described by Sgarbossa et al. (1996b) (p. 120). However this concept has to be reconsidered after the Wong's paper (2005) (p. 249).

(3) Presence of certain arrhythmias

–The presence of **persistent sinus tachycardia** is, in itself, a sign of poor prognosis (Adgey et al., 1982).

–The presence of **PVCs**, especially of the R on T type, may represent a real risk of **sudden death due to VF** during the acute phase of ischaemia. In post-infarction patient, when PVCs are found in a surface ECG of 1- or 2-minute duration, this generally implies that PVCs will be frequent in the Holter recording, which has prognostic implications (Bigger et al., 1984).

(4) The presence of ECG normal, nearly normal or unchanged or the presence in the ECG of changes that suggest small infarct (mild ST-segment elevation or depression) **is not an absolute guarantee of good prognosis**.

The following complications may appear:

(a) STE-ACS evolving to Q-wave MI with small ST-segment elevation due to occlusion of LCX may present **cardiac rupture** in spite of ECG signs of apparently small MI (Figure 8.28).

(b) The presence of normal ST during pain may be an expression of a pseudonormalisation (Figure 3.21B). Therefore it is advisable to record another ECG after pain (Figure 3.21A).

(c) The presence of normal ECG in the absence of pain may be accompanied by important changes during pain. This occurs even in case of LMT subocclusion (Figure 8.19).

(d) The evidence of **taller-than-usual T wave in V1–V3**. This morphology may

From the practical point of view, patients presenting with the following characteristics may be considered of high risk:

a. Repetitive anginal pain with persistentb ST-segment elevation or depression in several leads, along with clearly positive troponin levels.

b. In general, those with a high-risk score both in STE-ACS (Antman et al., 2000, 2004; Fiol et al., 1993; Hathaway et al., 1998a,b) and in NSTE-ACS (TIMI risk score 2000), especially when there is an ECG indicating a poor prognosis

(which have been already discussed), and/or dynamic ECG changes.

c. In the STE-ACS, fibrinolysis may be used as the first-choice therapy in the first 3 hours after the onset of symptoms. However, primary PCI is advised, whenever possible. Both treatments may be carried out, if necessary, on the same patient.

d. In all types of high-risk ACS, interventional procedures must be indicated and have to be performed if possible as an emergency.

evolve over a short time towards an ST-segment elevation, which evolves to infarction Q wave (Figure 8.9). Said evolution may be aborted if fibrinolytic therapy or PCI is performed immediately.

(e) **In patients with prior infarction and/or poor ventricular function, the risk may be high**, in spite of presenting minimal changes in the ECG, such as slight ST-segment deviations compared to prior ECGs or a taller-than-normal T wave, especially if chest pain is persistent.

(5) **The prognosis is worse** when **not only** leads many but **also Q waves present ST-segment** deviations. This generally implies that the infarct is already established when Q waves appear in the leads with ST-segment elevation. It may also mean that the patient has suffered a prior infarction (Hathaway et al., 1998a,b).

C. Enzymatic changes
Troponin I and/or T levels clearly increased.

D. Global risk score
High-risk score in cases of both ACS with or without ST-segment elevation, according to the TIMI risk score (6–7 points) (Antman et al., 2004; Morrow et al., 2000a,b) and in **thrombolysis MI risk index (TRI >70–80)** (Wiviott et al., 2006) **is predictive of high risk of mortality at 30 days and composite end point** (Figures 8.37 and 8.38). Also, recently, the importance of ST-segment depression compared with biomarkers in risk stratification in NSTEMI (Westerhout et al., 2006) and the importance to add information on co-

morbidity (Singh et al., 2002) and EF have been demonstrated.

Low-risk ACS
These are patients with an ACS evolving towards a low-risk UA or small infarction (Q-wave or non-Q-wave). Currently, the 30-day mortality rate is less than 3%.

The following characteristics are considered of low risk:

(A) Clinical

Non-persistent or recurrent anginal pain, especially in patients of less than 70 years of age. The atypical pain (referred to as 'prickly' and/or modified by movements or thoracic compression) is usually seen in low-risk patients.

(B) ECG changes

1. In case of STE-AMI, the following findings are signs of good prognosis: (a) the presence of small ST-segment elevation in a few leads; (b) an early inversion of terminal portion of the T wave is probably a better prognostic marker of reperfusion than ST resolution (Corbalan et al., 1999).

2. In case of NSE-ACS the presence of **negative T wave**, especially if it is not deep and is seen in few leads usually with a dominant R wave, is of better prognosis than ST-segment depression. Remember that, as we have previously pointed out, the presence of deep and negative T wave in V1–V4–V5 is considered an atypical pattern of STE-ACS (Figure 8.3).

(A)

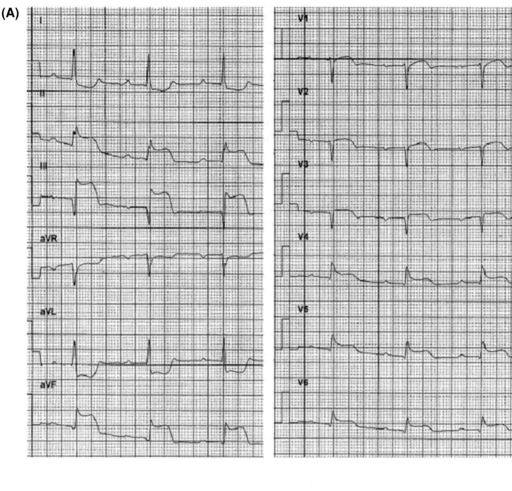

(B)

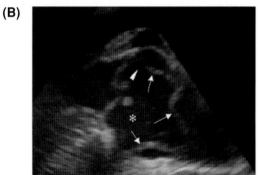 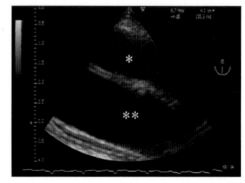

△ Intimal tear
→ Intimal flap
* True lumen
** False lumen

Figure 8.39 (A) A 61-year-old man with ST-segment elevation in all precordial leads II, III and VF (III > II) and ST-segment depression in I and VL with small rS in V1–V3 with sudden change to R in V4–V6. (B) The figure shows that the ECG changes are explained by very proximal occlusion of a very dominant RCA produced by a dissecting aneurysm type A affecting the RCA (see Table 4.2, p. 80 for differential diagnosis with ST-segment elevation in precordial and inferior leads due to distal LAD occlusion).

Low-risk patients are characterised by the following:
• Anginal pain is not intense and/or repetitive, and the ECG is normal with no changes in the follow-up or with flattened or mildly negative T wave in leads with dominant R wave. Sometimes, small Q waves of necrosis or mildly ST-segment depression may be seen.
• The TIMI global risk score is low.
• Optimal therapy should be individually assessed.
• A coronary angiogram may be advisable, especially in young patients.

3. **The 'q' wave (qr), if present, is limited to one or two leads**, generally in the inferior wall or in V1–V2.

4. **The ECG is often normal with a narrow QRS complex that does not change over time**. This occurs mainly in distal occlusions of a non-dominant LCX or RCA and in the enzymatic infarction (*necrosette*). **Sometimes an apparently normal or mildly abnormal ECG (positive and symmetrical T wave in V1–V2) may be seen in patients at high risk**. To take sequential recordings is mandatory to check the presence of ST-segment deviations.

(C) Enzymatic changes

Normal or slightly raised markers. The troponin level allows for the differentiation between unstable angina and a non-Q-wave infarction. In this group of low-risk patients, cases with negative or slightly raised troponin levels are included.

(D) Global risk score

A low-risk score in both ACS with and without ST-segment elevation, according to the **TIMI risk score (0–1 points) and the TRI index (<20)** (Figures 8.37 and 8.38) is predictive of **in-hospital mortality lower than 3%**. All other parameters (clinical, ECG and enzymatic) may help to stratify subgroup of even a lower risk.

Intermediate risk

Between these two options, many intermediate situations may be found. **A typical case** could be an ACS with anginal pain, even intense but not repetitive. The ECG shows mild ST-segment elevation that evolves to not very large Q-wave. The enzyme-level rise is moderate.

On other occasions, there is ST-segment depression not so striking and limited to a few leads with a dominant R wave, with enzymes moderately

elevated (non-Q-wave infarction). In these cases, conservative or interventional therapy will be indicated at individual level according to all the clinical and electrocardiographic characteristics of ACS.

We consider that ACS with deep negative T wave in V1–V4, as mentioned before (p. 212), is an atypical pattern of STE-ACS that usually does not imply an emergency because this ECG represents that probably the artery is at least partially open. The urgency depends on the clinical picture (repetitive pain) and on ECG dynamic changes. However, in all these cases, a coronary angiography has to be performed as soon as possible. Obviously, this ECG pattern when seen after reperfusion treatment represents a good marker of open artery (p. 230).

The aforementioned risk scores present intermediate values (TIMI risk score of 3/4 and TRI index between 30 and 50) (Figures 8.37 and 8.38).

ACS not due to coronary atherothrombosis: clinical and electrocardiographic characteristics

Patients with an ACS (new anginal pain and/or anginal pain of longer duration) that are not due to coronary atherothrombosis (which is generally related to a vulnerable plaque rupture or erosion) are included in this group (Figure 6.1 and Table 6.1;). In principle, clinical and electrocardiographic changes are usually similar or equal to the classical ACS secondary to coronary atherothrombosis, but some different nuances are seen in some of these, which should be highlighted. Frequently, 5% of all ACS and 20% in younger than 35 years, these cases present normal coronary arteriogram.

Hypercoagulation states

Hypercoagulation state may exist in many of the cases with ACSs that evolve to an infarction, in the presence of normal coronary arteries. This is explained by a coronary thrombosis, with no significant coronary atherosclerosis. The mechanisms that could cause a hypercoagulation state are (1) heavy smokers that may have lower endogenous fibrinolytic activity which predisposes to acute thrombosis usually in the presence of plaque rupture (Newby et al., 1999); (2) drug-induced states (contraceptive drugs, etc.); (3) pregnancy; (4) hereditary thrombophilia (genetic defects). Hypercoagulation state, as seen in smokers, often coincides with the presence of small atheromatous plaques.

In all these situations, ACS may occur, generally with ST-segment elevation, frequently followed by a Q-wave infarction that may be large. ECG characteristics are not helpful in differentiating these cases. The LAD artery is the most frequently involved one (Pinney and Rabbani, 2001).

These cases usually occur in relatively young people, often smokers, and the prognosis after the acute phase is usually good if the triggering factors that produced the hypercoagulation state are suppressed. We have followed a smoker for more than 40 years who presented a large anterior Q-wave infarction at the age of 39.

Angina secondary to a tachyarrhythmia

Frequently, especially in the elderly, **a paroxysmal arrhythmia crisis, especially atrial fibrillation, may cause chest pain**, which may have **anginal characteristics** and may be of long duration, in relation with the duration of the arrhythmia. In this case the possibility to be confused with ACS is high. Often, no concurrent coronary atherosclerosis is present, and basically, the impairment of diastolic properties due to the tachycardia may explain the clinical picture. In spite of the presence of severe symptoms, the lack of enzyme-level changes, in the presence of a long-duration thoracic pain and tachyarrhythmia, leads one to suspect that this is not a classical ACS, but rather pain of anginal characteristics and usually not due to ischaemia but to haemodynamic origin.

When an **ECG** is recorded during the crisis, **certain abnormalities, such as ST-segment depression or a negative T wave**, may be found and are usually reversible (Fig. 3.36). In spite of that and long duration of pain, the repeated enzyme levels are normal. The **ST-segment elevation evolving to Q-wave MI is never found**.

We would like to stress that this situation occurs frequently, especially in the elderly, and often the patient may not realise that he or she has had a crisis of tachyarrhythmia because the patient presents chest discomfort that may be considered as angina but does not have the feeling of palpitations.

Coronary dissection (Figures 8.39–8.41)

This is an ACS that occurs suddenly, usually in young multiparous women, during the postpartum period, and is due to a collagen abnormality that favours dissection. The LAD is the most frequently involved artery and it may be dissected from its origin, which commonly causes a quite large infarction. It is even more severe because it occurs in an area with no previous ischaemia and in which collateral circulation has not been developed.

In these cases, there is a **significant ST-segment elevation**, generally of the type found in LAD occlusion, proximal to S1 and D1, with mirror pattern in II, III and VF, or in the proximal RCA (Figure 8.39) or LCX occlusion. **If the coronary dissection affects LMT, ST-segment elevation ACS usually appears because there is no previous subendocardial ischaemia or collateral circulation.** Therefore, it is important to emphasise that although usually the ECG of LMT presents huge and diffuse ST-segment depression (Figure 4.59), in special circumstances even in ACS due to atherothrombosis, ST-segment elevation ACS may occur (see p. 98 and Figure 4.44).

These patients may present cardiogenic shock and may even need heart transplantation if VF has not triggered sudden death. In case of LMT involvement, there are usually no signs of occlusion proximal to S1 (ST↑ in VR, V1 and ST↓ in V6) because of the involvement of LCX that counterbalances the septal ischaemia (Figure 8.40). Often, in case of LAD involvement, advanced RBBB appears (Figure 8.41). Additionally, a significant sinus tachycardia is seen. However, when the case is controlled, evolution may be good (Roig, 2003).

(A)

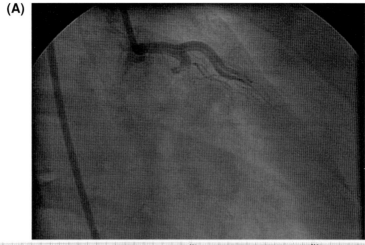

(B)

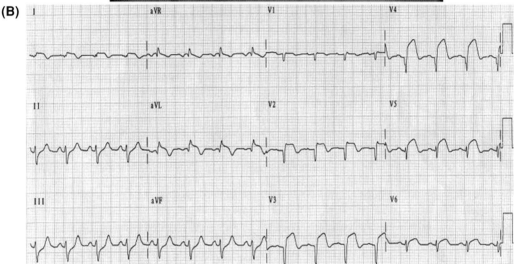

Figure 8.40 (A) Coronary angiography of a patient with dissection of the left main trunk. (B) The ECG shows an STE-ACS with ST-segment elevation from V2 to V6, I and VL, and ST-segment depression in inferior leads. The ECG does not show signs of occlusion of LAD proximal to S1 (ST↑ in V1 and ST↓ in V6) due to the involvement of LCX that counterbalances the septal ischaemia.

Transient left-ventricular apical ballooning (Tako–Tsubo syndrome)

(Figure 8.42)

Within the clinical setting of a potentially ACS, the existence of a significant and transient apical dyskinesia (transient apical ballooning) has been demonstrated by imaging techniques (Kurisu et al., 2002). **This anomaly that remember a pot used in Japan for fishing octopus (Tako-Tsubo), is accompanied by characteristic electrocardiographic changes.** The most interesting issue is that the pattern of apical dyskinesia is transient and that coronary arteries are normal or scarcely affected. Probably, it is ACS that may be explained by increase in coronary arteries tone and/or catecholamine storm release rather than an authentic spasm, without much involvement of the vessel but, probably, with lysis of a thrombus. It is known that catecholamines can induce, especially in women, an obstruction of left-ventricle outflow tract that may be related to powerful emotional stress, resulting in severe apical ischaemia. It has also been

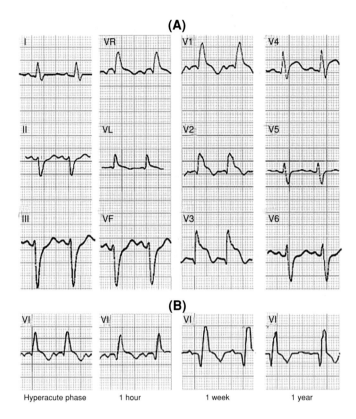

(A)

(B)

Hyperacute phase   1 hour   1 week   1 year

Figure 8.41 (A) ECG of a 35-year-old multiparous woman with a very serious ACS due to occlusion of LAD proximal to D1 and S1. Observe the morphology of the advanced RBBB + SAH together with evident ST-segment changes (ST elevation in precordials – occlusion in LAD), with ST-segment depression in II, III and VF (occlusion proximal to D1), and ST-segment elevation in VR and V1 with ST-segment depression in V6 (occlusion proximal to S1). (B) The ECG patterns of the evolution through time (V1).

considered as a type of catecholamine-induced cardiotoxicity with myocardial stunning in the apical part of left ventricle (Previtali, Repetto and Scuteri, 2005). Tako–Tsubo syndrome has been described more frequently in cases with long and sinuous coronary arteries (Ibañez et al., 2004). It has recently been hypothesised that this syndrome may be **a form of spontaneous aborted myocardial infarction due to autolysis of thrombus** (Ibañez et al., 2006). This syndrome, first described in Japan with the name of **Tako–Tsubo syndrome** (Kurisu et al., 2002), is rarely seen in the West (Peraira et al., 2002).

From the electrocardiographic standpoint a **pattern of STE-ACS** is usually evident, which evolves towards a deep negative T wave with the morphological characteristics of opened artery, which we have described previously (**reperfusion pattern**) (see p. 38). This pattern is accompanied by a transient 'Q' wave (QS morphology) (Figure 8.42). These changes especially seen in precordial leads occur concomitantly with a **transient lengthening** of the QTc interval. All the ECG changes usually normalise in a week.

Similar ECG patterns with transient ST-segment elevation and q wave may be seen in **myocarditis** (Figure 5.47). However, the QTc interval in myocarditis is usually normal, the voltage of QRS is also usually very low and there is usually sinus tachycardia. Furthermore, in myocarditis the angiographic features are not present. Also, recently, some cases of acute ST-segment elevation have been described in patients with catecholamine discharge and stroke, sometimes with chest pain. In these cases, a transient dyskinesia of basal part of the heart has been found (p. 274).

Congenital defects

The presence of congenital defects in the coronary arteries is infrequent (≈1% of the cases), but only a small proportion of them are accompanied by symptoms, generally angina or dyspnoea. The diagnosis of these anomalies has been facilitated by the frequent performance of multislice

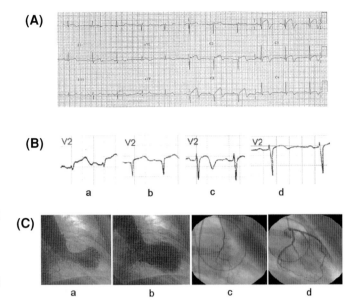

Figure 8.42 (A) Twelve-lead ECG in subacute phase in a patient with typical transitory apical ballooning (Tako–Tsubo syndrome). (B) Electrocardiographic changes in V2 during the period of 3–4 days (a–d). (C) The typical angiographic image (a,b) and normal coronary tree (c,d).

scanner. Coronary anomalies should be suspected when a very young person suffers from exertional anginal pain. The congenital defects causing more problems are the anomalous take-off of the left coronary artery, from the pulmonary artery (Figure 8.43), or the presence of atresia or severe congenital stenosis of any coronary artery (Angelini, Velasco and Flamm, 2002). These defects may explain cases of sudden death in children and young patients.

Cases of **Q-wave and non-Q-wave infarctions** due to atherothrombosis have also been described in patients with coronary artery anomalies. However, often the **resting ECG is normal, but repolarisation abnormalities, generally ST-segment depression, may be seen during exercise, with anginal pain** (Figure 8.44).

Cardiac surgery

Major cardiac surgery (CABG and valvular surgery) still poses a significant early morbidity and mortality. These have shown to be higher in patients with post-operative cardiogenic shock. This is related with a poor myocardial protection, myocardial stunning or development of ACS with Q-wave or non-Q-wave infarction. The ST/T changes are usually also present, but they are hard to assess due to the global patient's condition.

The **Q-wave infarction** is diagnosed by the development of a new Q wave plus enzyme-level increase (CPK or troponin-level rise). Because of the setting in which the Q-wave infarction occurs, repolarisation changes that precede it are sometimes difficult to assess, but sometimes a clear ACS with ST-segment elevation may be diagnosed.

Cumulative evidence has shown that the myocardial damage expressed by an enzyme-level increase, with no Q wave (non-Q-wave infarction) in the post-operative setting indicates poor prognosis. However, in the absence of reliable symptoms and of new Q wave, the diagnosis has to be based on the rise of the enzymes. The troponin I levels at 14 hours above 15 ng/mL in patients submitted to CABG and above 40 ng/mL in patients with valvular surgery[§] permit one to assure that, even in the absence of a new Q wave, this is explained by non-Q-wave infarction (Alyanakian et al., 1998, Gensini et al., 1998; Sadony et al., 1998).

Furthermore, the enzyme-level increase (CPK M3 > 61 μg/g) during the first post-operative day

---

[§] This figure is higher in these patients because there is a direct injury caused by cardiotomy. These figures are the result of the summing up of two standard deviations to the mean troponin level of patients with no complications (Alyanakian et al., 1998).

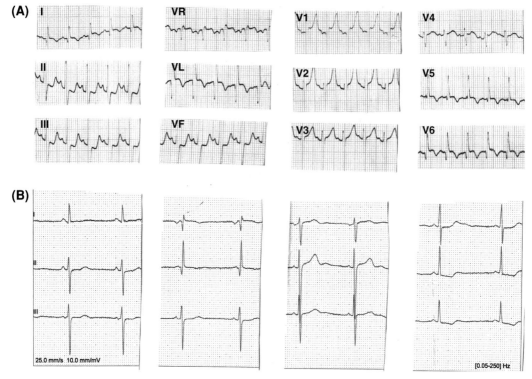

Figure 8.43 (A) A 3-year-old girl with abnormal origin of left coronary artery from pulmonary artery. ECG recording previous to a surgical intervention shows very abnormal Q wave especially in VL and V6. Ligature of left coronary artery was performed. (B) The same patient at 12 years of age. The abnormal q wave has practically disappeared. Currently, all the coronary perfusion depends on the huge RCA.

has recently been shown by Steuer et al. (2002) to be related with a high risk of early and late death. Ponce et al. (2001) have reported that 16% of patients who underwent valvular surgery suffered a perioperative infarction (6% Q-wave infarctions and 10% non-Q-wave infarctions), with the mortality rate being quite low in the group with no infarction (1%) and quite high in the group with infarction (>30%), regardless of the presence of a Q wave. It could be said that both Q-wave and non-Q-wave infarctions imply a poor prognosis compared with the prognosis of patients with no infarction, in whom the mortality rate is quite low.

Percutaneous coronary intervention

The sudden occlusion of a coronary artery during PCI prolongs QTc in 100% of cases according to Kenigsberg (2007). This change is usually accompanied by rectified ST segment and symmetric T wave that is often taller than normal. However, changes of T wave polarity (from negative to positive) and ST-segment deviations are very infrequent due to short time of ischaemia. The presence of ST-segment deviations represents a marker of worst prognosis (Bjorklund et al., 2005; Quyyumi et al., 1986) (see 2.3.1.1.2.4).

The cases with transient changes in the T wave and/or in the ST segment (sometimes changes from negative T wave to positive T wave, or even to ST elevation) during a PCI, usually occur when not much collateral circulation exists. When the presence of clear signs of localised wall motion abnormalities is noted during PCI, the ST-segment elevation in the ECG has been shown to be correlated with the extension of the asynergy (Cohen, Scharpf and Rentrop, 1987; Santoro et al., 1998). Occasionally, periprocedural infarctions occur, which are generally small but represent a marker of worst prognosis. A post-PCI infarction is considered to have occurred when at least a threefold increase in enzyme levels above

(A)

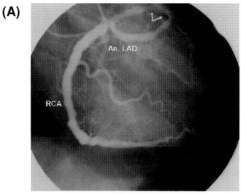

(B)

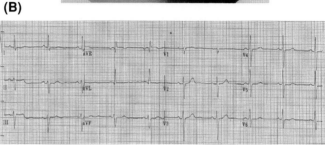

Figure 8.44 (A) Anomalous origin of LAD from a very big RCA. The LAD makes a loop and presents a long stenosis responsible for exercise anginal pain. (B) The basal ECG was practically normal but during exercise test the patient presents ST-segment depression and angina.

their maximum normal value is seen. Electrocardiographic changes, especially in the ST segment even sometimes with the development of an infarction Q wave, may be found.

During the PCI, especially during the balloon inflation, different types of ventricular arrhythmias may be observed, generally being self-limited and benign (isolated PVCs or short runs of non-sustained VT) (Meinertz et al., 1988).

The implantation of bioactive stents and the administration of new drugs, such as the IIb/IIIa inhibitors, have greatly decreased the incidence of post-PCI thrombosis and PCI-related infarct rate.

In STE-ACS, PCI is accompanied by the disappearance of the ST-segment elevation, sometimes in a short period of time, when the artery is completely opened. Especially in case of LAD proximal occlusion, the ECG sign of opened artery after PCI is usually a very deep and negative T wave (reperfusion pattern). In case of intrastent thrombosis the ECG may present changes from negative T wave to pseudonormalised T wave or even ST-segment elevation ACS (Figure 8.9). The persistence of the ST-segment elevation 30 minutes following a primary PCI is a specific marker of an incomplete reperfusion (Watanabe et al., 2001).

In the coronary spasm, which is a clinical situation similar to coronary artery occlusion during PCI but generally of longer duration, electrocardiographic changes are usually more striking (Bayés de Luna et al., 1985) (see below).

Coronary spasm: Prinzmetal variant angina (Figures 8.45 and 8.46)

This type of angina, due to coronary spasm, classically occurs at the same time daily, generally at night and at rest. It more frequently occurs in patients with evident coronary atherosclerosis, which 'triggers' the spasm but rarely there is any coronary anomaly or only small plaque is detected.

The coronary spasm may be present in any of the three epicardial arteries and the duration ranges from seconds to a few minutes (Figure 8.10). During the crisis sometimes a transient Q wave appears. Figure 8.45 shows a case of very striking coronary spasm of proximal LAD that is followed by very deep negative T wave in all precordial leads with Q wave in V1–V2 but without increase of enzymes (reperfusion pattern). After few days, the ECG normalises (see Figure 8.45C).

On certain occasions, in the presence of significant coronary artery atherosclerosis, repeated

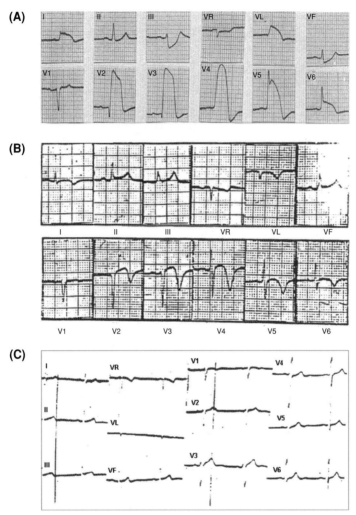

Figure 8.45 (A) Surface ECG of 65-year-old patient with typical crisis of Prinzmetal angina that presents in the peak of pain an ST-segment elevation like a TAP. This case corresponds to a transitory complete proximal occlusion of LAD above D1 (ST-segment elevation from V1 to V6, I and VL with ST-segment depression in inferior leads especially III and VF). The lack of ST-segment elevation in VR, the small ST-segment elevation in V1 and the clear ST-segment elevation in V6 – if the placement of V6 is well done – is against that the occlusion is also above S1 (see Fig. 4.43). This is the first case of Prinzmetal angina seen by us in early 1970s. Coronariography was not performed but enzymes were normal. (B) ECG after some hours of the crisis with a typical pattern of very negative T wave in all precordial leads (reperfusion pattern). (C) After 1 week the ECG was normal even with the recovery of rS morphology in V1–V2.

Prinzmetal angina crises occur during a typical ACS. On the other hand, several pharmacological agents (antimigraine tablets, chemotherapy drugs, amoxicillin and illicit drugs) have been identified as potential trigger of coronary spasm, especially in young people.

Sometimes, even very evident electrocardiographic signs are not accompanied by pain (silent ischaemia), as has been demonstrated by Holter monitoring (Bayes de Luna, 1985). In the trend of ST segment and heart rate the crisis of cardiac spasm presents different features than crisis of exercise angina (Figure 11.2). **On other occasions, pain may occur with minor or absent electrocardiographic signs** (Bayés de Luna et al., 1985). **The electrocardiographic changes typical of a coronary**

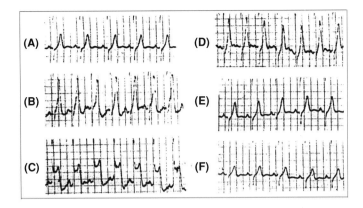

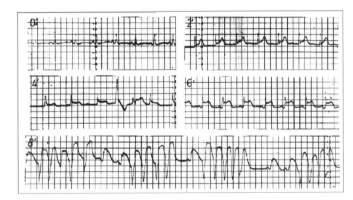

Figure 8.46 Above: Crisis of coronary spasm (Prinzmetal angina) recorded by Holter ECG. (A) Control. (B) Initial pattern of a very tall T wave (subendocardial ischaemia). (C) Huge pattern of ST-segment elevation. (D–F) Resolution towards normal values. Total duration of the crisis was 2 minutes. Below: Sequence of a crisis of Prinzmetal angina with the appearance of ventricular tachycardia runs at the moment of maximum ST-segment elevation.

spasm described by Prinzmetal (variant angina) **the very brisk development of an ST-segment elevation, sometimes quite striking,** may disappear within a few seconds. However, occasionally, ST-segment depression may be sometimes seen, probably in patients with previous very important subendocardium ischaemia, and also minor changes of T wave, which generally become negative or more peaked, or even U-wave changes may appear (Figure 3.25).

In almost half of the cases the **ST-segment elevation is preceded by a tall and peaked T wave** indicative of subendocardial ischaemia (Figure 8.46; Bayés de Luna et al., 1985). In other occasions, repolarisation changes of T wave are also very dynamic and transient usually accompanied by prolongation of QTc, but the ST-segment elevation does not develop. When the basal T wave is negative, a pseudonormalisation of the T wave may appear, sometimes with negative U wave (Figure 3.25).

When coronary spasm persists longer, an ST-segment/TQ-interval alternance may occur (Figure 8.11), and also ventricular arrhythmias may appear (Figure 8.46).

The importance of ventricular arrhythmias is related to the degree of ST-segment elevation and the duration of the crisis (Bayés de Luna et al., 1985). In spite of the presence of electrocardiographic signs of severe ischaemia, such as ST-segment/TQ-interval alternance (Figure 8.11) and runs of ventricular tachycardia (Figure 8.46), rarely VF and sudden death are triggered (Bayés de Luna et al., 1985).

Others

There are other situations that may cause atypical ACS (Braunwald, Zipes and Libby, 1998). Among these are the following:

–**Cocaine:** During the last 20 years the association of cocaine abuse with myocardial ischaemia, acute myocardial infarction and stroke has been known to exist (Coleman et al., 1982). In fact, in patients using cocaine, the risk of suffering an acute myocardial infarction shows a 24-fold increase during the first hour after the use of the drug. Therefore, this possibility should be borne in mind in a patient, especially if young, with chest pain. The mechanism is multifactorial. The increase in oxygen demand plus a generalised marked vasoconstriction of the coronary arteries, as well as the increase in platelet aggregation that could lead to thrombus formation, intervene in the pathophysiology. Naturally, when atherosclerosis is associated and the patients are smokers, the possibility to suffer MI is much higher.

The electrocardiographic changes, when present, are of STE-ACS type and, frequently, with evolving Q-wave infarction. Furthermore, **there is a risk for a false-positive diagnosis**, since in the young population consuming cocaine, **the pattern of early repolarisation is also frequently seen**.

• **Carbon monoxide poisoning**: Patients with carbon monoxide intoxication, whether or not in the presence of coronary atherosclerosis, may have an ACS and sometimes a silent Q-wave myocardial infarction and arrhythmias of different types. Carbon monoxide poisoning may cause chronic angina (see p. 301). According to Satran et al. (2005) the most frequent ECG changes are sinus tachycardia (40%) and ST/T changes, especially ST-segment depression (30%).

• **Anaphylactic crisis**: Cases of **ACS with Q- or non-Q-wave infarction** have been described in patients with different types of anaphylactic crises, including scorpion bites. On other occasions, the anaphylactic crisis has been the consequence of the administration of a drug. It is probable that an associated spasm may also have some influence (Massing et al., 1997).

• **Acute anaemia**: It may cause a clinical picture that may be confounded with an ACS. The ECG shows generally diffuse and frequently slight ST-segment deviations, especially ST-segment depression that may also be seen in chronic anaemia (see p. 300). Sometimes, anginal exercise pain is found. However, in most cases, anaemia in patients with no coronary atherosclerosis causes no anginal pain or striking electrocardiographic changes.

• **Transient dyskinesia of the mid- and basal part of LV**: Recently, **transient dyskinesia of the mid- and basal part of LV** in patients presenting striking ST-segment deviations sometimes has been described (Hurst et al., 2006). Catecholamine discharge and stroke are frequently associated. Often the patient presents chest pain. Although this atypical ACS seems related to high catecholamine release, it is difficult to understand why dyskinesia of all basal part of left ventricle is present because this area does not correspond to any specific myocardial territory perfusion (see p. 267).

• **X syndrome**: Sometimes patients with X syndrome may present chest pain at rest that may be considered an atypical ACS (see p. 298).

• **Other situations**: Situations such as a **pheochromocytoma and coronary arteritis** secondary to **systemic diseases**, as **Takayasu's disease, Kawasaki's disease, Churg–Strauss syndrome, etc.**, may generate myocardial ischaemia, ACS and even a myocardial infarction. This is also the case for patients with **AIDS** that often present diffuse and severe atherosclerotic lesions.

CHAPTER 9

Myocardial infarction with Q wave

We will now deal with the importance of ECG, especially from a clinical and prognostic standpoint, in patients with Q-wave myocardial infarction.

Myocardial infarctions with and without Q waves: new concepts

Classically, the electrocardiographic pattern of the established transmural infarction was associated with the presence of a pathological Q wave, generally accompanied by a negative T wave (Q wave of necrosis) (Horan, Flowers and Johnson, 1971; Table 4.6). This concept includes the presence of equivalents of Q wave. These are R waves in V1 greater than normal as a mirror pattern of myocardial infarction of lateral wall and also the presence of "r" wave of low voltage (≤ 5 mm) in lateral leads. In the first part (p. 131) (Figures 5.2–5.6), the mechanisms that explain the origin of Q wave of necrosis are discussed in detail. Until not so many years ago it was thought that the cases of subendocardium localisation were electrically 'mute' (non-Q-wave infarction). Thus, it was considered that myocardial infarctions with Q waves implied a transmural involvement, while non-Q-wave infarctions implied a subendocardium compromise.

Significant advances have been made during the last years in the knowledge of the relationship between the acute and chronic infarctions and their electrocardiographic manifestation (Bayés de Luna, 1999; Gersh and Rahimtoola, 1991; Sclarovsky, 1999; Wellens, Gorgels and Doevendans, 2003). The most important advances, some of them already commented in Chapter 5 are the following:

(a) It is known from **pathological point of view** that **exclusively subendocardium infarctions do not exist**. Nevertheless, there are infarctions that compromise a great portion of the wall, but with subendocardium predominance, which may or may not develop a Q wave (Maisel et al., 1985). Additionally, there are infarctions that may be transmural

(such as some infarctions involving some basal areas of left ventricle), which do not exhibit a Q wave (Goodman, Langer and Ross, 1998; Phibbs et al., 1999; Spodick, 1983).

(b) Cardiovascular MRI with gadolinium injection (CE-CMR) is currently the gold-standard technique not only for infarct identification, but also for transmurality characterisation (Mahrhold, 2005a,b; Moon et al., 2004; Wu et al., 2001). Therefore, it is the ideal technique for infarct location, size and correlation of the area of infarction with Q wave in different leads (ECG patterns of infarction). Thanks to CE-CMR, the precise size of infarction (grams of infarcted tissue) (see later 'Quatification of the infracted area') (see Figures 9.1 and 9.2) and the correlation between Q waves and location of the infarcted areas are much better known (Bayés de Luna et al., 2006a–c; Cino et al., 2006). This correlation has allowed us to propose a **new classification for Q-wave infarctions** according to the infarcted myocardial areas/ECG patterns correlation (Bayés de Luna et al., 2006b) (see p. 137 and Figure 5.9).

Mahrholdt et al. (2005a,b) have demonstrated with CMR that in the following coronary occlusion the myocardial function falls immediately throughout the region of ischaemia. However, till 15 minutes after occlusion no cellular infarction is found. From this point a 'wavefront' of infarction begins in the subendocardium and grows towards the epicardium over the next few hours, increasing continuously towards a transmural infarction (Figure 8.4). Therefore, there are infarctions predominantly, although probably not exclusively, in the subendocardium or transmural, but never exclusively in the subepicardium or in the middle part of the wall (Figures 1.5 and 5.2). This allows defining the non-ischaemic and ischaemic hyperenhancement patterns.

Moon et al. (2004) showed in a correlation study with CE-CMR that infarctions with predominantly

Table 9.1 Complete 50-Criteria. 31-Point QRS Scoring System*

Lead	Maximum Lead Points	Criteria	Points
I	(2)	Q ≥ 30 ms	(1)
		{ R/Q ≤ 1	(1)
		{ R ≤ 0,2 mV	(1)
II	(2)	{ Q ≥ 40 ms	(2)
		{ Q ≥ 30 ms	(1)
aVL	(2)	Q ≥ 30 ms	(1)
		R/Q ≤ 1	(1)
aVF	(5)	{ Q ≥ 50 ms	(3)
		{ Q ≥ 40 ms	(2)
		{ Q ≥ 30 ms	(1)
		{ R/Q ≤ 1	(1)
		{ R/Q ≤ 2	(2)

Lead	Region	Max	Criteria	Points
V1	Anterior	(1)	Any Q	(1)
V1	Posterior	(4)	R/S ≥ 1	(1)
			{ R ≥ 50 ms	(2)
			{ R ≥ 1,0 mV	(2)
			{ R ≥ 40 ms	(1)
			{ R ≥ 0,6 mV	(1)
			Q and S ≤ 0,3 mV	(1)
V2	Anterior	(1)	{ Any Q	(1)
			{ R ≤ 10 ms	(1)
			{ R ≤ 0,1 mV	(1)
			{ R ≤ R V1 mV	(1)
V2	Posterior	(4)	R/S ≥ 1,5	(1)
			{ R ≥ 60 ms	(2)
			{ R ≥ 2,0 mV	(2)
			{ R ≥ 50 ms	(1)
			{ R ≥ 1,5 mV	(1)
			Q and S ≤ 0,4 mV	(1)

Lead	Max	Criteria	Points
V3	(1)	{ Any Q	(1)
		{ R ≤ ms	(1)
		{ R ≤ 0, 2mV	(1)
V4	(3)	Q ≥ 20 ms	(1)
		{ R/S ≤ 0,5 mV	(2)
		{ R/Q ≤ 0,5 mV	(2)
		{ R/S ≤ 1	(1)
		{ R/Q ≤ 1	(1)
		{ R ≤ 0,6 mV	(1)
V5	(3)	Q ≥ 30 ms	(1)
		{ R/S ≤ 1	(2)
		{ R/Q ≤ 1	(2)
		{ R/S ≤ 2	(1)
		{ R/Q ≤ 2	(1)
		{ R ≤ 0,7 mV	(1)
V6	(3)	Q ≥ 30 ms	(1)
		{ R/S ≤ 1	(2)
		{ R/Q ≤ 1	(2)
		{ R/S ≤ 3	(1)
		{ R/Q ≤ 3	(1)
		{ R ≤ 0,67 mV	(1)

*The maximal number of points that can be awarded for each lead is shown in parentheses following each lead name (or left-ventricular region within a lead for leads V1 and V2) and the number of points awarded for each criterion is indicated in parentheses after each criterion name. The QRS criteria from 10 of the 12 standard ECG leads are indicated. Only one criterion can be selected from each group of criteria within a bracket. All criteria involving R/Q or R/S ratios consider the relative amplitudes of these waves. (Modified from Selvester1985). (Taken from Wagner GS, 2001).

subendocardium involvement exhibit an infarction Q wave of necrosis in approximately 30% of the cases. Furthermore, they demonstrated that a similar figure of transmural infarctions was found in non-Q-wave infarctions. From the CE-CMR standpoint, 50% of the infarctions had been at some point transmural, but almost all of them had sometimes predominantly subendocardium extension. From a comprehensive point of view, and though Q waves of necrosis may be seen in small infarctions, **Q-wave infarctions in comparison to non-Q-wave infarctions are not 'more' transmural, but they are larger. Therefore, differentiating between an MI with and without Q wave is important because the former involves a larger area and not because it is or is not transmural** (Moon et al., 2004).

Very recently Kwong et al. (2006) in a group of patients with clinical suspicion of CHD but without history of MI demonstrated that the presence of areas of the LV with gadolinium enhancement carries a high cardiac risk. In addition, the presence of gadolinium enhancement areas has prognostic implications beyond the common clinical, angiographic and functional predictors.

In spite that the CE-CMR is the 'gold standard' for identification, location and quantification of MI (Figures 9.1 and 9.2), recently it has been published (Engblom et al., 2003) that the QRS score

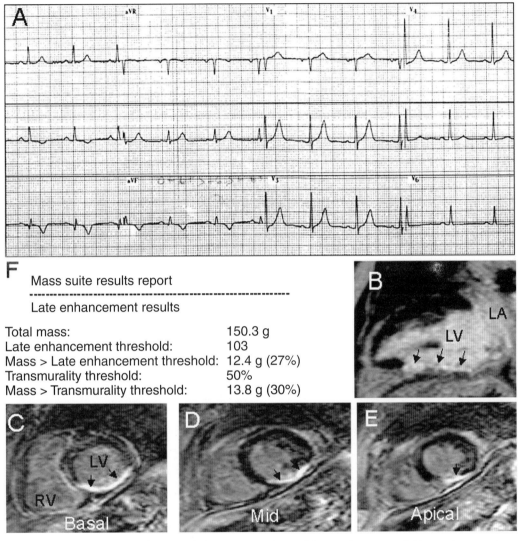

Figure 9.1 Inferior myocardial infarction. (A) The ECG shows Qr in leads DIII and VF and rS in V1. (B) CE-CMR image in a vertical long-axis (sagittal-like) view confirming inferior myocardial infarction as showed by delayed hyperenhancement (arrows). (C–E) Contrast-enhanced short-axis images show myocardial hyperenhancement (arrows) at basal, mid and apical levels of the inferior wall, indicating transmural myocardial infarction. (F) Quantification of myocardial necrotic mass.

(Selvester–Wagner) is significantly related to both MI size and transmurality in post-MI patients assessed by CE-CMR.

(c) Though the terms Q-wave MI and non-Q-wave MI are no longer accepted in the acute phase, it is true that in the **subacute and especially in chronic phases of MI**, there are **infarctions with and without Q wave**. The higher the number of Q waves or their equivalent, the worse the prognosis is.

(d) From the electrocardiographic point of view, the **Q wave has been considered the only specific finding in chronic myocardial infarction**. MI without Q wave does not present in chronic phase any specific electrocardiographic sign that allows for its identification. However, in coronary patients it is already known from many years (Horan, Flowers and Johnson, 1971) that some changes in the mid-late part of QRS are also specific signs of chronic

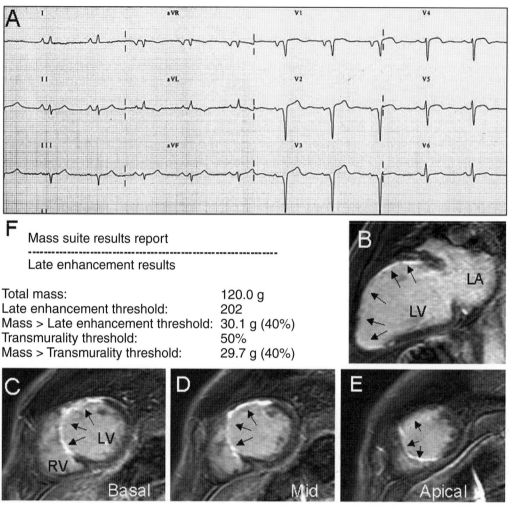

Figure 9.2 Apical-anterior MI. (A) ECG showing Q waves in V1–V3 with rS V4–V5 corresponding to an apical-anterior myocardial infarction. (B) CE-CMR image in a sagittal view: myocardial hyperenhancement (arrows) shows a non-transmural necrosis of the anterior wall. (C–E) Transversal images show myocardial hyperenhancement (arrows) at low basal, mid and apical levels of the anterior MI. and septal wall, and at apical level in inferior wall but without evident lateral involvement. Therefore it is not extensive infarction (type A-3) but an apical anterior with anteroseptal extension (type A-2)(see Figure 1.14). Due to that there is only Q in precordial leads but not in VL and I. (F) Quantification of myocardial necrotic mass.

MI. These changes have now been reviewed (Das et al., 2006), named **fractioned QRS**, including **morphologies** such as low R in V6, rsr in some leads (I, II, precordial leads), notches and slurrings in the QRS, etc. (see Figures 9.3 and 9.4 and p. 129).

(e) Since **new treatments during the acute phase may greatly reduce the final infarcted area**, it is difficult to know in Q-wave infarction the exact location of the acute occlusion that has led to the infarction. Furthermore, sometimes revascularisation therapy may virtually cause the occlusion to disappear (lysis of the thrombus), though unfortunately this may occur when the infarction is already established (Figure 2.3).

(f) Furthermore, **the recent consensus on MI diagnosis of the ESC/ACC** (European Society of Cardiology / American College of Cardiology – (Alpert et al., 2000) **accepts the diagnosis of infarction**

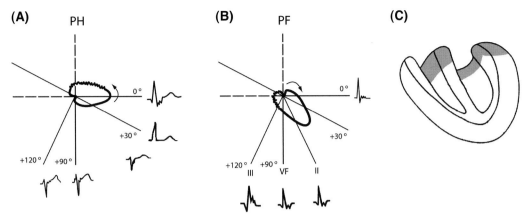

Figure 9.3 If the necrosis affects the areas of late ventricular depolarisation (in grey (C)), instead of pathologic Q wave, it will result in a change of the direction of the vectors of the second part of QRS, which is presented as 'slurrings' in the terminal part of QRS in II, III, VF and V5–V6 or as rr' or r' of a very low voltage in precordial leads and/or I or II, or even slurrings in the beginning of ST segment (A, B). These morphologies are considered as fractioned QRS (Das et al., 2006) (p. 131).

if a troponin-level increase is found, accompanied by any of the rest of the factors that are listed in Table 6.2, **not requiring the presence of electrocardiographic changes**. Consequently, there are infarctions that produce less than the amount of infarcted tissue needed to modify an ECG (Wagner et al., 2000). That implies that many UAs evolve into infarctions (**microinfarctions or 'necrosettes'**). Until this definition was accepted it was infrequent to find a normal ECG in the acute phase of an infarction. Generally, they were small infarctions secondary to the occlusion of short LCX, or obtuse marginal branch (OM), or small branches of the LAD or RCA. Nowadays, with this consensus the diagnosis of small MI is more frequently made. **(g) In the following, we will discuss in particular the prognostic implications of the different types of Q-wave infarctions according to the new classification that we have proposed, on the basis of the correlation with CMR** (see Figure 5.9). Also, we will comment on the utility and limitations of the ECG for the quantification of infarction in the era of CE-CMR, as well as all the types of MIs without Q wave. Finally, prognostic markers in post-infarction patients and electrocardiographic characteristics in patients with stable anginal pain and other clinical settings outside ACS will also be discussed.

Myocardial infarction with Q wave or equivalents and normal intraventricular conduction

Q wave secondary to a single infarction

Introduction

Let us now summarise what has been explained previously (p. 128).

(a) There is often a multivessel involvement, but just one infarction, which is the result of the generally total occlusion of an epicardial coronary artery. However, currently, with the new treatments available, the artery may be reopened, and consequently,

–The **distinction between transmural (Q-wave infarctions) and subendocardium (non-Q-wave infarctions) cannot be supported any longer.**
–Infarction occurring in areas of late depolarisation (>40 ms from the onset of the depolarisation) does not produce Q wave or equivalent. However, it could exhibit minimal changes in the mid-final portion of ventricular depolarisation (**fractioned QRS**) (Figures 9.3 and 9.4).

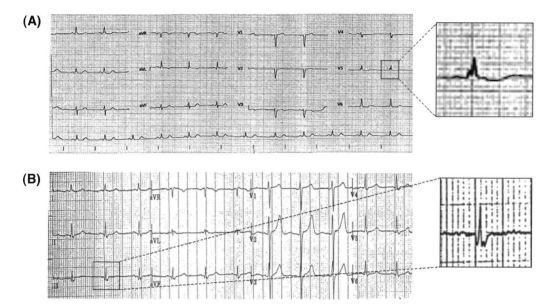

Figure 9.4 (A) A 55-year-old patient with previous MI due to LCX occlusion that presents a nearly normal ECG with low-voltage R wave in V5–V6 with evident 'slurrings'. (B) Sixty-year-old patient who suffered MI 8 months ago. The coronary angiography demonstrated occlusion of the LCX.

Striking final 'slurrings' in II, III, VF, VL and right precordial leads (V2–V3). The Q wave in inferior leads and the 'r' wave in V1 are narrow, and additionally the R/S ratio <0.5. This is an evident case of MI presented by striking final 'slurrings' of QRS.

the infarction is sometimes smaller than expected, since the amount of area at risk in the acute phase does not coincide with the final infarction (Figure 2.3).

(b) The first electrocardiographic change recorded in Q-wave infarction, form both experimental (Figure 3.3) and clinical (Figure 3.18) point of view, is ST-segment elevation. This is frequently preceded in the hyperacute phase by T wave that is taller than normal and, if much ischaemia is present, by decrease and even abolition of the S wave (Figure 8.9). The subsequent development of the Q wave and the negative T wave is accompanied by a decrease in the ST-segment elevation. **The Q wave corresponds to an area that is electrically mute, but which is not necessarily dead yet.** This explains why sometimes, shortly after the infarction, the Q wave may disappear if perfusion of the involved area suddenly improves. In some cases, NSTE-ACS may generate Q-wave infarction if ischaemia involves the subepicardium area located close to the subendocardium (Figures 5.2C(2–8)).

(c) In cases with transmural and homogeneous involvement of ventricular wall (Figure 5.2B) and also

in some cases of practically transmural infarction, but with a subendocardium predominance (Figure 5.2C), there will be more or fewer leads that will face the tail of infarction vector and thus different Q wave morphologies (QS, QR and qR complexes), according to which the extension of the infarction will be recorded. The infarction vector changes the normal onset of ventricular depolarisation; thus, the QRS loop presents a different direction and sometimes rotation. This change in loop direction and morphology explains, thanks to loop–hemifield correlation, the presence of an abnormal Q wave or its equivalent (R in V1–V2) (Figures 5.4–5.6) when the infarcted area is depolarised within the first 40 milliseconds of ventricular activation. This occurs throughout the entire ventricle, with the exception of the most basal areas of the left ventricle.

(d) The normal cardiac activation sequence of left ventricle (Durrer et al., 1970) depicted in the form of isochrone plot is shown in Figure 9.5. The basal areas are shown to depolarise after 40 milliseconds. Thus, infarction of these areas (areas of activation after 40 ms) does not generate Q waves or equivalent,

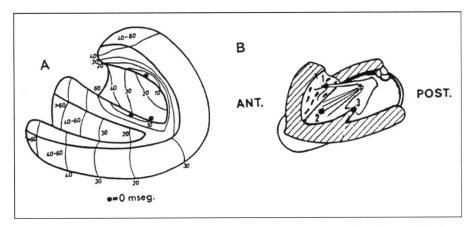

Figure 9.5 (A) Three approximate starting points (*) and the isochronal sequential lines of the ventricular depolarisation (Durrer et al., 1970). (B) Left lateral view of the correlation between the endocardial areas of initial ventricular activation and the divisions of the left branch (1, superoanterior; 2, media septal fibers and 3 inferoposterior).

but may explain the presence of minor changes in the final portion of the QRS complex (fractioned QRS).

(e) Occlusion of the first diagonal branch (D1) generates infarction that may be expressed by QS morphology in VL (Warner et al., 1986). It is currently known that this infarction does not involve the high lateral wall, as has been thought for more than 50 years. The infarction due to occlusion of D1 affects predominantly mid-anterior wall and also a part of the mid-lateral wall, but not of high lateral wall that is perfused by LCX. **Thus, the association Q wave in VL/high lateral infarction is not certain** (see Figure 5.9).

(f) The presence of RS morphology in coronary patients that have suffered an STE-ACS is due to infarction of the lateral wall and not to infarction of inferobasal segment (old posterior wall) (see Figure 5.9).

Criteria of diagnosis and location: prognostic implications of different patterns

Although it was thought that there is no clear evidence that the presence of Q waves has independent influence on long-term outcome, CMR has demonstrated that the presence of Q waves is more related to the extension of MI, more larger area, than to its transmurality (Moon et al., 2004). Also, different studies (Petrina, Goodman and Eagle, 2006) have shown higher in-hospital mortality with Q-wave MI than with non-Q-wave MI.

To diagnose a chronic Q-wave infarction, **the criteria that define a Q wave of necrosis should be identified**. The criteria used for the diagnosis of an infarction involving the different walls into which the left ventricle may be divided have been discussed on page 135 (Tables 5.2 to 5.4). Measurement and assessment of Q and R waves may be made according to the Minnesota code (Blackburn et al., 1960) (Figure 5.1). All these aspects have been commented on in Chapter 1.

We will just remind (see p. 137) that **seven areas of MI detected by CE-CMR have good correspondence with seven ECG patterns (four in anteroseptal zone – septal, apical-anterior, extensive anterior and mid-anterior – and three in the inferolateral zone – inferior, lateral and inferolateral)** (Figure 5.9; Cino et al., 2006). We have also demonstrated that in clinical practice **the presence of these seven ECG patterns correlates well with the corresponding infarction areas detected by CE-CMR, and therefore these have real value in clinical practice** (Bayés de Luna et al., 2006a–c) (Table 5.3). Therefore, **in chronic infarction** the correlation between ECG changes (Q waves of necrosis) and involved area (CE-CMR) is clearly good (88% global concordance). However, the infarcted area of apical infarction (A-2 type), mid-anterior infarction (A-3 type) and lateral infarction (B-1 type) presents the lower concordance.

However, with the current treatment available in developed countries, the ECG–CMR correlation in chronic phase is not useful for assessing, on the basis of the leads with a Q wave in the ECG, the coronary occlusion site that caused the infarction. In pre-reperfusion era an occlusion of a coronary artery, e.g. the proximal part of the LAD, would have generated an STE-ACS that would evolve to Q-wave MI, involving the entire area perfused by the LAD distal to the occlusion. In this case it would correspond to a large area of the anterior, the septal anterior, part of the inferior and part of the lateral walls. However, with the new treatments available currently any occlusion that would manifest a relatively large area at risk in the acute phase may turn, in the chronic phase, into smaller infarcted area (chronic infarction) (Figure 2.3), or in some cases, infarction may even be aborted (Figure 8.9). Occasionally, treatment has reopened artery, but that has not been enough to avoid large infarcted area. Therefore, **Q wave of necrosis will be useful to know the infarcted area but not how the arterial occlusion is at this time**, although we can presume where was the occlusion that have produced the MI (Figure 5.9).

Each of the seven electrocardiographic patterns with a Q wave of necrosis or its equivalent that we find in daily clinical practice is shown in Figure 5.9. In the first part of this book (p. 141) we have commented on the diagnostic clues for each of the seven ECG patterns, based on the CE-CMR correlations (Figures 5.10–5.36). Now, we will briefly discuss first the comparative prognosis of ECG pattern of anteroseptal versus inferolateral pattern and later the most important prognostic implications of each pattern.

Anteroseptal versus inferolateral MI: prognostic implications. It is known that the **MI involving LAD presents for similar area of necrosis, increased myonecrosis, reduced early and late left-ventricular function and high mortality compared with infarction in other vascular territories.** However, the mechanisms underlying a worse prognosis are not completely characterised. Recently, it has been demonstrated (Kandzari et al., 2006) that prognosis after primary PCI in patient with ACS, the majority with ST-segment elevation, is different in patients with LAD occlusion than in RCA or LCX. Acute myocardial infarction due to LAD is associ-

ated with reduced EF, less frequent collateral flow, impaired myocardial perfusion and reduced perfusion success. All these factors may explain the increase of major cardiac events, including mortality, which presents the group of patients with acute myocardial infarction with LAD occlusion compared with other group (RCA or LCX). Thus efforts to enhance post-reperfusion microcirculatory function after PCI especially in anteroseptal MI have to be made.

The importance of other factors additional to amount of necrosis has also been studied. In patients with first acute MI treated with PCI, LAD-related MI show for a similar amount of myocardial necrosis as determined by enzymatic infarct size, lower left-ventricular ejection fraction (LVEF) when compared to non-LAD-related MI. LVEF-measured 6-month post-MI showed a decrease, for every 1000 cumulative lactate dehydrogenase release, of 4.8% for LAD and 2.4% for non-LAD-related infarcts ($p < 0.0001$), and these results remain in the multivariate analysis (Elsman et al., 2006).

The prognostic implications of MI location have been recently reviewed (Petrina, Goodman and Eagle, 2006). The most relevant finding is that anterior MI compared with inferior MI, both with and without Q waves, presents an independent higher risk factor for short-term mortality and probably also for long-term mortality.

ECG patterns of the anteroseptal and inferolateral zones: prognostic implications. Before commenting on the prognosis implications of different ECG patterns, we would like to remind the following: (1) as we have already stated for similar area of necrosis, the MI of anteroseptal zone presents worst prognosis and higher mortality, and (2) in both zones, anteroseptal and inferolateral, the prognosis is worst in case of larger MI. However, we would like to make some considerations about some ECG characteristics that may give specific clues of the outcome and prognosis of the seven different ECG patterns. Only the long follow-up of these patients will give the real information in the future.

1. Electrocardiographic pattern type A-1 (Figure 5.9-A1): **Q waves in V1–V2** (Figures 5.10–5.12). This corresponds to **septal infarction** and is generally due to a LAD occlusion involving the septal branches but not the diagonal branches (p. 141).

–Prognostic implications

Frequently, isolated septal infarctions are small and present a good prognosis (Figures 5.10). If early revascularisation is attained, a large evolving extensive anterior infarction secondary to LAD occlusion proximal to S1 and D1 may sometimes be reduced and limited to an exclusively septal infarction if the areas dependent on the diagonal branches have been reperfused. In these cases, infarction that had been threatening large area (extensive anterior) has been limited to small infarction (septal). An example is shown in Figure 2.3. In the top, during the hyperacute phase, large ST-segment elevation is seen in V1–V5 with isoelectric ST segment in V6. The sum of ST-segment elevations in the precordial leads was greater than 30 mm, which implies a large area at risk. Fibrinolytic therapy was begun, and at 30 minutes the sum of ST-segment deviations was reduced to 14 mm and was limited to V1–V4, with a clear depression in V5–V6. The area at risk was reduced to the myocardial area depending on septal perfusion, since an electrocardiographic pattern typical of septal involvement (ST-segment elevation in V1 and depression in V6) had appeared, as is seen in cases of ACS due to an occlusion proximal to the S1 but not D1. In this case the occlusion changed from proximal to S1 and D1 to proximal to S1, with the diagonal branches having been spared from the occlusion, as is shown for the presence of small ST-segment elevation in inferior leads. The infarction was reduced but still fairly large, although exclusively septal, with a moderately impaired LVEF (50%) and good functional capacity (Figure 5.11). In other cases the infarction may be much more limited than expected and on occasion may even become an **aborted infarction** (Figures 8.2 and 8.9).

The prognosis is specially related with the infarction size. Even in cases of large septal infarction (Figure 5.11) the EF is usually only moderately reduced. In the majority of septal infarctions the EF is over 50%.

2. Electrocardiographic pattern type A-2 (Figure 5.9-A2): Q wave in V1–V2to V4–V6 (Figures 5.13–5.17). This corresponds to **apical-anterior infarction**. At times, the extension of the infarction involves upper areas especially of the anterior and

septal walls. We remind that, compared with the A-1 pattern, Q waves (QS or qr) may be seen beyond V3 but not in leads I and VL. This is generally due to a LAD occlusion distal to S1 and D1 or to a LAD incomplete occlusion involving the septal branches more than the diagonal branches (p. 142).

–Prognostic implications

To recognise the extension of the apical-anterior myocardial infarction it is important to check carefully small ECG details because the typical patterns of this infarction in the precordial leads (QS from V1–V2to V5–V6) do not recognise the amount of anterolateral involvement. However, it has already been said (p. 145) that if a 'q' wave is seen in II, III and VF, the inferior wall involvement is probably more important than the anterior wall involvement because this represents that the LAD is long and the inferior involvement is rather large (Figure 5.16B) or, at least, it is larger than the anterior involvement (Figure 5.16A). In these cases the inferior vector of infarction is dominant with respect to the anterior vector of infarction and generates the Q wave in II, III and VF. These data support that probably the anteroseptal involvement is small. If, in turn, the presence of an 'R' wave or an R/S pattern is seen in II, III and VF, this indicates that the anterior involvement is larger than the inferior involvement, and the anterior vector of infarction is dominant over the inferior vector of infarction. Thus, Q waves are not seen in II, III and VF (Figure 5.16C).

Most infarctions with type A-2 pattern (QS from V1 to V4–V5), especially cases without too much anteroseptal involvement, **have usually a good prognosis because they are not very extensive**. However, the infarctions with the best prognosis are the apical-anterior infarctions due to very distal, not very long, LAD occlusion since these are the smallest (Figure 5.16A). These may be considered 'true apical' infarctions.

In turn, **there are rare cases of infarctions with this pattern that present a poorer prognosis because they are caused by the proximal occlusion of a quite long LAD**. In this situation (Figure 5.8) the inferior and anterior infarction vector may cancel each other, and therefore the Q in I and VL and inferior leads are not present, but significant haemodynamic impairment and heart failure may exist (Takatsu, Osugui and Nagaya, 1986). Consequently, **this rare possibility (proximal occlusion of a very long LAD) should be considered when the clinical picture and the patient's haemodynamic status are very poor and the ECG presents a pattern of apical-anterior MI (A-2 type)** (Q in precordial leads beyond V2 without Q wave in VL).

3. Electrocardiographic pattern type A-3 (Figure 5.9-A3): Q waves from V1 to V5–V6, I and VL (Figures 5.18–5.19). **This pattern corresponds to extensive anterior infarction.** Compared to the A-2 pattern, this infarction also exhibits a Q wave (QS and QR patterns) in VL and, sometimes, lead I. It is usually due to a very proximal LAD occlusion (p. 148).

–Prognostic implications

It has been shown that **infarctions presenting with Q waves in the precordial leads and in I and VL (sometimes with new pattern of RBBB) have a larger infarcted ventricular mass (more segments involved) and a lower EF.** Consequently, these patients must undergo more complex evaluations after the acute phase, with the aim of better stratifying their prognosis and treating residual ischaemia, if present (Warner et al., 1988). It is especially important to check for the presence of ECG signs of proximal LAD occlusion in the acute phase, such as the specific ST-segment deviations seen in occlusion proximal to D1 and S1 (ST-segment elevation in V1–V4–V5 and VR, and ST-segment depression in II, III, VF and V6) (see Figures 4.10, 4.12 and 4.18) and the development of an RBBB. As may happen with other MI but more often in this type there are frequently signs of a larger myocardial area at risk, such as the sum of ST-segment elevations and depressions greater than 15 mm, or the patterns of severe ischaemia, with ST-segment elevation concave with respect to the isoelectric baseline and a J point/R-wave ratio greater than 0.5 mm (see p. 224). In all these circumstances, we must act extremely rapidly (i.e. urgent coronary angiogram). **The appearance of a systolic murmur is a sign of very bad prognosis** in a patient with extensive anterior MI (proximal occlusion) **because there is probably a sign of septal rupture, which is a very severe complication** (see p. 245). However, though the infarction involves the entire anterior and septal walls, it does not involve the high lateral wall (which is perfused by the LCX), but rather the low-middle lateral one. The presence of a

QS (Qr) pattern in VL had been considered as due to a high lateral infarction, but in fact it is generated by an infarction due to first diagonal occlusion, in this case included in the LAD occlusion proximal to S1 and D1.

Also the presence of R wave in inferior leads suggests that the involvement of inferior wall is lesser than the involvement of anterior wall. This is explained, because the occlusion of LAD is proximal but the artery is short and does not wrap the apex (Figure 5.18 and 5.38).

4. (Electrocardiographic pattern type A-4 (Figure 5.9-A4): Q wave in I and VL with, at times, a 'q' wave in V2–V3 (sometimes QS just in V2) (Figures 5.20–5.22). **It corresponds to mid-anterior infarction.** It is due to a selective occlusion of D1 or LAD involving the diagonal branches, but not the septal branches (p. 154).

–Prognostic implications

These are generally small infarctions that frequently cause slight electrocardiographic changes, especially in the chronic phase. Therefore, **usually the prognosis is good.** We have demonstrated that often the typical and very specific, although with a lower sensitivity, low-voltage QS pattern in VL normalises over time, and the ECG becomes normal. In the acute phase a slight ST-segment elevation is generally seen in several precordial leads with often small 'q' in V2–V3. When a slight ST-segment depression is found, it generally occurs because ischaemia is caused not only by the D1 occlusion, but also by RCA involvement or, more frequently, LCX involvement. These cases due to multivessel disease present a worst prognosis.

5. Electrocardiographic pattern type B-1 (Figure 5.9-B1): tall and/or wide R wave in V1 and/or low-voltage 'qr' or 'r' pattern in V5–V6, I and/or VL (Figures 5.23–5.26). This corresponds to lateral infarction. It is caused by OM occlusion, and sometimes by a proximal but quite small LCX occlusion (p. 154).

–Prognostic implications

Generally, they are not large infarctions, especially when the ECG is normal or near normal (Figure 10.2). However, **in presence of normal ECG recording in some cases, the myocardial mass involved may be relatively important, because a great part of the lateral wall depolarises after 40 milliseconds** and, therefore, does not generate

Q wave or equivalent. Therefore, **it is necessary to check carefully the ECG to detect small changes in the mid-late part of QRS as low-voltage 'r'in V6, 'r' in V1 ≥ 3 mm and small 'q' wave in II, III and VF, rsr' in some leads (II, precordial leads) and other morphologies included in the concept of fractioned QRS** (p. 129).

The prognosis is worst in spite that there are usually small infarctions in cases **that present (a)persistence of ST-segment elevation even small**, without appearance of negative T wave. This sign **is a marker of cardiac rupture** (see Figures 8.27 and 8.29; see Plate 2.2); (b) **appearance of systolic murmur as a sign of mitral regurgitation**. This appears in case of posteromedial papillary muscle dysfunction or rupture (Figure 8.29A; see p. 245).

6. Electrocardiographic pattern type B-2 (Figure 5.9-B2): Q wave in at least two contiguous inferior leads II, III and VF (Figures 5.27–5.30). This corresponds to inferior infarction. It is secondary to the occlusion of a non-dominant RCA or sometimes to very distal occlusion of long LCX (p. 159).

–Prognostic implications

An isolated inferior infarction detected by the presence of Q waves in any inferior lead (II, III and VF) is often not too large and, **generally, of good prognosis.** This is especially true when the QR pattern in II, III and VF is not very apparent and, primarily, if diagnostic doubts arise. In case of doubt it is advisable to rule out that the Q wave is caused by positional changes, which happens especially when it is recorded only in III. The fact that it disappears or is significantly reduced during inspiration supports its benign nature (Figure 5.42). **The cases of inferior MI of worst prognosis** correspond to (a) **the proximal non-dominant RCA involving AV node branch** (AV block may be seen) **and/or RV branches.** (RV infarction in acute phase may be present.) **The prognosis is worst when the RCA is dominant** (type B-3) because the area at risk is higher; (b) **the cases associated with** SAH (Figure 5.54) because this association suggests multivessel disease.

7. Electrocardiographic pattern (type B-3) (Figure 5.9-B3): Q wave in II, III and VF and R wave in V1–V2 and/or Q wave in V5–V6 and/or I and VL (Figures 5.31–5.34). This corresponds to an infarction involving the inferior and lateral walls.

It is due to occlusion of dominant RCA or LCX (p. 1.161).

–Prognostic implications

The presence of many electrocardiographic criteria showing inferior and lateral involvement **represents generally a large infarction that encompasses the cases of worst prognosis of MI of inferolateral zone, especially in case of MI due to very dominant RCA or LCX.** The ejection fraction is usually diminished. Therefore, **in the acute phase**, quick decision should be taken (urgent PCI) to avoid haemodynamic complications.

An example of this type of infarction due to an **occlusion proximal to the take-off of the RV branches in a dominant RCA** is shown in Figure 9.6. In the acute phase (Figure 9.6A) all the electrocardiographic signs supporting this diagnosis are seen (↑ST III > II, ↓ST in I < VL, isodiphasic ST segment in V1 and ↑ in V5–V6 and V4R). Complications such as a complete AV block may occur in the acute phase. **In the chronic phase**, clear signs of a large inferolateral infarction due to RCA occlusion are seen (QR in II, III and aVF (III > II), R > S in V1 and QR in V6 with a low-voltage R wave in lead I, but without Q in I and aVL). In the chronic phase, on the contrary to what happens in the acute phase (Figure 9.6), there are no ECG criteria of associated RV infarction.

Proximal occlusion of very dominant LCX also corresponds to a large area at risk (Figure 4.42).**In chronic phase** most typical ECG patterns of inferolateral MI due to proximal LCX occlusion are Q in II, III and VF, and sometimes with Q in II > III, Rs or RS in V1 and q in I, aVL and/or V5–V6 (Figure 2.2D).

Quantification of the infarcted area

Myocardial damage and viability may be approximately quantified in the chronic phase of a Q-wave infarction. Different scores have been described, to know with a greater or lesser accuracy the amount of myocardium involved and, indirectly, the LV function (EF) (Palmeri et al., 1982). Selvester, Wagner and Hindman (1985) described a 31-point scoring system, on the basis of 50 criteria (presence of Q wave in different leads, R wave in V1–V2 as mirror pattern, etc.). This score quantifies the amount of infarcted tissue (3% of the left-ventricular mass for each point). Also, the reduction of the EF due to the infarction may be

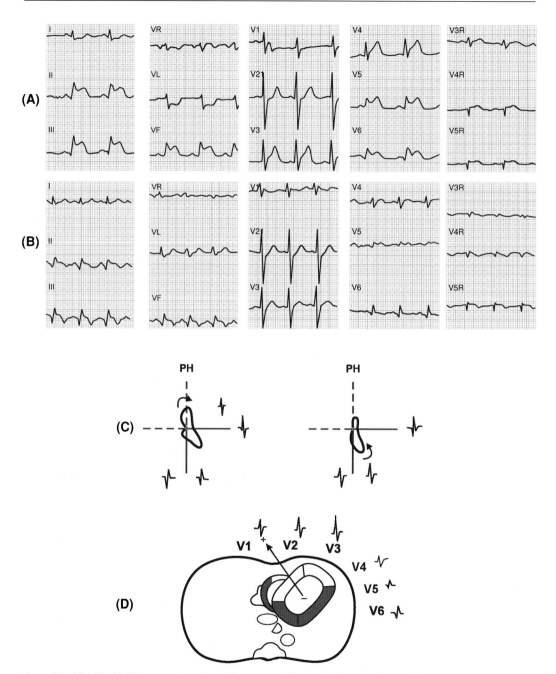

Figure 9.6 (A) ACS with ST-segment elevation of the inferolateral area due to proximal occlusion (involving RV) of a superdominant RCA (ST ↑ III > II, ST↓ in I, ST isoelectric in V1–V2, ST↑ in V4R and ST↑ > 2 mm in V6). (B) In the chronic phase an MI type B-3 (inferolateral) is confirmed. Observe QR in II, III and VF, and RS in V1 with qr in V6. (C) VCG loop in the chronic phase and (D) drawing of the involved area in a horizontal axial transection with infarction vector facing V1, what explains the RS pattern in V1 and the qr pattern in V6.

performed by using the formula (EF = 60 − 3 × no. of points in the QRS) (Hinohara et al., 1984; Table 9.1). Its reliability has been demonstrated in patients with single chronic infarctions and also in cases of multiple infarctions. It is also useful as a prognostic marker (Pahlm et al., 1998; Sevilla et al., 1990).

However, at the individual level, the standard error of myocardial damage quantification using this score is large, such that its clinical usefulness is limited. The most important cause of errors of this score is produced by the method's inability to quantify basal infarcted areas, mainly the septal and lateral areas.

Nowadays, **CMR** has demonstrated great accuracy in estimating infarcted mass (Horáček et al., 2006; Moon et al., 2004) (Figures 9.1 and 9.2), which makes this technique the '**gold standard**' for the quantification of infarction mass. However, recently, Engblom (2006) has reported that in patients with first time reperfused MI the QRS score is significantly related to both MI size and transmurality. Also, recently, it has been published that high QRS Selvester score is an independent predictor of incomplete ST recovery and complications in STE-ACS treated with primary PCI (Uyarel et al., 2006).

ECG changes from the acute to chronic phase

Before the era of reperfusion with fibrinolytics or PCI it was relatively easy to predict the final Q-wave infarction pattern according to the acute phase STE-ACS. Aldrich et al. (1988) described a score (see p. 224) for estimation of the extent of myocardium at risk of infarction in the absence of reperfusion therapy. However, currently with the new strategies of treatment, this is impossible because if the treatment is started on time, the infarction may be aborted (Figure 8.2) or at least decreased.

Therefore, in chronic patients it is impossible to know the exact degree of occlusion of the coronary artery culprit of ACS in this moment, although, probably, it can be predicted what the type and location of the occlusion that produced the MI were. For example, a case of proximal occlusion to D1 and S1 of LAD (Figure 2.3A) after treatment presented an ECG of non-complete occlusion of LAD, encompassing the septal branches, but not the diagonal branches (Figure 2.3B). These result in a large but exclusive septal MI (Figure 5.11). However, in the chronic phase the coronarography of this patient was nearly normal, because the treatment that was unable to abort the infarction finally has completely opened the artery.

The ECG in multiple infarctions: prognostic implications

In Chapter 1 we have discussed (see 'The ECG in multiple infarctions') the ECG changes that may occur in case of more than one MI. Now we would like to emphasise that **the prognosis in case of multiple Q-wave infarcts is usually worst because the infarcted area is often larger than that in case of single Q-wave MI, and therefore the EF is more reduced than that in case of single infarction**. Also if the MIs are involving more anteroseptal areas, they will represent a worst prognosis (see p. 282). However, with the current classification of MI (consensus ACC/ESC; Alpert et al., 2000) two or more small MIs of necrossette type may be present without too much myocardial area being infarcted.

Myocardial infarction with Q wave and wide QRS

On some occasions patients with ACS and wide QRS present ST-segment elevation evolving to a Q-wave myocardial infarction. The ECG criteria to diagnose Q-wave infarction in presence of ACS with wide QRS have been explained in the first part (see p. 170).

The patients with **STE-ACS evolving to Q-wave infarction that presents wide QRS have worst prognosis** (see p. 247). As a matter of fact, the patients with ACS and LBBB pattern with or without a normal ST-segment deviation present worst prognosis and are candidates to fibrinolysis. However this concept has to be reconsidered after the Wong's paper (2005) (p. 249). On the other hand, the appearance of new RBBB in STE-ACS appears in case of LAD occlusion proximal to S1 and D1 and represents a huge area at risk and worst prognosis. As we have already commented (p. 247), the prognosis of MI with RBBB is also related to the width of QRS and to the evidence that the RBBB is new. Even the presence of SAH that does not have very wide QRS (<0.120 ms) has worst prognosis (Biagini et al., 2005) than control group.

Electrocardiographic signs of poor prognosis in post-infarction patient

The following electrocardiographic signs are of poor prognosis:

(a) **Sinus tachycardia**: Its presence in isolated ECG recording and, especially, its confirmation in 24-hour Holter monitoring are markers of poor prognosis.

(b) **Long QT interval**: Its presence has been considered a marker of poor prognosis (Schwartz et al., 1985).

(c) **Atrial wave changes**: The presence of electrocardiographic signs of left atrial enlargement has been described as marker of poor prognosis (Rios, 1997).

(d) **Residual persistence of ST-segment elevation or depression** (in both in Q-wave and non-Q-wave infarctions): Different studies have shown that persistence of ST-segment elevation is a marker of left ventricular aneurysm (LVA). However, the sensitivity and specificity of this ECG sign are poor (p. 304).

(e) **Very abnormal QRS complexes, with Q waves of necrosis** in many leads as an indirect marker of poor ventricular function.

(f) **The presence of fractioned QRS morphologies** including RSR' pattern and its variants in the absence of LBBB (QRS < 120 ms): These ECG signs are very specific (>90%) of LVA, although their sensitivity is much lower (Reddy et al., 2006) (see Figure 13.2 and p. 304).

(g) Pattern of **bundle branch block, especially of the left bundle,** when the QRS complex is very wide (Moss et al., 2002).

(h) **Exercise stress test**: The presence of ST-segment depression (see Table 4.4) and the appearance of important ventricular arrhythmias are markers of poor prognosis (Theroux et al., 1979). Especially if angina appears, it is compulsory to proceed for a coronary angiography and take the appropriate solution.

(i) **Holter technology**: It includes not only **arrhythmias and ischaemia**, but also late potentials and **ANS assessment** (Malik and Camm, 2004), such as RR variability, dynamic study of repolarisation, heart rate turbulence, etc. **The presence of frequent PVCs** in Holter recording is a marker of poor prognosis in the post-infarction patient, in the presence of low EF (Bigger et al., 1984; Moss et al., 1979). However, the presence of PVC in elderly patients with echocardiographically normal heart is not increased by significant coronary artery disease (Shandling et al., 2006). The presence of peaks of QT interval greater than 500 milliseconds in Holter ECG (Homs et al., 1997) is a marker of bad outcome. With respect to the QT dispersion, the results are not concordant. Recently, it has been demonstrated that QT-dispersion decrease following PCI is a marker of better reperfusion.

(j) **Electrophysiological studies**: Electrophysiological studies for risk stratification are not often performed, because except in special cases they are not useful.

(k) **Sudden death**: Sudden death in the post-infarction setting occurs (1) **in relation to a sustained ventricular tachycardia around the post-infarction scar**, which triggers VF. This is most frequent, especially, in patients with poor ventricular function, or (2) **as a consequence of a new acute ischaemic syndrome**.

Other data of clinical and prognostic interest with regard to the usefulness and the limitations of the ECG in the patients with chronic CHD are discussed later (see p. 304).

CHAPTER 10

Myocardial infarction without Q waves or equivalent: acute and chronic phase

In probably more than 50% of cases, an MI with normal intraventricular conduction and narrow QRS **does not show a Q wave of necrosis or equivalent (R in V1–V2). However, it may show anomalies in the mid-late part of QRS** (as low 'r' in lateral leads, rsr', slurrings, etc. (**fractioned QRS**)). **Also repolarisation changes may be recorded** especially in the acute phase. The incidence of MI without Q wave is variable depending on whether it is detected. In the emergency department it is higher and in the CCU lower.

All the types of MI without Q waves or equivalent are summarised in Table 10.1. This also includes the cases of MI without Q wave that present abnormal ventricular activation as BBB, WPW and pacemaker. These different types of MI without Q wave will be now discussed in detail.

Non-Q-wave myocardial infarction: ST-segment depression and/or negative T wave (Table 10.1)

Non-Q-wave MI presents occlusion of the coronary artery generally incomplete and the patient usually has significant previous ischaemia, even transmural but mainly at the subendocardial zone. Consequently, when the ischaemia increases (ACS), a TAP of poor quality is generated in the subendocardium, which explains the development of a subendocardial injury pattern (**ST-segment depression**) (Figures 4.5 and 4.8). Though the extension of the injury and, later, the infarction involve all or a large portion of the wall, it will not generate Q wave if the subepicardial inner area (close to the subendocardium), which is where begins the generation of infarction vector, is not involved by infarction (Figure 5.2D).

Sometimes the abnormality of repolarisation is an **isolated negative or flattened T wave**. These patterns are probably more related with partial or total reperfusion than with 'active' ischaemia. This may be an explanation of the best prognosis having non-Q-wave MI with negative T wave (p. 239). Furthermore, often **the levels of troponine are decisive to assure that an ACS has evolved to an MI** because the ECG pattern may not give the correct answer (see Figure 8.2, and Tables 2.1 and 8.1).

On the contrary, in **Q-wave infarction** the coronary artery occlusion is usually complete, and classically it was considered that the MI was transmural and often presents homogeneous wall involvement (QS pattern) or at least the infarction involves the subendocardium and also part of the subepicardium in contact with the subendocardium (QR pattern) (Figure 5.2C). CMR has demonstrated that often Q-wave MIs are not transmural and, on the contrary, often are transmural non-Q-wave MIs (Moon et al., 2004). The Q-wave MI often appear in a patient without very much prior ischaemia (first infarction). Consequently, an acute ischaemia (ACS) generates a poor-quality TAP in the entire wall that is recorded, from the precordium, as subepicardial injury pattern (ST-segment elevation) (Figures 4.5 and 4.8). Later, the myocardium becomes non-excitable and Q wave of necrosis develops (Figures 5.2B and 5.3).

Clinical and electrocardiographic presentation (Sclarovsky, 1999; Wellens, Gorgels and Doevendans, 2003)

Large infarctions exist within the non-Q-wave group of infarctions, including cases secondary to involvement of LMT that have not generated an

Table 10.1 Myocardial infarction without Q wave or equivalent.

1. **Non Q wave MI:** ST depression and/or negative T wave
2. **Other types of MI without Q wave**
    2.1 **Infarction located in an area, which does not generate Q wave of necrosis.**
        a) **Atria** (never single infarction): anteroseptal or more often extensive inferoposterior involvement. Usually present Q wave due to associated MI.
        b) **Right ventricle.** It is usually associated with an inferior wall MI. It is due to an occlusion of a proximal RCA before the RV branches and usually presents Q wave of inferior MI.
        c) **MI of basal areas of LV** (distal occlusion of the LCX or RCA). Usually without Q wave, but often with fractioned QRS pattern (see fig. 9.3, 9.4).
        d) **Microinfarction** (enzymatic). ECG usually normal.
    2.2 **Q wave MI, with Q that disappears during the follow-up (fig 5.46)**
    2.3 **Aborted MI with Q wave: Acute coronary syndrome (ACS) with ST elevation** (infarction in evolution) with early and efficient reperfusion. Rarely spontaneous thrombus resolution. Troponine level is decisive to separate unstable angina from MI without Q wave.
    2.4 **Masked Q wave.**
        a) Left bundle branch block
        b) Wolff-Parkinson-White syndrome } Often can present an abnormal Q wave
        c) Pacemaker

infarction Q wave. However, most of them are small infarctions. Currently, they likely represent more than 50% of all infarctions.

In acute phase, non-Q-wave infarction shows repolarisation changes (ST-segment depression and/or negative T wave)with non-pathological Q waves. Therefore, it is not accompanied by the electrocardiographic infarction Q-wave pattern (Figures 4.59–4.64). In the first part the diagnostic clues of ST-segment depression and negative T wave that are necessary to be considered as a criteria of NSTE-ACS have been discussed (p. 40 and 111) and also the prognostic implications of these patterns have already been commented on (p. 234). **Once the acute phase is past, some repolarisation changes can persist in the ECG, but these are generally less evident.** Sometimes the ECG can even return almost to normal despite quite marked repolarisation changes (Figure 10.1). **Table 8.1B shows the electrocardiographic patterns that may be seen in the NSTE-ACS** – ST depression and/or flat or negative T wave, or even a normal ECG.

It has classically been considered that non-Q-wave infarctions are not an indication for fibrinolytic therapy, although there is some controversy about it (Braunwald and Cannon, 1996; Table 8.2). They must undergo intensive medi-

cal antithrombotic therapy (AAS, heparin, IIB–IIIA inhibitors, etc.). The invasive treatment is necessary especially for cases of circumferential subendocardium involvement. For cases of regional involvement it may also be advisable (PURSUIT Trial, 1998), although there is some debate and the final decision has to be taken at individual level (p. 239).

In chronic phase, ECG of patients that have had non-Q-wave infarction is usually normal or presents mild abnormalities (flat T wave, slight ST-segment depression, etc.) (Figs. 4.60 and 4.63). Even the group of patients that present important occlusion of LMT may present normal or nearly normal ECG in approximately 30% of the cases (Fig. 8.19). Around 30% of the cases may present evident ST-segment depression in some leads, with ST-segment elevation in VR in not more than 15–20% of the cases.

Other types of MI without Q wave

On occasions, as it happens in MI of areas of late depolarisation, RV, atria or when the infarcted area is very small, the ECG does not generate Q wave of necrosis and may be completely normal or presents changes only in the last part of QRS or subtle

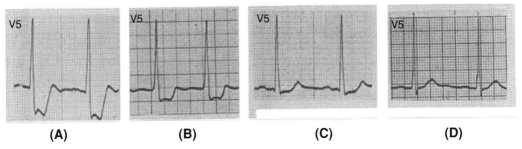

Figure 10.1 Evolution of non-Q-wave MI with important ST-segment depression at the beginning which normalises in few weeks (A–D).

changes of repolarisation. Now we will describe the most important ECG characteristics of these types of MIs.

Infarction of the basal parts of the left ventricle (areas of late depolarisation)

We have to remind that basal areas of LV depolarise after 40 milliseconds (Durrer et al., 1970; Figure 9.5), and therefore this MI does not generate Q wave or equivalent. On the contrary, different changes of mid-late part of QRS may appear (**fractioned QRS**) (Das et al., 2006). The most frequent isolated MIs involving the basal part of LV are lateral MI.

Isolated lateral infarction involving especially the inferior portion of the lateral wall is generally due to distal occlusion (posterobasal branch)of a non-dominant LCX or OM branch. Sometimes Q-wave infarction, which is seen as a tall R wave in V1 and/or V2, may be generated if the MI involves more than basal segment. It is useful to record the posterior leads in ECG (V7–V9) for the purpose of seeking the 'q' wave of this area (Casas, Marriott and Glancy, 1997; Matetzky et al., 1999). However, often when the infarction is localised in the more laterobasal portions, or even if it is more extensive, the ECG may be virtually normal (Figure 10.2, p. 292), or only showing small changes in the mid-late part of QRS (fractioned QRS) or small changes in repolarisation (Figures 9.3 and 9.4). The

usefulness of the new cardiac mapping techniques for the diagnosis of this type of infarctions has been published (Menown, McKenzie and Adgey, 2000).

Other isolated infarctions of basal segments of the anterior, septal and inferior walls are uncommon. Sometimes we have realised that MI of isolated segment 4, which was considered a typical posterior MI in the classical classification, presents a very low voltage of QRS in frontal plain with 'rsr' or 'qrs' patterns and a very small r wave in V1. The latter clearly demonstrates that the RS morphology in V1 is not due to necrosis of inferobasal segment (posterior wall) (Figure 10.3). In acute phase, STE-ACS involving the upper part of the septum generates apparent ST-segment changes (Figure 4.12), but not infarction Q waves, since the first depolarisation vector is generated in the mid-low septal portion, the high portion being electrically mute. Furthermore, especially the basal septal, inferior and also basal lateral walls may receive double perfusion (LAD + RCA in case of septal and RCA + LCX in case of inferior and LCX + LAD in case of lateral wall). This explains that often there is no transmural infarction in these segments in spite of complete occlusion.

An apparently normal or near-normal ECG in chronic phase may be considered probably abnormal if the following subtle changes are present:

A non-Q-wave infarction is an NSTE-ACS that presents increased enzyme levels. Some Q-wave infarctions are not transmural and on the contrary, some non-Q-wave infarctions are .

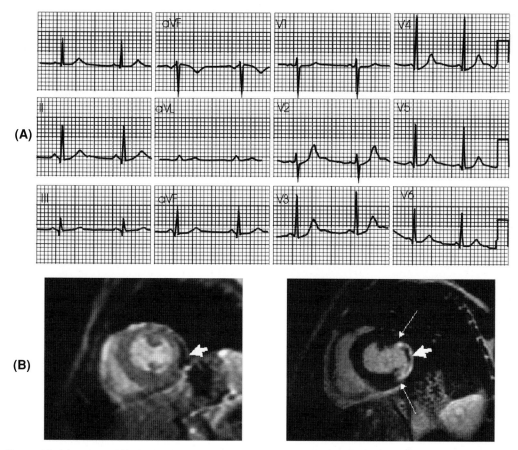

(A)

(B)

Figure 10.2 (A) A 46-year-old patient who had suffered an MI 2 years ago. The ECG does not show any abnormality in the QRS morphology and only the mild ST-segment depression and positive and symmetric T wave in V2 with rS morphology can suggest lateral ischaemia. (B) The CE-CMR demonstrated the presence of a lateral infarction without any clear abnormality in the ECG.

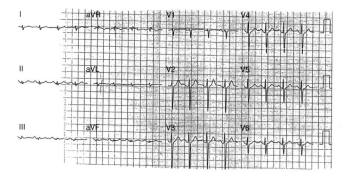

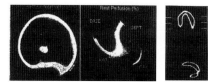

Figure 10.3 A 60-year-old patient that presented MI some months ago. According to the SPECT imaging (below) the MI affects predominantly segment 4 (inferobasal). In the FP cannot be seen evident Q wave, neither tall R in V1, although the low voltage of QRS in frontal plane with qrs or rSr′ pattern in inferior leads in a man without COPD suggests ischaemic heart disease.

(a) There is evidence of amputation of the R wave in I and VL (sequential ECG) (Figure 8.22).

(b) There is development of 'slurrings' or 'notches' of the final portions of the QRS complex in different leads (sometimes a 'slurred' S wave in II, III and VF or an r' wave in V1 or rsr' in II and V4–V6) (Figures 9.3 and 9.4).

(c) There is a very striking low voltage of QRS in frontal plane (Figure 10.3) with dubious 'q' wave (qrs, rsr'), in the inferior leads, in the absence of COPD, emphysema or other factors that may decrease the voltage of QRS.

(d) The presence in V1–V2 of a peaked tall T wave or mild ST-segment depression (<0.5 mm) with normal QRS complex (Figure 10.2).

Right-ventricular infarction (Figures 9.6 and 10.4)

This is secondary to **proximal occlusion of the right coronary artery** before the take-off of the marginal branches of the RV. Usually, this occlusion produces not only RV infarction, but also large left-ventricular infarction, more or less important, depending on the RCA being dominant or not (Figure 9.6) (Candell-Riera et al., 1981; López-Sendon et al., 1985). **Rarely, isolated RV infarctions have been described**, generally related to occlusion of very small right coronary artery. In this case ST-segment elevation in right precordial leads (V1–V3) is sometimes more striking than that in II, III and VF (Finn and Antman, 2003; Figure 10.4).

In the acute phase of STE-ACS of inferior wall (ST-segment elevation in II, III and VF), RV involvement may be suspected due to the presence of ST-segment elevation in the extreme right precordial leads (V3–V4R) with a positive T wave in V4R (Wellens and Connover, 2006). Changes in the extreme right precordial leads in STE-ACS of inferior wall are of value for the differential diagnosis between very proximal RCA occlusion with RV involvement (ST-segment elevation), non-proximal RCA occlusion (positive T wave) or LCX occlusion (negative T waves) (Figure 4.32).

These repolarisation changes in the extreme right precordial leads are seen only in the hyperacute phase of infarction. Therefore, their absence does not rule out the diagnosis of an RV infarction in the subacute phase. According to our experience,

the ST-segment isoelectric or elevated in V1 is also very useful for diagnosing extension of inferior MI to RV wall (Fiol et al., 2004a) (Figures 4.31 and 9.6).

In the presence of an ECG with chronic infarction of inferolateral wall (Q wave in II, III and VF, RS morphology in V1 and/or Q wave in I, VL and V6), there are no signs that suggest RV involvement in the standard leads (Figure 9.6). On certain occasions, an RV infarction may generate Q waves in the extreme right precordial leads, though in general these leads are not recorded.

From the prognostic standpoint, MIs of inferolateral zone with RV involvement – proximal occlusion of RCA – especially when the artery is dominant, have worst prognosis in the acute phase, as they potentially involve a very large myocardial area at risk. Consequently, carrying out an urgent coronary angiogram is mandatory (Figures 4.31 and 9.6).

Atrial infarction (Figures 10.5 and 10.6)

The atrial infarction occurs because an atrial branch, taking off usually from the RCA or LCX, is involved by occluded artery.

This infarction **never occurs in isolation** (Zimmerman, 1968). In acute phase of large inferolateral infarctions or, less frequently, of anteroseptal infarctions, the presence of PR-segment deviations, atrial arrhythmias and/or abnormal P waves (notched, irregular shape) suggests that atrial involvement has occurred. This probably occurs rarely, although this has to be studied with new image techniques (CE-CMR).

Regarding the most important ECG changes **in the acute phase, the atrial injury** (infarction) is expressed in different leads as PR depression and/or PR elevation (Figures 10.5 and 10.6). In 1961 Liu, Greenspan and Piccirillo (1961) published the following diagnostic criteria of atrial infarction: (a) PR-segment elevation ≥0.5 mm in leads V5–V6 with reciprocal depression in V1–V2; (b) PR-segment elevation ≥0.5 mm in lead I with reciprocal change in II and III; (c) PR-segment depression >1.5 mm in precordial leads and ≥1.2 mm in I, II and III associated with any atrial arrhythmias. Also, PR-segment elevation in VR is frequently seen in the presence of PR-segment depression in II

(A)

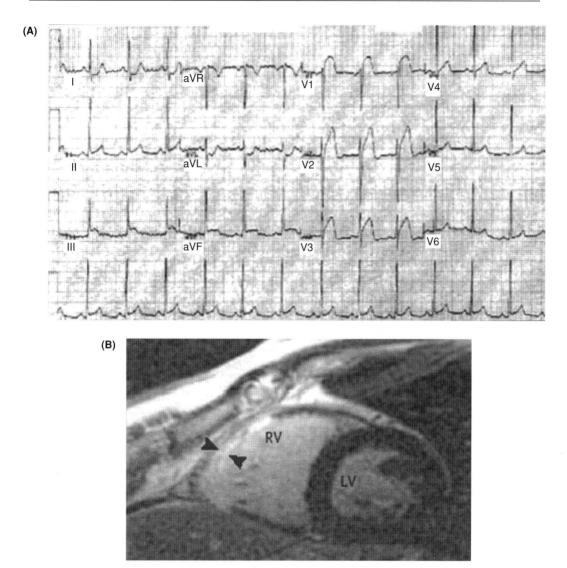

(B)

Figure 10.4 The occlusion of a short RCA produces an MI of the RV without any repercussion in LV. The ST-segment elevation in V1–V3 in the acute phase can be attributed to an ACS of the LAD, but the slight ST-segment elevation in II, III and VF suggests involvement of a short RCA. The cases of a distal LAD involvement (Figure 4.23) with ST-segment elevation in II, III and VF present ST-segment elevation in V3–V4 > V1, contrary to the RCA involvement proximal to RV branches, where ST-segment elevation in V1 > V3–V4. Additionally, in general, in an occlusion of a distal LAD is not seen ST-segment elevation in V1. (Taken from Finn and Antman, 2003.)

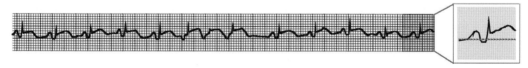

Figure 10.5 Lead II of a patient with acute inferior MI. Note the depression of the PR interval as a manifestation of atrial lesion (alteration of the atrial repolarisation) due to atrial infarction extension. Atrial arrhythmias, frequent in the atrial extension of an infarction, may also be seen.

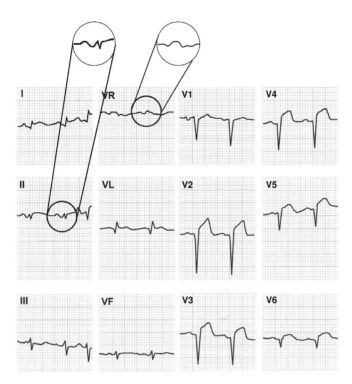

Figure 10.6 Patient with an extensive anterior MI in the subacute phase (QS- and ST-segment elevation in all the anterior leads and, additionally, a QR complex in I and VL). A PR-segment depression in II, with PR interval elevation in VR, is seen. These changes and the presence of frequent atrial arrhythmias suggest the atrial extension of the infarction.

(Figure 10.6). **However, no signs are present in the chronic phase that suggests the presence of atrial infarction.**

From the prognostic point of view, these usually correspond to large anteroseptal or inferolateral infarctions. In case of acute inferior MI the presence of PR-segment depression ≥1.2 mm in inferior leads has been demonstrated to be a marker of higher risk of in-hospital mortality and cardiac rupture (Jim et al., 2006) (Figure 10.6). Often these cases present supraventricular arrhythmias, especially atrial fibrillation.

Enzymatic myocardial infarction (necrosette)

The ESC/ACC (Alpert et al., 2000) consensus of the new definition of MI considers that an MI exists when enzymatic-level increase (troponins) is found in presence of anginal pain or its equivalent, even when no changes are found in the ECG (sub-ECG MI) (Wagner et al., 2000; Table 6.2). Therefore, more infarctions will be diagnosed than before. In our opinion, we should accept this new classification, though it implies some social, economic and

legal problems, because, although false-positive troponin cases exist (heart and renal failure, etc.), troponin levels increase in an adequate clinical context means myocardial infarction. However, the prognosis of infarctions, which present narrow QRS complex and normal ECG, even in the acute phase, is generally very good.

The Q-wave MI with Q that disappears during the follow-up

Some Q-wave infarctions may exhibit normal or near-normal ECG recordings in the chronic phase. They are usually but not always small septal, mid-anterior, inferior or lateral infarctions that, generally, in the acute phase exhibit ST-segment elevation in the corresponding leads, accompanied by a Q wave. Relatively often, especially in the inferolateral zone or in septal or mid-anterior infarction, the Q wave disappears over time (Figure 8.12; Bayés de Luna et al., 2006a–c).

On other occasions, Q wave disappears because it is cancelled out by the infarction vectors generated by an infarction that occurred in the opposite area, or because an intraventricular conduction defect developed, masking the Q wave (Figure 5.39).

Aborted MI with Q wave (Figure 8.9)

This is an ACS with ST-segment elevation that, due to early and efficient treatment, or perhaps, in some occasions due to spontaneous thrombus autolysis does not generate an infarction and consequently does not present Q wave (see p. 219, Figures 8.2 and 8.9, and Table 10.1).

Myocardial infarction with wide QRS

Many cases of MI in presence of wide QRS usually do not present Q waves or equivalents. However, the RBBB do not interfere with the presence of Q waves (see p. 170), and on the contrary in case of LBBB usually the Q waves are masked. The diagnosis of the electrocardiographic patterns of ischaemia, injury and infarction in the presence of a wide QRS complex has already been described in detail in pages 54 (ischaemia), 120 (injury) and 170 (infarction).

We have already commented (see 'MI with Q wave and wide QRS') (see p. 287) that the development of complete RBBB in STE-ACS involving the anteroseptal wall is due to very proximal occlusion of LAD. These are patients with a worse prognosis and should be closely followed (Figure 4.66). The presence of complete LBBB, especially when the QRS complex is very wide (Moss et al., 2002), is in itself a very poor prognostic sign. However this concept has to be reconsidered after the Wong's paper (2005) (p. 249).

CHAPTER 11

Clinical settings with anginal pain, outside the ACS

Here we are referring Tables 6.1-2, p. 197), to situations in which patients generally refer stable exertional anginal pain or, to certain situations, which, though they sometimes may present as an ACS, generally does not lead to urgent hospitalisation of patients. However, it is necessary to evaluate the situation as soon as possible, firstly to confirm if the pain is ischaemic in nature and secondly to know the pathophysiological explanation in order to decide which is the best therapeutic approach.

Classic exercise angina

Patients with stable angina chest pain are not included within the ACS. In most cases they correspond to classic exercise angina (Tables 2.1–2), and electrocardiographic changes are explained by the presence of a fixed – stable plaque – coronary artery stenosis limiting blood flow, which frequently presents smaller lumen but thicker fibrous cap than the plaque that produce an ACS (Figure 6.1A). The exercise decreases the already existing impaired subendocardium perfusion that however is not so important to change the basal ECG. We have to remind that the subendocardium is more vulnerable to myocardial ischaemia since its vasodilatory capacity is less. Therefore, during an exertional test an ST-segment depression may appear (subendocardial injury pattern) with or without angina (Figures 4.8A and 4.64). In these cases of stable angina the atherosclerotic plaque is stable, although the stenosis is frequently more important than the obstruction resulting from a vulnerable plaque before its rupture (Figure 6.1). However, it is less likely that an occlusion due to coronary thrombosis occurs, since the fibrous wall is usually thick and the risk of plaque rupture and exposure of the lipid core to the circulating blood is much lower (Figure 6.1); see Plate 5).

Therefore, **patients with chronic stable exercise angina are not an ACS**. However, at any given moment, their clinical situation may deteriorate and evolve to an ACS (pre-infarction angina). The electrocardiographic changes during and outside of anginal crises are the following:

• **The ECG at rest**: In 50% of the cases the ECG recording is normal, even in the presence of three-vessel disease. Evidence of a prior myocardial infarction in the ECG (infarction Q wave or equivalent) may or may not exist. The most frequent findings are a **negative or flattened T wave** (ECG pattern of subepicardial ischaemia) (Figure 4.64) or **ST-segment depression**, which usually is not evident (ECG pattern of subendocardial injury). Minor electrocardiographic changes (T-wave flattening or ST-segment rectification) may be explained by other causes, such as the early phase of left-ventricular enlargement, and may be frequently seen with no underlying cardiac disease. Also, sometimes, mixed patterns may be recorded (Fig. 3.27).

• **The ECG during exercise**: The ECG changes may be detected during exercise test (Figs. 4.62 and 4.64) or with Holter ECG (Figure 11.1). Holter technology may give the opportunity, as happens with the exercise test, to record the duration of the crisis and its relation with heart rate (Figure 11.2). Also, Holter technology records the crisis of angina due to anxiety, sympathetic overdrive, etc.

In patients with exercise angina in over 80–90% of cases, angina pain appears and the ECG is very often abnormal being the most frequent change an **ST-segment depression usually appearing in leads with predominant R wave** (Table 4.4) (Figures 4.57, 4.62 and 4.64). During both Holter monitoring

(A)   **(B)**

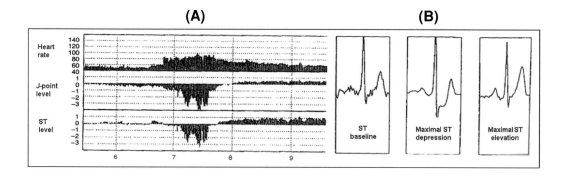

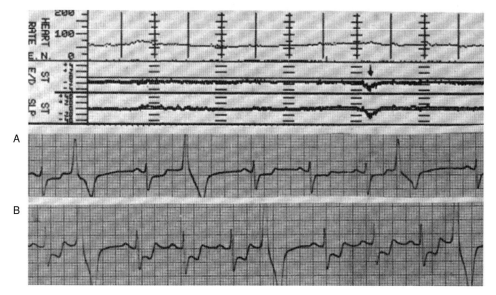

Figure 11.1 Above: Changes of the ST segment in a patient with exercise angina. (A) The trend of ST-segment changes and heart rate; (B) the different morphologies of ST. Below: Increase of ST-segment depression during angina (arrow and B) without increase in the number of PVC.

and exercise testing often the ECG changes appear without pain (see p. 302). On certain occasions, electrocardiographic changes are very mild, such as subtle T-wave changes. Their ischaemic origin may only be suggested if prior ECG recordings are available for comparison. The presence of ischaemia may be demonstrated by imaging techniques. Currently, the most used are isotopic studies (SPECT) (Figure 1.3). However, promising results may be obtained with CMR, and probably in the future the role of CMR in the detection of perfusion defects will be greater.

On rare occasions an ST-segment elevation due to coronary spasm may be seen during exercise test (Prinzmetal phenomenon) (Figure 11.3).

X syndrome

This syndrome is defined as a chest pain frequently of anginal characteristics that is related to small-vessel disease, in the absence of atherosclerotic lesions. It is more frequently seen in the female population, and probably but not always ischaemia is the origin of the chest pain (Kaski, 2004).

The resting ECG recording may be normal, or it may have non-specific ST-segment/T-wave changes. Often, typical X syndrome presents new electrocardiographic changes during the exercise test, with often perfusion defects (SPECT) (Figure 11.4). Sometimes the chest pain occurs at rest and may be considered an atypical ACS (see

(A)

(B)

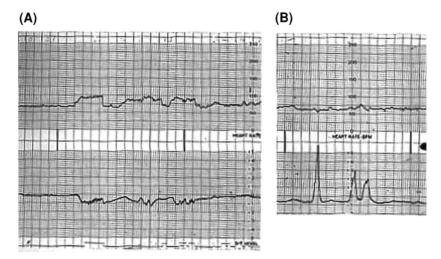

Figure 11.2 Trend of heart rate and ST-segment deviations in case of exercise angina (A). See the increase of heart rate and decrease of ST, and the plateau shape of the crisis. In case of Prinzmetal angina (B) the heart rate does not change and the crisis is shorter (triangle shape).

(A)

(B)

(C)

(D)

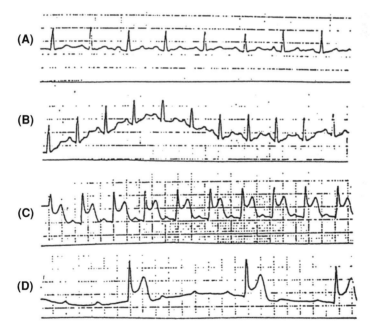

Figure 11.3 Exercise test in a patient with precordial pain. Before the exercise test (A) and during it (B), ST segment is normal. At the end, there is an important ST-segment elevation, accompanied by precordial pain (C), which was followed by advanced AV block (D).

Table 6.1, p. 274). Rarely, ST-segment elevation may occur, which is probably explained by multiple microcirculatory spasms. The prognosis is generally good and, in general, does not evolve to myocardial infarction.

Myocardial bridging

This is an anomaly of the course of the coronary arteries, especially the LAD, which partly penetrates epicardial muscular mass. It is frequently, though

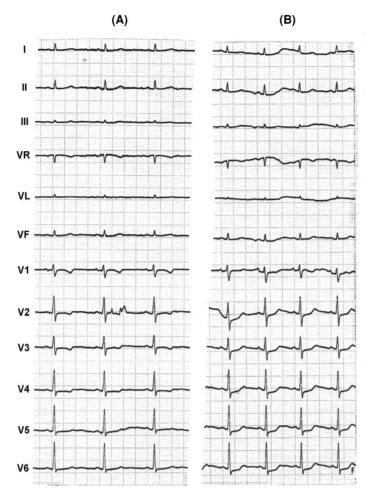

Figure 11.4 (A) A 60-year-old patient with typical X syndrome and normal coronary arteries. Observe the diffuse but moderate alterations of ST segment in the majority of the leads of the horizontal plane and the flattened T wave in the frontal plane. (B) After exercise testing an increase of ST-segment depression in HP may be seen.

not always, accompanied by atherosclerosis and/or coronary spasm.

The clinical picture is often stable exercise angina that may appear without ECG changes in a patient with usually normal basal ECG. On other occasion the anginal pain appears at rest probably in relation with coronary spasm related with myocardial bridging. Rarely, cases of ACS with or without myocardial infarction (with and without Q wave) have also been described. It has been linked exceptionally to sudden death, although in general the prognosis is good (Mohlenkamp et al., 2002).

Miscellaneous

Among the other causes that may induce chronic exercise anginal pain are the following:

1. Pulmonary hypertension: In this anginal pain is probably secondary to RV ischaemia.

2. The presence of anaemia: The most frequent ECG changes in chronic anaemia are unspecific ST-segment and T-wave changes, as well as tachycardia. **Chronic anaemia** is a marker of poor prognosis in the presence of heart failure (Mozafarrian, 2003). Additionally, **acute anaemia** may mimic true ACS (see p. 274).

3. Carbon monoxide poisoning: It may sometimes present chronic, anginal pain of non-atherothrombotic origin. On occasion it is presented as an ACS (see p. 274).

4. LVH and coronary perfusion: An imbalance between **LVH** and coronary perfusion may be the cause of anginal pain in AS and hypertrophic cardiomyopathy.

5. AIDS: Patients with AIDS frequently present with ischaemic heart diffuse, often very diffuse, which may originate exercise angina or myocardial infarction (p. 274).

CHAPTER 12

Silent ischaemia

There is no doubt that silent ischaemia, a term introduced by Stern and Tzivoni (1974), exists and represents lack of myocardial perfusion before the presence of pain or equivalents (Nesto and Kowaldruk, 1987) (ischaemic cascade – Figure 12.1). It is frequently seen in both patients with ACS and those with chronic IHD (Cohn, 1980, 2001; Cohn, Fox and Daly, 2003; Deanfield et al., 1984; Stern, 1998; Stern and Tzivoni, 1974).

Two types of silent ischaemia have been described. **Type I is when anginal pain is never present**, even during acute infarction. The Framingham study (Aguilar et al., 2006; Guidry et al., 1999; Kannel and Abbott, 1984) showed that half of the patients (20%) that in routine reviews performed every 2 years have presented new Q waves of necrosis never have had any type of chest pain suggesting angina. Thus, they were truly asymptomatic. These MIs have similar prognosis than MIs that are clinically recognised.

Type II represents that in **the global burden of ischaemia there are crises with and without anginal pain.** This is why the concept of 'total ischaemic burden' involving the sum of different periods of time with symptomatic (ST-segment changes plus pain) and asymptomatic (exclusively ST-segment changes) ischaemia was coined.

Silent ischaemia is present in different clinical setting of IHD. We have already commented that MI may be completely silent (Kannel and Abbott, 1984). **In patients with ACS admitted to the coronary care unit**, the presence of asymptomatic ST-segment changes has been shown by means of the Holter technique to be a marker of poor prognosis (Gottlieb et al., 1986). Other later studies confirmed these results. With Holter ECG we have demonstrated (Bayés de Luna et al., 1985) that **transient painless ST-segment elevation may also occur during a Prinzmetal crisis**. Sometimes in the same patient, different crises with ST-segment elevation or depression with or without pain are recorded (Figure 12.2).

In the chronic patient, silent ischaemia is very frequent during exercise (positive exercise stress test from an electrocardiographic standpoint, with no clinical manifestation), as well as in daily life (Holter ECG monitoring) (Bayés de Luna, Camacho and Guindo, 1989; Camacho, Guindo and Bayés de Luna, 1992; Theroux et al., 1979). ST-segment depressions, horizontal or of down-sloping greater than 0.5 mm for some authors or 1 mm for others, lasting for over 30 seconds, have been shown to correspond to myocardial ischaemia. In general they are not striking and are unaccompanied by arrhythmias. The prognostic significance in chronic patients of silent ischaemia detected by exercise testing or Holter technique is better than ischaemia with anginal pain. However, there is no doubt that it

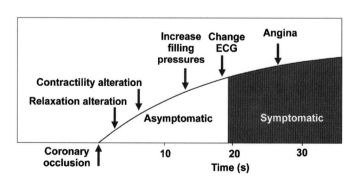

Figure 12.1 Ischaemic cascade. The figure shows the sequence of events in asymptomatic period before angina starts.

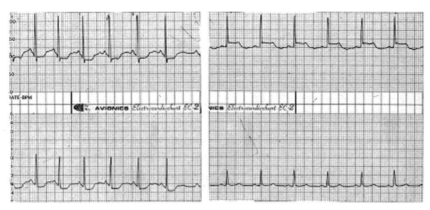

Figure 12.2 During Holter monitoring in a patient with ischaemic heart disease, crises often silent with ST-segment elevation or depression may be recorded.

should be treated and reduced as much as possible with drugs or even PCI if necessary. In the presence of very striking positive stress test, especially if is suggestive of LMT occlusion or three-vessel disease, an urgent coronary angiography may be recommended. On other occasions usually other non-invasive tests (SPECT and multislice scanning) and a global study of each case have to be performed.

However, it is necessary to remind that, with some frequency, the presence of an asymptomatic ST-segment depression at rest, or its development with no symptoms during daily life (Holter), or during exercise, even with evident ST-segment depression, may be seen in patients with normal coronary arteries (false positives) (Figure 4.58). Therefore, in these cases it is compulsory to perform a coronarography or multislice scanning in case of doubt to confirm the diagnosis.

CHAPTER 13

Usefulness and limitations of the ECG in chronic ischaemic heart disease

The **presence of wide QRS complexes** (bundle branch block and pacemaker), especially when the bundle branch block has developed during an ACS, is **in itself a poor prognosis marker, especially when the QRS is very wide**. New RBBB in ACS is suggestive of LAD occlusion proximal to S1 and D1. Furthermore, a chronic infarction in the presence of LBBB, Wolff–Parkinson–White syndrome or pacemaker is often impossible to diagnose by ECG. However, occasionally, there are evident suggestive electrocardiographic signs (see p. 172 and 197 and Figures 5.51 and 5.65). We have recently reported (Bayes-Genis, 2003) that patients with ischaemic DCM and complete LBBB exhibit QRS pattern in V2–V3 with low-voltage S wave and evident notches that are different from idiopathic DCM, which exhibit an rS morphology with deep S waves and without notches (Figure 13.1). Finally, the presence of inferior infarction plus SAH suggests two-vessel disease.

Left ventricular aneurysms (LVA) occurs currently in less than 4% of the cases of myocardial infarction. However, it is important to detect its presence because it is associated with ventricular arrhythmias and heart failure. In the past it has been associated with persistent ST-segment elevation and prominent R in VR (Bhatnagar, 1994; Cooley et al., 1958). However, the sensitivity and specificity of these findings are poor. The presence in coronary patients with narrow QR or fractioned QRS morphologies (rSR' pattern or its variants), especially in II and V3–V6 (Figure 13.2), has been considered a marker of LVA (Sherif, 1970). Recently Reddy et al. (2006) demonstrated that the specificity of these findings for LVA in patients with IHD is very high (>90%), although its sensitivity is much lower (50%).

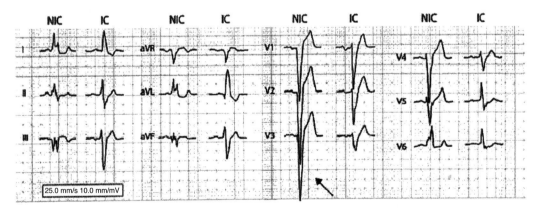

Figure 13.1 ECGs of two patients, one with non-ischaemic (NIC) and the other with ischaemic cardiomyopathy (IC). Both ECGs have a similar QRS width, LVEF and LVEDD. Note the pronounced voltages of right precordial leads, particularly V2 and V3 (arrow), in non-ischaemic cardiomyopathy compared with ischaemic cardiomyopathy.

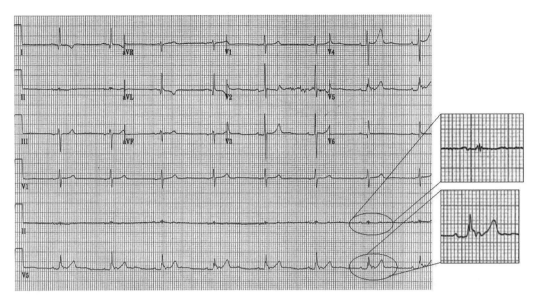

Figure 13.2 The ECG of a patient that has suffered two MIs of inferolateral zone and a two-bypass grafting surgery. The patient presents important left ventricular aneurysm. Observe the presence of RS in V1, q in lateral leads and abnormal morphology of QRS (fractioned QRS) in several leads (see amplified leads II and V5).

ECG recordings with **QS morphology in V1–V2 may be seen due to septal fibrosis** or in elderly patients. This pattern most probably corresponds to an old infarction when this is recorded in patients with chronic IHD and is accompanied by changes of repolarisation suggestive of ischaemia. **The presence of Q waves in certain leads does not rule out the presence of viability** in the correlated cardiac segments (Schinkel et al., 2002).

Different score systems have been developed to estimate, following a Q-wave infarction, its size and ventricular function (Hinohara et al., 1984; Pahlm et al., 1998; Palmeri et al., 1982; Selvester, Wagner and Hindman, 1985; Wagner and Hinohara, 1984). However, currently CE-CMR is the gold standard for measurement and characterisation of infarcted area (see 'Quantification of the infarcted area').

MRI has also demonstrated that there are transmural infarctions without Q waves and Q-wave infarctions that are not transmural (Moon et al., 2002) (see 'MI with or without Q waves or equivalents' p. 275). Furthermore, thanks to ECG–MRI correlations, we have published **a new classification of Q-wave MI** (Bayés de Luna et al., 2006a–c; Cino et al., 2006). Also, we have demonstrated that the presence of RS pattern in V1 in coronary patients is

due to lateral MI and not to posterior (inferobasal) MI and that QS pattern in VL without Q in V6 is due to mid-anterior MI and not due to high lateral MI (Figure 5.9).

In a patient with chronic coronary artery disease, normal ECG is frequently found. The ECG is normal in 25% patients with three-vessel disease (Figure 8.24). Also in patients with Q-wave infarction the Q wave may disappear over time. This may be explained by the following causes: (a) normalisation of ECG in the follow-up even in a case of extensive anterior infarction due to improved perfusion in the peri-infarction area provided by collateral circulation (Figure 8.12); (b) development of MI in opposite areas with cancellation of two vectors of infarction (Figures 5.38 and 5.39); (c) the presence of new intraventricular block, especially LBBB. Lastly, there are many cases of non-Q-wave MI that present in chronic phase a normal ECG or only with mild abnormality.

In a patient with chest pain **the presence of a tall and peaked T wave in V1–V2** has to be considered as possible expression of the hyperacute phase of STE-ACS (Figure 8.7).

The correlation between clinical presentation and electrocardiographic changes has shown (Framingham study) that **10–20% of the patients with**

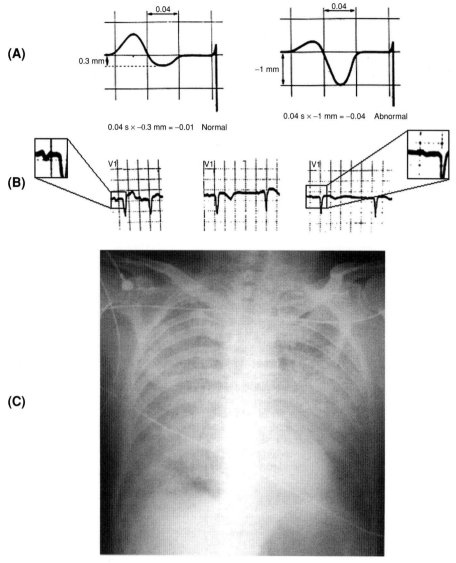

Figure 13.3 (A) A diagram showing a normal and an abnormal negative component of the P wave in V1. When the product of the width in seconds by the height in millimetres of the negative mode exceeds (in negativity) – 0.03, it is considered abnormal. (B) An example of pulmonary oedema (a) in acute phase of myocardial infarction (see X-ray in (C)). Twelve hours (b) and 3 days later (c), the ECG shows the reduction of the negative P mode in V1 with the clinical improvement is evident. This can be properly evaluated only when V1 lead is taken at the same site. In the hospital environment this can be insured by marking the site on patient's skin.

clinical evidence of myocardial infarction do not present suggestive electrocardiographic signs. Therefore, a normal ECG does not exclude the presence of an old infarction. In turn, around **10–20% of the patients with an ECG indicative of a Q-wave infarction had no history of prior infarction** (p. 302). This indicates the potential reversibility of the ECG pattern of myocardial infarction in the first group and the possibility that clinically silent myocardial infarctions may have occurred in the second group.

In patients with coronary artery disease, electrocardiographic evidence of **abnormal P wave**, similar to left atrial enlargement, is a marker of poor left ventricular function and prognosis (Rios, 1977).

We have recently shown that left atrial enlargement is a predictor of total and sudden death in patients with heart failure, of both ischaemic and idiopathic origin (Bayés-Genis et al., 2007). The electrocardiographic P-wave pattern of the left atrial enlargement (LAE) may be seen as a reversible pattern in acute pulmonary oedema (Figure 13.3). Likewise, the incidence of P-wave abnormalities is higher in coronary patients with multivessel disease.

The existence of a **negative U wave** in I, VL and/or V2–V6 in a patient with coronary artery disease with or without prior infarction in the ECG is very suggestive (90%) of significant LAD involvement (Figures 3.24–3.26).

In this book **the 'bull's-eye' view has been used**, dividing the heart into 17 segments (Cerqueira, Weissman and Disizian, 2002) to easily recognise the site of occlusion and anatomic location of the injury areas in the STE-ACS and infarction areas in chronic Q-wave infarction (Figures 1.14 and 5.9). We consider that the use of this approach is useful to realise at first glance the importance of myocardial area at risk in acute phase and of infarcted area in chronic phase.

CHAPTER 14

The ECG as a predictor of ischaemic heart disease

The ECG may be used for detecting CHD in the general population or predicting the presence of CHD in the future. The presence of depolarisation and repolarisation changes is of special importance (Cedres et al., 1982; Knutsen et al., 1988). In the Framingham study and in others, such as in the Charleston study, the **association between non-specific changes in ST segment and T wave with increased risk of CHD** has been demonstrated (Kannel et al., 1987; Sutherland et al., 1993). However, the ST segment and the T wave may be altered due to many causes other than CHD, e.g. alcohol intake, hyperventilation, etc. All this limits the usefulness of the isolated changes seen in the ST segment/T wave for the screening of the general population.

Therefore, **the association of other factors to the ST-segment/T-wave changes may be of great value.** The combination of high cholesterol levels alone or associated with other risk factors, such as tobacco use, left ventricular hypertrophy in the ECG, glucose intolerance, etc., better identifies male patients at risk of developing coronary artery disease and sudden death (Kannel and Abbott, 1984; West of Scotland Coronary Prevention Study, 1996; Figure 14.1). Multivariate logistic analysis in the Framingham study (Kannel and Abbott, 1984; Kannel et al., 1987), including all coronary risk factors, indicates that in males, age, systolic pressure, cigarette smoking, and relative body weight are all independently related to the incidence of sudden death. In females, aside from age, only hypercholesterolaemia and vital capacity are independently associated with an increased risk of sudden death (Figure 14.1). Using these parameters, there is a wide variation in the risk of sudden death. Forty-two per cent of sudden deaths in males and 53% in females occur in the tenth of the population in the top decile of multivariate risk. Furthermore,

microalbuminuria in patients with ST-segment/T-wave changes in the resting ECG has been reported to identify a subgroup of individuals at a higher risk of IHD and death from any cause (Diercks et al., 2002).

The isolated presence of **minor T-wave abnormalities has been considered a potential risk marker for future cardiovascular events.** This includes, among others, the following:

(a) Presence of flattened T wave in lead I: Its presence is a marker of bad prognosis (McFarlane and Coleman, 2004).

(b) presence of a TV1 > TV6 and TI < TIII: The TV1 > TV6 criterion in patients with chest pain with or without other ECG changes had been considered to be specific, but not very sensitive for one or more vessel diseases. However, prognostic value of TV1 > TV6 criterion is controversial. For some authors it may only be used as a marker of CHD and, especially, of LAD involvement in patients with chest pain or in those undergoing a coronary angiogram. Furthermore, the presence of a TV1 > TV6 did not have any statistically significant prognostic value for other authors.

In a recent study carried out on more than 10,000 patients who presented risk factors for CHD, and who were followed during more than 20 years (MRFIT study; Prineas et al., 2002), the presence of a flattened or minimally negative T wave in lateral or inferior lead (corresponding to the Minnesota Code 5, 3, 5, 4) has been shown to have prognostic value for future cardiovascular events.

• **Gender differences**: In spite of the fact that it is well known that women present significantly longer QT than men and that also other gender differences in QRS and ST/T parameters exist, few ECG criteria routinely use gender-specific diagnostic criteria (Okin, 2006). Recently (Rautaharju, 2006), the value of the computer-based ECG measurements

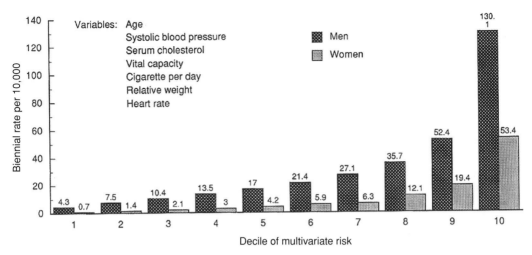

Figure 14.1 Risk of sudden death according to the multivariable risk decile.

for risk stratification in women has been demonstrated. This study shows that repolarisation abnormalities in post-menopausal women are important predictors of IHD events and mortality and of congestive heart failure.

• **Value of exercise test**: The response to exercise test has been studied for many years as a marker of ischaemic events in the future. Ellestad and Wen (1975) reported that the presence of ST-segment depression ≥ 1.5 mm predicted an incidence of new coronary event of 9.5% a year, as compared with 1.7% in those with a negative test. Furthermore, early onset of ECG abnormality or the presence of angina occurring during the exercise was associated with a higher incidence of coronary event, and therefore makes it compulsory to start the appropriate treatment, including the practice of coronariography.

References

Adgey AA, Oevlin JE, Webb SW, Mulholland HC. Initiation of ventricular fibrillation outside hospital in patients with acute ischaemic heart disease. Br Heart J 1982; 47: 55.

Akkerhuis KM, Klootwijd PA, Lindeboom W et al. Recurrent ischaemia during continuous multilead ST-segment monitoring identifies patients with acute coronary syndromes at high risk of adverse cardiac events: meta-analysis of three studies involving 995 patients. Eur Heart J 2001; 22: 1997.

Aldrich HR, Wagner NB, Boswick J et al. Use of initial ST-segment deviation for prediction of final electrocardiographic size of acute myocardial infarcts. Am J Cardiol 1988; 61(10): 749–53.

Alpert JS, Thygesen K, Antman E, Bassand JP. Myocardial infarction redefined – a consensus document of the Joint European Society of Cardiology/American College of Cardiology Committee for the redefinition of myocardial infarction. J Am Coll Cardiol 2000; 36: 959; Eur Heart J 2000; 21: 1502.

Alyanakian MA, Oehoux M, Chatel O et al. Cardiac troponin I in diagnosis of perioperative myocardial infarction after cardiac surgery. J Cardiothorac Vasc Anesth 1998; 12: 288.

Anderson RH, Razavi R, Taylor AM. Cardiac anatomy revisited. J Anat 2004; 205(3): 159–77.

Angelini P, Velasco JA, Flamm S. Coronary anomalies: incidence, pathophysiology, and clinical relevance. Circulation 2002; 105: 2449.

Anguera L, Miranda-Guardiola F, Bosch X et al. Elevation of serum levels of the anti-inflammatory cytokine interleukin-10 and decreased risk of coronary events in patients with unstable angina. Am Heart J 2002; 144: 811.

Antman EM, Anbe DT, Armstrong PW et al. ACCC/AHA guidelines for the management of patients with ST-elevation myocardial infarction: a report of the American College of Cardiology/American Heart Association Task Force on Practice Guidelines (Committee to Revise the 1999 Guidelines for the Management of patients with acute myocardial infarction). J Am Coll Cardiol 2004; 44: E1–211.

Antman EM, Cohen M, Bernink PJ et al. The TIMI risk score for unstable angina/non-ST elevation MI: a method for prognostication and therapeutic decision making. JAMA 2000; 284: 835.

Arbane M, Goy JJ. Prediction of the site of total occlusion in the left anterior descending coronary artery using admission electrocardiogram in anterior wall acute myocardial infarction. Am J Cardiol 2000; 85: 487.

Aros F, Boraita A, Alegria E et al. Guidelines of the Spanish Society of Cardiology for clinical practice in exercise testing. Rev Esp Cardiol 2000; 53: 1063. Article in Spanish.

August T, Mazzeleni A, Wolff L. Positional and respiratory changes in precordial lead patterns simulating acute myocardial infarction. Am Heart J 1958; 55: 706.

Bairey CN, Shah PK, Lew AS, Hulse S. Electrocardiographic differentiation of occlusion of the left circumflex versus the right coronary artery as a cause of inferior acute myocardial infarction. Am J Cardiol 1987; 60: 456.

Bar FW, Volders PG, Hoppener P et al. Development of ST-segment elevation and Q- and R- wave changes in acute myocardial infarction and the influence of thrombolytic therapy. Am J Cardiol 1996; 77: 337.

Barold SS, Falkoff MO, Ong LS, Heinle RA. Electrocardiographic diagnosis of myocardial infarction during ventricular pacing. Cardiol Clin 1987; 5: 403.

Barrabes J, Figueras J, Moure C, Cortadellas J, Soler Soler J. Prognostic significance of ST depression in lateral leads on admission ECG in patients with first acute myocardial infarction. J Am Coll Cardiol 2000; 35: 1813.

Bassan R, Potsch A, Maisel A et al. B-type natriuretic peptide: a novel early blood marker of acute myocardial infarction in patients with chest pain and no ST-segment elevation. Eur Heart J 2005; 26: 234.

Bayés de Luna A. Clinical Electrocardiography: A Textbook, 2nd edn. New York: Futura. Spanish version: Tratado de electrocardiografía clínica. Barcelona: Editorial Espaxs, 1999.

Bayés de Luna A (ed.). Electrocardiología Clínica. Barcelona: Editorial Científico-Médica, 1977.

Bayés de Luna A, Batchvarov V, Malik M. The morphology of the electrocardiogram. In: Camm J, Serruys P, Luscher J (eds.) Textbook of Cardiology. London: Blackwell, 2006b: 1.

Bayés de Luna A, Borras Torrada J, Gaursí Gené C, Balaguer Vintró I, Bentalbol G. Angina de pecho invertida. Rev Esp Cardiol 1971; 24: 305–10.

Bayés de Luna A, Camacho AM, Guindo J. Silent myocardial ischemia and ventricular arrhythmias. Isr J Med Sci 1989; 25: 542.

Bayés de Luna A, Carreras F, Cladellas M, Oca F, Sagues F, Garcia Moll M. Holter ECG study of the electrocardiographic phenomena in Prinzmetal angina attacks with emphasis on the study of ventricular arrhythmias. J Electrocardiol 1985; 18: 267.

Bayes de Luna A, Cino JM, Pujadas S et al. Concordance of electrocardiographic patterns and healed myocardial infarction location detected by cardiovascular magnetic resonance. Am J Cardiol 2006a; 97: 443.

Bayes de Luna A, Cino J, Kotzeva A et al. New ECG criteria of inferolateral myocardial infarction assessed by contrast enhanced-cardiovascular magnetic resonance based on the morphology of QRS in V1. Eur Heart J Supl 2006b; 27: 871. Abstract.

Bayés de Luna A, Coumel P, Leclercq JF. Ambulatory sudden cardiac death: mechanisms of production of fatal arrhythmia on the basis of data from 157 cases. Am Heart J 1989; 117: 151.

Bayés de Luna A, Fiol M, Antman E. The 12-Lead ECG in ST Elevation Myocardial Infarction: A Practical Approach for Clinicians. London: Blackwell, 2006.

Bayes de Luna A, Serra Grima HR, Oca Navarro F. Electrocardiografia de Holter. Barcelona: Editorial Científico-Médica, 1983.

Bayés de Luna A, Wagner G, Birnbaum Y et al. A new terminology for the left ventricular walls and for the location of myocardial infarcts that present Q wave based on the standard of cardiac magnetic resonance imaging: a statement for healthcare professionals from a committee appointed by the International Society for Holter and Non Invasive Electrocardiography. Circulation 2006c; 114: 1755.

Bayés-Genis A, Lopez L, Vinolas X et al. Distinct left bundle branch block pattern in ischemic and non-ischemic dilated cardiomyopathy. Eur J Heart Fail 2003; 5: 165–70.

Bayés-Genis A, Santalo-Bel M, Zapico-Muniz E et al. N-terminal probrain natriuretic peptide (NT-proBNP) in the emergency diagnosis and in-hospital monitoring of patients with dyspnoea and ventricular dysfunction. J Eur J Heart Fail 2004; 6: 301–8.

Bayes-Genis A, Vazquez R, Bayes de Luna A et al. For the MUSIC Study Group. Left atrial enlargement and NT-proBNP as predictors of sudden cardiac death in patients with heart failure. Eur J Heart Fail. 2007 Jun 12; [Epub ahead of print]

Bayley RH, La Due JS. Electrocardiographic changes of impending infarction, and the ischemia-injury pattern produced in the dog by total and subtotal occlusion of a coronary artery. Am Heart J 1944; 28: 54a.

Bayley RH, La Due JS, York DJ. Further observations on the ischemia-injury pattern produced in the dog by tempo-rary occlusion of a coronary artery, incomplete T diversion patterns, theophylline T reversion, and theophylline conversion of the negative T pattern. Am Heart J 1944; 27: 657b.

Bell J, Fox A. Pathogenesis of subendocardial ischemia. Am J Med Sci 1974; 268: 2.

Ben-Gal T, Herz I, Solodky A, Birnbaum Y, Sclarovsky S, Sagie A. Acute anterior wall myocardial infarction entailing ST elevation in V1: electrocardiographic and angiographic correlations. Clin Cardiol 1998; 21: 399.

Bertrand ME, Simoons ML, Fox KA et al. Management of acute coronary syndromes in patients presenting without persistent ST-segment elevation. Eur Heart J 2002; 23: 1809; Eur Heart J 2003; 24: 485.

Bertrand M, Spencer B. Acute Coronary Syndromes: A Handbook for Clinical Practice. Oxford: Blackwell, 2006.

Bhatnagar SK. Observations of the relationship between left ventricular aneurysm and ST segment elevation in patients with a first acute anterior Q wave myocardial infarction. Eur Heart J 1994; 15: 1500.

Biagini E, Elhendy A, Schinkel AF et al. Prognostic significance of left anterior hemiblock in patients with suspected coronary artery disease. J Am Coll Cardiol 2005; 46: 858.

Bigger JT, Fleiss JL, Kleiger R, Miller JP, Rolnitzky LM. The relationships among ventricular arrhythmias, left ventricular dysfunction, and mortality in the 2 years after myocardial infarction. Circulation 1984; 69: 250.

Birnbaum Y. The burden of nonischemic ST-segment elevation. J Electrocardiol 2007; 40: 6–9.

Birnbaum Y, Atar S. Electrocardiogram risk stratification of non ST elevation acute coronary syndrome. J Electrocardiol 2006; 39: 558.

Birnbaum Y, Hasdai D, Sclarovsky S, Herz I, Strasberg B, Rechavia E. Acute myocardial infarction entailing ST segment elevation in lead AVL: electrocardiographic differentiation among occlusion of the left anterior descending, first diagonal and first obtuse marginal coronary arteries. Am Heart J 1996a; 131: 38.

Birnbaum Y, Herz I, Sclarovsky S et al. Prognostic significance of the admission electrocardiogram in acute myocardial infarction. J Am Coll Cardiol 1996b; 27: 1128.

Birnbaum Y, Sclarovsky S, Blum A, Mager A, Gabbay U. Prognostic significance of the initial electrocardiographic pattern in a first acute anterior wall myocardial infarction. Chest 1993; 103: 1681.

Birnbaum Y, Solodky A, Herz I et al. Implications of inferior ST segment depression in anterior acute myocardial infarction: electrocardiographic and angiographic correlation. Am Heart J 1994; 127: 1467.

Bjorklund E, Stenestrand U, Lindback J, Svensson L, Wallentin L, Lindahl B; the RIKS-HIA Investigators Prehospital diagnosis and start of treatment reduces time delay and mortality in real-life patients with STEMI. J Electrocardiol 2005; 38: 186.

Blackburn H, Keys A, Simonson E, Rautaharju P, Punsar S. Electrocardiogram in population studies: a classification system. Circulation 1960; 21: 1160.

Blackwell GB, Cranney GB, Pohost GM. Slide Atlas of MRI: Cardiovascular System. London: Gower Medical, 1993.

Bogaty P, Boyer L, Rousseau L, Arsenault M. Is anteroseptal myocardial infarction an appropriate term? Am J Med 2002; 113: 37.

Bonnefoy E, Godon P, Kirkorian G, Fatemi M, Chevalier F, Touboul P. Serum cardiac troproponin I and ST-segment elevation patients with acute pericarditis. Eur Heart J 2000; 21: 798.

Bough E, Boden W, Kenneth K, Gandsman E. Left ventricular asynergy in electrocardiographic 'posterior' myocardial infarction. J Am Coll Cardiol 1984; 4: 209.

Brandt RR, Hammill ST, Higano ST. Images in cardiovascular medicine: electrocardiographic diagnosis of acute myocardial infarction during ventricular pacing. Circulation 1998; 97: 2274.

Braunwald E, Antman EM, Beasley JW et al. ACC/AHA guidelines for the management of patients with unstable angina and non-ST-segment elevation myocardial infarction: executive summary and recommendations: a report of the American College of Cardiology/American Heart Association task force on practice guidelines (Committee on the Management of Patients with Unstable Angina). Circulation 2000; 102: 1193.

Braunwald E, Cannon CP. Non-Q wave and ST segment depression myocardial infarction: is there a role for thrombolytic therapy? J Am Coll Cardiol 1996; 27: 1333.

Braunwald E, Zipes DP, Libby P. A Textbook of Cardiovascular Medicine. Philadelphia: WB Saunders, 1998.

Brodie BR, Hansen C, Stuckey TD et al. Door-to-balloon time with primary percutaneous coronary intervention for acute myocardial infarction impacts late cardiac mortality in high-risk patients and patients presenting early after the onset of symptoms. J Am Coll Cardiol 2006; 47: 289.

Burnes JE, Ghanem RN, Waldo AL, Rudy Y. Imaging dispersion of myocardial repolarization, 1. Comparison of body-surface and epicardial measures. Circulation 2001; 104: 1299.

Cabrera E. Teoría y práctica de la electrocardiografía. México DF: La Prensa Médica Mexicana, 1958.

Camacho AN, Guindo J, Bayés de Luna A. Usefulness of silent subendocardial ischemia detected by ST-segment depression in postmyocardial infarction patients as a predictor of ventricular arrhythmias. Am J Cardiol 1992; 69: 1243.

Camm AJ, Lüscher TF, Serruys PW (eds.). The ESC Textbook of Cardiovascular Medicine. Oxford: Blackwell, 2006.

Candell-Riera F, Figueras J, Valle V et al. Right ventricular infarction: relationships between ST segment elevation in V4R and hemodynamic, scintigraphic and echocardiographic findings in patients with acute inferior myocardial infarction. Am Heart J 1981; 101: 281.

Candell-Riera J, Rodriguez J, Puente A, Pereztol-Valdes O, Castell-Conesa J, Aguade-Bruix S. Myocardial perfusion (SPECT) in patients with non-Q-wave myocardial infarction. Med Clin (Barc) 2005; 125: 574. Spanish.

Cannon CP. Defining acute myocardial infarction by ST segment deviation. Eur Heart J 2000; 21: 266.

Cannon CP. Management of Acute Coronary Syndromes. New Jersey: Humana, 2003.

Casas RE, Marriott HJ, Glancy DL. Value of leads V7–V9 in diagnosing posterior wall acute myocardial infarction and other causes of tall R waves in V1–V2. Am J Cardiol 1997; 80: 508.

Castellanos A, Zoble R, Procacci PM, Myerburg RJ, Serkovits SV. St-qR pattern: new sign for diagnosis of anterior myocardial infarction during right ventricular pacing. Br Heart J 1973; 35: 1161.

Cedres SL, Liu K, Stamler J et al. Independent contribution of electrocardiographic abnormalities to risk of death from coronary heart disease, cardiovascular diseases and all causes: findings of three Chicago epidemiologic studies. Circulation 1982; 65: 146.

Cerqueira MD, Weissman NJ, Disizian V. Standardized myocardial segmentation and nomenclature for tomographic imaging of the heart: a statement for healthcare professionals from the Cardiac Imaging Committee of the Council on Clínical Cardiology of the American Heart Association. Circulation 2002; 105: 539.

Chiladakis JA, Karapanos G, Davlouros P, Aggelopoulos G, Alexopoulos D, Manolis AS. Significance of R-on-T phenomenon in early ventricular tachyarrhythmia susceptibility after acute myocardial infarction in the thrombolytic era. Am J Cardiol 2000; 85: 289.

Chou TCH, Helm R, Kaplan S. Clinical Electrocardiography. New York: Grune & Stratton, 1974.

Cinca J, Janse MJ, Morena H et al. Mechanism and time course of the early electrical changes during acute coronary artery occlusion. Chest 1980; 77: 499.

Cino JM, Pujadas S, Carreras F et al. Utility of contrast-enhanced cardiovascular magnetic resonance (CE-CMR) to assess how likely is an infarct to produce a typical ECG pattern. J Cardiovasc Magn Reson 2006; 8: 335.

Cohen M, Scharpf SJ, Rentrop KP. Prospective analysis of electrocardiographic variables as markers for extent and location of acute wall motion abnormalities observed during coronary angioplasty in human subjects. J Am Coll Cardiol 1987; 10: 17.

Cohn PF. Silent myocardial ischemia in patients with a defective anginal warning system. Am J Cardiol 1980; 45: 697.

Cohn PF. The value of continuous ST segment monitoring in patients with unstable angina. Eur Heart J 2001; 22: 1972.

Cohn PF, Fox KM, Daly C. Silent myocardial ischemia. Circulation 2003; 108: 1263.

Coksey J, Massie E, Walsh T. Clinical ECG and Vectocardiography. Chicago: Year Book Medical, 1960.

Coleman DL, Ross TF, Naughton JL. Myocardial ischemia and infarction related to recreational cocaine use. West J Med 1982; 136: 444.

Collinson J, Flather MO, Fox KA et al. Clinical outcomes, risk stratification and practice patterns of unstable angina and myocardial infarction without ST elevation: Prospective Registry of Acute Ischaemic Syndromes in the UK (PRAIS-UK). Eur Heart J 2000; 21: 1450.

Cooley DA, Collins HH, Morris GC, Jr, Chapman DW. Ventricular aneurysm after myocardial infarction: surgical excision with use of temporary cardiopulmonary bypass. J Am Med Assoc 1958; 167: 557.

Cooper HA, de Lemos JA, Morrow DA et al. Minimal ST-segment deviation: a simple, noninvasive method for identifying patients with a patent infarction-related artery after fibrinolytic administration. Am Heart J 2002; 144: 790.

Corbalan R, Prieto JC, Chavez E, Nazzal C, Cumsille F, Krucoff M. Bedside markers of coronary artery patency and short-term prognosis of patients with acute myocardial infarction and thrombolysis. Am Heart J 1999; 138: 533.

Correale E, Sattista R, Ricciardíello V, Martone A. The negative U wave: apathogenetic enigma but a useful, often overlooked bedside diagnostic and prognostic clue in ischemic heart disease. Clin Cardiol 2004; 27: 674.

Crimm A, Severance HW, Coffey K et al. Prognostic significance of isolated sinus tachycardia during first three days of acute myocardial infarction. Am J Med 1984; 76: 983.

Curtis JP, Portnay EL, Wang Y et al.; National Registry of Myocardial Infarction-4. The pre-hospital electrocardiogram and time to reperfusion in patients with acute myocardial infarction, 2000–2002: findings from the National Registry of Myocardial Infarction-4. J Am Coll Cardiol 2006; 47(8): 1544.

Das MK, Khan B, Jacob S, Kumar A, Mahenthiran J. Significance of a fragmented QRS complex versus a Q wave in patients with coronary artery disease. Circulation 2006; 113: 2495.

Davies MJ. Stability and instability: two faces of coronary atherosclerosis. The Paul Dudley White Lecture 1995. Circulation 1996; 94(8): 2013.

De Chantal M, Diodati JG, Nasmith JB et al. Progressive epicardial coronary blood flow reduction fails to produce ST-segment depression at normal heart rates. Am J Physiol Heart Circ Physiol 2006; 291(6): H2889–96.

De Winter RJ, Windhausen F, Cornel JH et al.; Invasive versus Conservative Treatment in Unstable Coronary Syndromes (ICTUS) Investigators. Early invasive versus selectively invasive management for acute coronary syndromes. N Engl J Med 2005; 353: 1095.

De Zwan C, Bär H, Wellens HJ. Characteristic ECG pattern indicating a critical stenosis high in left anterior descending coronary artery in patients admitted because of an impending infarction. Am Heart J 1982; 103: 730.

Deanfield JE, Shea M, Ribiero P et al. Transient ST-segment depression as a marker of myocardial ischemia during daily life. Am J Cardiol 1984; 54: 1195.

Dellborg M, Topol EJ, Swedberg K et al. Dynamic QRS complex and ST segment vectorcardiographic monitoring can identify vessel patency in patients with acute myocardial infarction treated with reperfusion therapy. Am Heart J 1991; 122: 943.

Demoulins J, Kulbertus H, Histopathologic correlates of the left posterior fascicular block. Am J Card 1979; 44: 1083.

Denes P, Pick A, Muller R, Pieetros R, Rosen KM. A characteristic precordial repolarization abnormality in patient with intermittent left bundle branch block. Ann Intern Med 1978; 89: 55.

Diderholm E, Andren B, Frostfeldt G et al. ST depression in ECG at entry indicates severe coronary lesions and large benefits of an early invasive treatment strategy in unstable coronary artery disease: the FRISC II ECG substudy. The fast revascularisation during instability in coronary artery disease. Eur Heart J 2002; 23: 41.

Diercks GF, Hillege HL, van Boven AJ et al. Microalbuminuria modifies the mortality risk associated with electrocardiographic ST-T segment changes. J Am Coll Cardiol 2002; 40: 1401.

Doevendans PA, Gorgels AP, van der Zee R, Partouns J, Bar FW, Wellens HJ. Electrocardiographic diagnosis of reperfusion during thrombolytic therapy in acute myocardial ifnarction. Am J Cardiol 1995; 75: 1206–10.

Dowdy L, Wagner GS, Birnbaum Y et al. Aborted infarction: the ultimate myocardial salvage. Am Heart J 2004; 147: 390.

Dressler W, Roesler H, Higb T. Waves in the earliest stage of myocardial infarction. Am Heart J 1947; 34: 627.

Dumont CA, Monserrat L, Soler R et al. Interpretation of electrocardiographic abnormalities in hypertrophic cardiomyopathy with cardiac magnetic resonance. Eur Heart J 2006; 27(14): 1725–31.

Dunn W, Edwards J, Pruitt R. The electrocardiogram in infarction of the lateral wall of the left ventricle: a clinicopathological study. Circulation 1956; 14: 540.

Dunn RF, Newman HN, Bernstein L et al. The clinical features of isolated left circumflex coronary artery disease. Circulation 1984; 69: 477.

Durrer D, Van Dam R, Freud G, Jame M, Meijler F, Arzbaecher R. Total excitation of the isolated human heart. Circulation 1970; 41: 899.

East T, Oran S. The ECG in ventricular aneurysm following acute infarction. Br Heart J 1952; 14: 125.

Edmond JJ, French JK, Stewart RA et al.; HERO-2 Investigators. Frequency of recurrent ST-elevation myocardial infarction after fibrinolytic therapy in a different territory as a manifestation of multiple unstable coronary arterial plaques. Am J Cardiol 2006; 97: 947.

Ellestad H. Stress testing: problems and appropriate use in acute coronary syndromes. Am J Cardiol 2004; 94: 1534.

Ellestad M, Wen M. Predictive implications of stress testing: follow-up of 2700 subjects after maximum treadmill stress testing. Circulation 1975; 51(2): 363.

Elsman P, Van't Hof AW, de Boer MJ et al. Impact of infarct location on left ventricular ejection fraction after correction for enzymatic infarct size in acute myocardial infarction treated with primary coronary intervention. Am Heart J 2006; 151: 1239.e9–14.

Engblom H, Wagner G, Setser R et al. Development and validation of techniques for quantitative clinical assessment of myocardial infarction by electrocardiography and MRI. J Electrocardiol 2002; 35: 203.

Engblom H, Wagner G, Setser R et al. Quantitative clinical assessment of chronic anterior myocardial infarction with delayed enhancement magnetic resonance imaging and QRS scoring. Am Heart J 2003; 146: 359.

Engelen DJ, Gorgels AP, Cheriex EC et al. Value of the electrocardiogram in localizing the occlusion site in the left anterior descending coronary artery in acute anterior myocardial infarction. J Am Coll Cardiol 1999; 34: 389.

Erhardt L, Herlitz J, Bossaert L et al. Task force on the management of chest pain. Eur Heart J 2002; 23: 1153.

Eskola MJ, Nikus KC, Niemela KO, Sclarovsky S. How to use ECG for decision support in the catheterization laboratory: cases with inferior ST elevation myocardial infarction. J Electrocardiol 2004; 37: 257.

Figueras J, Curos A, Cortadellas J, Sans M, Soler-Soler J. Relevance of electrocardiographic findings, heart failure, and infarct site in assessing risk and timing of left ventricular free wall rupture during acute myocardial infarction. Am J Cardiol 1995; 76: 543.

Finn A, Antman E. Images in clinical medicine: isolated right ventricular infarction. N Engl J Med 2003; 349: 17.

Fiol M (ed.). Arritmias cardíacas en el paciente crítico. Barcelona: Edika-med SA, 2001.

Fiol M, Barcena JP, Rota JI et al. Sustained ventricular tachycardia as a marker of inadequate myocardial perfusion during the acute phase of myocardial infarction. Clin Cardiol 2002; 25: 328.

Fiol M, Carrillo A, Cygankiewicz I et al. New criteria based on ST changes in 12 leads surface ECG to detect proximal vs distal right coronary artery occlusion in case of an acute inferoposterior myocardial infarction. Ann Noninvasive Electrocardiol 2004a; 9: 383.

Fiol M, Cino J. Carrillo A, et al. The value of an algorithm based on ST segment deviations to locate the place of occlussion in left anterior descending coronary artery 2007. Submitted.

Fiol M, Cino J, Carrillo A, I et al. The value of an algorithm based on ST segment deviations to locate the place of occlussion in left anterior descending coronary artery in case of ST-segment elevation-myocardial infarction 2007. Submitted.

Fiol M, Cygankiewicz I, Bayés-Genis A et al. The value of ECG algorithm based on 'ups and downs' of ST in assessment of a culprit artery in evolving inferior myocardial infarction. Am J Cardiol 2004b; 94: 709.

Fiol M, Cygankiewicz I, Guindo J et al. The value of ECG algorithm based on 'ups and downs' of ST in assessment of a culprit artery in evolving inferior myocardial infarction. Ann Noninvasive Electrocardiol 2004c; 9: 180.

Fiol M, Marrugat J, Bayes de Luna A, Bergada J, Guindo J. Ventricular fibrillation markers on admission to the hospital for acute myocardial infarction. Am J Cardiol 1993; 71: 117.

Fiol M, Marrugat J, Bergada J, Guindo J, Bayés de Luna A. QT dispersion and ventricular fibrillation in acute myocardial infarction. Lancet 1995; 346: 1424.

Flugelman MY, Flugelman AA, Rozenman J et al. Prediction of atrial and ventricular fibrillation complicating myocardial infarction from admission data: a prospective study. Clin Cardiol 1987; 10: 503.

Friedman HH. Diagnostic electrocardiography and vectorcardiography. New York: McGraw-Hill, 1985: 241.

Fuster V, Topol E. Atherosclerosis and Coronary Artery Disease. Philadelphia: Lippincott-Raven, 1996.

Gallik DM, Obermueller SD, Swarna US, Guidry GW, Mahmarian JJ, Verani MS. Simultaneous assessment of myocardial perfusion and left ventricular dysfunction during transient coronary occlusion. J Am Coll Cardiol 1995; 25: 1529.

Gardner PI, Ursell PC, Fenoglio JJ, Wit AL. Electrophysiologic and anatomic basis for fractionated electrograms recorded from healed myocardial infarcts. Circulation 1985; 72: 596.

Gensini GF, Fusi C, Conti AA et al. Cardiac troponin I and Q-wave perioperative myocardial infarction after coronary artery bypass surgery. Crit Care Med 1998; 26: 1986.

Gersh B, Rahimtoola SH. Acute Myocardial Infarction. New York: Elsevier, 1991.

Giannuzzi P, Imparato A, Luigi P, Santoro F, Tavazzi L. Inaccuracy of various proposed electrocardiographic criteria in the diagnosis of apical myocardial infarction – a critical review. Eur Heart J 1989; 10: 880.

Gibbons RJ, Balady GJ, Timothy Bricker J et al. ACC/AHA 2002 guideline update for exercise testing: summary article. J Am Coll Cardiol 2002; 40: 1531.

Goldman MJ. Principles of Clinical Electrocardiography. San Fracisco: LPM, 1964.

Gomez-Hospital JA, Cequier A. The reality of invasive strategies in non-ST-elevation acute coronary syndrome. Rev Esp Cardiol 2004; 57: 1133.

Goodman SG, Langer A, Ross AM. Non-Q-wave versus Q-wave myocardial infarction after thrombolytic therapy: angiographic and prognostic insights from the global utilization of streptokinase and tissue plasminogen activator for occluded coronary arteries-I angiographic substudy. GUSTO-I Angiographic Investigators. Circulation 1998; 97: 444.

Gorgels AP, Engelen DJHJ. Lead aVR, a mostly ignored but very valuable lead in clinical 2003; 38: 1355.

Gottlieb SO, Weisfeldt ML, Ouyang P, Mellits ED, Gerstenblith G. Silent ischemia as a marker for early unfavorable outcomes in patients with unstable angina. N Engl J Med 1986; 314: 1214.

Guidelines for Interpreting rest ECG. Arq Bras Card 2003; 80: 1.

Guidry UC, Evans JC, Larson MG, Wilson PW, Murabito JM, Levy D. Temporal trends in event rates after Q-wave myocardial infarction: the Framingham Heart study. Circulation 1999; 100: 2054.

Guizton LE, Lacks MM. The differential diagnosis of acute pericarditis from normal variant: new ECG criteria. Circulation 1982; 65: 1004.

Haraphongse M, Tanomsup S, Jugdutt BI. Inferior ST segment depression during acute anterior myocardial infarction: clinical and angiographic correlations. J Am Coll Cardiol 1984; 4: 467.

Harpaz D, Behar S, Gottlieb S et al. Complete atrioventricular block complicating acute myocardial infarction in the thrombolytic era. SPRINT Study Group and the Israeli Thrombolytic Survey Group. Secondary Prevention Reinfarction Israeli Nifedipine Trial. J Am Coll Cardiol 1999; 34: 1721.

Hasdai D, Behar S, Wallentin L et al. A prospective survey of the characteristics, treatments and outcomes of patients with acute coronary syndromes in Europe and the Mediterranean basin: the Euro Heart Survey of Acute Coronary Syndromes (Euro Heart Survey ACS). Eur Heart J 2002; 23: 1190.

Hathaway W, Peterson E, Wagner G et al. Prognostic significance of the initial electrocardiogram in patients with acute myocardial infarction. Clin Cardiol 1998a; 279: 387.

Hathaway WR, Peterson ED, Wagner GS et al. Prognostic significance of the initial electrocardiogram in patients with acute myocardial infarction. GUSTO-I Investigators. Global Utilization of Streptokinase and t-PA for Occluded Coronary Arteries. JAMA 1998b; 279: 387.

Hazinsky M, Cummis R, Field J. Handbook of Emergency Cardiovascular Care for Healthcare Providers. Dallas, TX: American Heart Association, 2000.

Hecht HS. Practice guidelines for electron beam tomography: a report of the Society of Atherosclerosis Imaging. Am J Cardiol 2000; 86: 705.

Heeschen E, Hamm CW, Mitrovic V, Lantelme NH, White HO. N-terminal pro-B-type natriuretic peptide levels for dynamic risk stratification of patients with acute coronary syndromes. Circulation 2004; 110: 3206.

Hellertein A, Katz C. The electrical effects of injury at various myocardial locations. Am Heart J 1948; 36: 184.

Henry TD, Atkins JM, Cunningham MS et al. ST-segment elevation myocardial infarction: recommendations on triage of patients to heart attack centers: is it time for a national policy for the treatment of ST-segment elevation myocardial infarction? J Am Coll Cardiol 2006; 47: 1339–45.

Herman MV, Ingram DA, Levy JA et al. Variability of electrocardiographic precordial lead placement: a method to improve accuracy and reliability. Clin Cardiol 1991; 14: 469.

Herz I, Assali AR, Adler Y, Solodky A, Sclarovsky S. New electrocardiographic criteria for predicting either the right or left circumflex artery as the culprit coronary artery in inferior wall acute myocardial infarction. Am J Cardiol 1997; 80: 1343.

Hindman NB, Schocken DD, Widmann M et al. Evaluation of a QRS scoring system for estimating myocardial infarct size. V: specificity and method of application of the complete system. Am J Cardiol 1985; 55: 1485.

Hinohara T, Hindman NB, White RO, Ideker RE, Wagner GS. Quantitative QRS criteria for diagnosing and sizing myocardial infarcts. Am J Cardiol 1984; 53: 875.

Hoffman I, Mehta J, Hilserath J et al. Anterior conductions delay: A possible cause for prominent anterior QRS forces. J Electrocardiology 1976; 9: 15.

Holmvang L, Clemmensen P, Wagner G, Grande P. Admission standard electrocardiogram for early risk stratification in patients with unstable coronary artery disease not eligible for acute revascularization therapy: a TRIM substudy. Thrombin inhibition in myocardial infarction. Am Heart J 1999; 137: 24.

Holper EM, Antman EM, McCabe CH et al. A simple, readily available method for risk stratification of patient with unstable angina and non-ST elevation myocardial infarction. Am J Cardiol 2001; 87: 1008.

Homs E, Martí V, Guindo J et al. Automatic measurement of corrected QT interval in Holter recordings: comparison of its dynamic behavior in patients after myocardial infarction with and without life-threatening arrhythmias. Am Heart J 1997; 134: 181.

Hopenfeld B, Stinstra JG, Macleod RS. Mechanism for ST depression associated with contiguous subendocardial ischemia. J Cardiovasc Electrophysiol 2004; 15: 1200.

Horáček BM, Warren JW, Albano A et al. Development of an automated Selvester Scoring System for estimating the size of myocardial infarction from the electrocardiogram. J Electrocardiol 2006; 39(2): 162–8.

Horan L, Flowers N. Diagnostic value of the Q wave. In: Schlant R, Hurst J (eds.) Advances in Electrocardiography. New York: Grune & Stratton, 1972: 321.

Horan L, Flowers N, Johnson J. Significance of the diagnostic Q wave of myocardial infarction. Circulation 1971; 63: 428.

Hoshino Y, Hasegawa A, Nakano A et al. Electrocardiographic abnormalities of pure posterior myocardial infarction. Intern Med 2004; 43(9): 883.

Huey B, Beller G, Kaiser O, Gibson R. A comprehensive analysis of myocardial infarction due to left circumflex artery occlusion: comparison with infarction due to right coronary and left anterior descending artery occlusion. J Am Coll Cardiol 1988; 12: 1156.

Hurd HP, Starling MR, Crawford MH, Dlabal PW, O'Rouke RA. Comparative accuracy of electrocardiographic and vectorcardiographic criteria for inferior myocardial infarction. Circulation 1981; 63: 1025–1029.

Hurst RT, Askew JW, Reuss CS et al. Transient midventricular ballooning syndrome: a new variant. J Am Coll Cardiol 2006; 48(3): 579–83.

Hyde TA, French JK, Wong CK et al. Four-year survival of patients with acute coronary syndromes without ST-segment elevation and prognostic significance of 0.5-mm ST-segment depression. Am J Cardiol 1999; 84: 379.

Ibañez B, Choi BG, Navarro F, Farre J. Tako-tsubo syndrome: a form of spontaneous aborted myocardial infarction? Eur Heart J 2006; 27: 1509.

Ibáñez B, Navarro F, Farré J et al. Tako-Tsubo transient left ventricular apical ballooning is associated with a left anterior descending coronary artery with a long course along the apical diaphragmatic surface of the left ventricle. Rev Esp Cardiol 2004; 57: 209.

Jacobs DR, Jr, Kroenke C, Crow R et al. PREDICT: a simple risk score for clinical severity and long-term prognosis after hospitalization for acute myocardial infarction or unstable angina: the Minnesota heart survey. Circulation 1999; 100(6): 599–607.

Jacobsen MO, Wagner GS, Holmvang L et al. Clinical significance of abnormal T waves in patients with non-ST-segment elevation acute coronary syndromes. Am J Cardiol 2001; 88: 1225.

Janse MJ. Electrophysiological changes in acute myocardial ischemia. In: Julian DG, Lie KI, Wihelmsen L (eds.) What is Angina? Suecia: Astra, 1982: 160.

Jemberg T, Lindahl B. A combination of troponin T and 12-lead electrocardiography: a valuable tool for early prediction of long-term 'mortality in patients with chest pain without ST-segment elevation'. Am Heart J 2002; 144: 804.

Jennings R. Early phase of myocardial ischemia, injury, and infarction. Am J Cardiol 1969; 24: 753.

Jensen JK, Ovrehus K, Moldrup M, Mickley H, Hoilund-Carlsen PF. Redefinition of the Q wave: is there a clinical problem? Am J Cardiol 2006; 97: 974.

Jim M-H, Siu C-W, Chan A O-O, Chan R H-W, Lee S W-L, Lau C-P. Prognostic implications of PR-segment depression in inferior leads in acute inferior myocardial infarction. Clin Cardiol 2006; 29(8): 36.

Johanson P, Jernberg T, Gunnarsson G et al. Prognostic value of ST-segment resolution – when and what to measure. Eur Heart J 2003; 24: 337.

Kabakci G, Yildirir A, Yildiran L et al. The diagnostic value of 12-lead electrocardiogram in predicting infarct-related artery and right ventricular involvement in acute inferior myocardial infarction. Ann Noninvasive Electrocardiol 2001; 6(3): 229–35.

Kandzari DE, Tcheng JE, Gersh BJ et al.; CADILLAC Investigators. Relationship between infarct artery location, epicardial flow, and myocardial perfusion after primary percutaneous revascularization in acute myocardial infarction. Am Heart J 2006; 151: 1288.

Kannel WB, Abbott RD. Incidence and prognosis of unrecognized myocardial infarction: an update on the Framingham study. N Engl J Med 1984; 311: 1144.

Kannel WB, Anderson K, McGee OL, Oegatano LS, Stampfer MJ. Nonspecific electrocardiographic abnormality as a predictor of coronary heart disease: the Framingham study. Am Heart J 1987; 113: 370.

Kannel WB, Cupples LA, Gagnon DR. Incidence, precursors and prognosis of unrecognized myocardial infarction. Adv Cardiol 1990; 37: 202.

Kaski JC. Pathophysiology and management of patients with chest pain and normal coronary arteriograms (cardiac syndrome X). Circulation 2004; 109: 568.

Kenigsberg D, Khanol S, Kowalski M, Krishnan S. Prolongation of the QTc interval is seen uniformly during early transmural ischaemia. JACC 2007; 49: 1299.

Kennedy RJ, Varriale P, Alfenito JC. Texbook of Vectocardiography. New Jersey: Harper and Row, 1970.

Kerwin AJ, McLean R, Tegelaar H. A method for the accurate placement of chest electrodes in the taking of serial electrocardiographic tracings. Can Med Assoc J 1960; 82: 258.

Khaw K, Moreyra AE, Tannenbaum AK, Hosler MN, Brewer TJ, Agarwal JB. Improved detection of posterior myocarodial wall ischemia with the 15-lead electrocardiogram. Am Heart J 1999; 138: 934–40.

Knutsen R, Knutsen SF, Curb JD et al. The predictive value of resting electrocardiograms for 12-year incidence of coronary heart disease in the Honolulu Heart Program. J Clin Epidemiol 1988; 41: 293.

Kontos M, McQueen R, Jesse R, Tatum J, Ornato J. Can myocardial infarction be rapidly identified in emergency department patients who have left bundle branch block? Ann Emerg Med 2001; 37: 431.

Kosuge M, Kimura K, Ishikawa T et al. New electrocardiographic criteria for predicting the site of coronary artery occlusion in inferior wall acute myocardial infarction. Am J Cardiol 1998; 82: 1318.

Kosuge M, Kimura K, Ishikawa T, Toshiak E, Setoshi V. Predictors of left-main or three vessel disease in patients who have acute coronary syndromes with non ST segment elevation. Am J Cardiol 2005; 95: 1366.

Kurisu S, Sato H, Kawagoe T et al. Tako-tsubo-like left ventricular dysfunction with ST-segment elevation: a novel cardiac syndrome mimicking acute myocardial infarction. Am Heart J 2002; 143: 448.

Kurum T, Oztekin E, Ozcelik F, Eker H, Ture M, Ozbay G. Predictive value of admission electrocardiogram for multivessel disease in acute anterior and anterio-inferior myocardial infarction. Ann Noninvasive Electrocardiol 2002; 7: 369.

Kwong RY, Chan AK, Brown KA et al. Impact of unrecognized myocardial scar detected by cardiac magnetic resonance imaging on event-free survival in patients presenting with signs or symptoms of coronary artery disease. Circulation 2006; 113: 2733.

Lamfers EJ, Hooghoudt TE, Herzberger DP, Schut A, Stolwijk PW, Verheugt FW. Abortion of acute ST segment elevation myocardial infarction after reperfusion: incidence, é~íáÉåíé characteristics and prognosis. Heart 2003; 89: 496.

Lee HS, Cross SJ, Rawles JM, Jennings KP. Patients with suspected myocardial infarction who present with ST depression. Lancet 1993; 342: 1204.

Lee KL, Woodlief LH, Topol EJ et al. Predictors of 30-day mortality in the era of reperfusion for acute myocardial infarction: results from an international trial of 41,021 patients. GUSTO Investigators. Circulation 1995; 91: 1659.

Lee TH, Cook EF, Weisberg M et al. Acute chest pain in the emergency room: identification and examination of low-risk patients. Arch Intern Med 1985; 145: 65.

Leibrandt PN, Bell SJ, Savona MR et al. Validation of cardiologist's decisions to initiate reperfusion therapy with ECG viewed on liquid crystal displays of cellular phones. Am Heart J 2000; 140: 747.

Lemberg L, Castellanos A, Jr, Arcebal AG. The vectorcardiogram in acute left anterior hemiblock. Am J Cardiol 1971; 28(4): 483–9.

Lengyel L, Caramelli Z, Monfort J, Guerra JC. Initial ECG changes in experimental occlusion of the coronary arteries in non-anesthetized dogs with closed thorax. Am Heart J 1957; 53: 334.

Levy L, Jacobs J, Chastant P, Strauss H. Prominent R wave and shallow S wave in lead V1 as a result of lateral myocardial infarction. Am Heart J 1950; 40: 447.

Lew AS, Hod H, Cercek B, Shah PK, Ganz W. Inferior ST segment changes during acute anterior myocardial infarction: a marker of the presence or absence of concomitant inferior wall ischaemia. J Am Coll Cardiol 1987; 10: 519.

Lew AS, Laramee P, Shah PK, Maddahi J, Peter T, Ganz W. Ratio of ST-segment depression in lead V2 to ST-segment elevation in lead aVF in evolving inferior acute myocardial infarction: an aid to the early recognition of right ventricular ischemia. Am J Cardiol 1986; 57: 1047.

Lie KI, Wellens HJ, Downar E, Durrer D. Observations on patients with primary ventricular fibrillation complicating acute myocardial infarction. Circulation 1975; 52: 755.

Liu CK, Greenspan G, Piccirillo RT. Atrial infarction of the heart. Circulation 1961; 23: 331.

López-Sendón J, Coma-Canella L, Alcasena S, Seoane J, Gamayo C. Electrocardiographic findings in acute right ventricular infarction: sensitivity and specificity of electrocardiographic alterations in right precordial leads V4R, V3R, V1, V2, and V3. J Am Coll Cardiol 1985; 6: 1273.

López-Sendón J, González A, López de Sa E et al. Diagnosis of subacute ventricular wall rupture after acute myocardial infarction: sensitivity and specificity of clinical, hemodynamic and echocardiographic criteria. J Am Coll Cardiol 1992; 19: 1145.

Lown B, Fakhro AM, Hood WB, Thorn GW. The coronary care unit: new perspectives and directions. JAMA 1967; 199: 188.

MacAlpin RN. Significance of abnormal Q waves in the electrocardiograms of adults less than 40 years old. Ann Noninvasive Electrocardiol 2006; 11: 203.

MacLeod RS, Shome S, Stinstra J, Punske BB, Hopenfeld B. Mechanisms of ischemia-induced ST-segment changes. J Electrocardiol 2005; 38: 8.

Madias JE. Difficulties in assessing the presence, duration, severity, extent, and evolution of acute myocardial ischemia and infarction: ischemic ST-segment counterpoise as a plausible explanation. J Electrocardiol 2006; 39: 156.

Madias JE, Mahjoub M, Valance J. The paradox of negative exercise stress ECG/positive thallium scintigram: ischemic ST-segment counterpoise as the underlying mechanism. J Electrocardiol 1996; 29: 243.

Madias JE, Manyam B, Khan M, Singh V, Tziros C. Transient disappearance of Q waves of previous myocardial infarction due to exercise-induced ischemia of the contralateral noninfarcted myocardium. J Electrocardiol 1997; 30: 97.

Madias J, Sinha A, Ashtiani R. A critique of the new ST-segment criteria for the diagnosis of acute myocardial infarction in patients with left bundle-branch block. Clin Cardiol 2001; 24: 652.

Madias JE, Win M. Incomplete ECG expression of acute true posterior myocardial infarction, owing to an antecedent anterior infarction. J Electrocardiol 2000; 33: 189.

Mahrholdt H, Wagner A, Judd RM, Sechtem U. Assessment of myocardial viability by cardiovascular magnetic resonance imaging. Eur Heart J 2002; 23: 602.

Mahrholdt H, Wagner A, Judd RM, Sechtem U, Kim RJ. Delayed enhancement cardiovascular magnetic resonance assessment of non-ischaemic cardiomyopathies. Eur Heart J 2005a; 26: 1461.

Mahrholdt H, Zhydkov A, Hager S et al. Left ventricular wall motion abnormalities as well as reduced wall thickness can cause false positive results of routine SPECT perfusion imaging for detection of myocardial infarction. Eur Heart J 2005b; 26: 2127.

Maisel AS, Ahnve S, Gilpin E et al. Prognosis after extension of myocardial infarct: the role of Q wave or non-Q wave infarction. Circulation 1985; 71: 211.

Malik M, Camm AJ (eds.). Dynamic Electrocardiography. Oxford: Blackwell, 2004.

Mandelzweig L, Battler A, Boyko V et al.; Euro Heart Survey Investigators. The second Euro Heart Survey on acute coronary syndromes: characteristics, treatment, and outcome of patients with ACS in Europe and the Mediterranean Basin in 2004. Eur Heart J 2006; 27(19): 2285–93.

Martinez-Dolz L, Arnau MA, Almenar L et al. Utilidad del ECG en la predicción del lugar de la oclusión en el infarto agudo de miocardio en el síndrome coronario agudo debido a oclusión de la arteria descendente anterior aislada. Rev Esp Cardiol 2002; 55: 1036.

Massing JL, Bentz MH, Schlesser P, Dumitru C, Louis JP. Myocardial infarction following a bee sting: apropos of a case and review of the literature. Ann Cardiol Angeiol (Paris) 1997; 46: 311–15.

Matetzky S, Barabash GI, Shahar A et al. Early T wave inversion after thrombolytic therapy predicts better coronary perfusion: clinical and angiographic study. J Am Coll Cardiol 1994; 24: 378.

Matetzky S, Freimark D, Feinbergt MS et al. Acute myocardial infarction with isolated ST-segment elevation in posterior chest leads V7-9: 'hidden' ST-segment elevations revealing acute posterior infarction. J Am Coll Cardiol 1999; 34: 748.

Mauri F, Maggioni AP, Franzosi MG et al. A simple electrocardiographic predictor of the outcome of patients with acute myocardial infarction treated with a thrombolytic agent. A Gruppo Italiano per lo Studio della Sopravvivenza nell'Infarto Miocardico (GISSI-2)-derived analysis. J Am Coll Cardiol 1994; 24: 600.

Mavric L, Laputovic L, Matana A et al. Prognostic significance of complete atrioventricular block in patients with acute inferior myocardial infarction with and without right ventricular involvement. Am Heart J 1990; 119: 823.

McConahay D, McCallister B, Smith R. Post exercise ECG: correlations with coronary arteriography. Am J Cardiol 1971; 28: 1.

McFarlane PW, Coleman EN. Resting 12-lead ECG electrode placement and associated problems. J Electrocardiol 2004; 94: 1534.

McFarlane P, Veitch Lawrie TD (eds.). Comprehensive Electrocardiography. Oxford: Pergamon, 1989.

Medrano G, Brenes C, De Micheli A et al. Bloqueo simultáneo de las divisiones anterior y posterior de la rama izquierda: Estudio clínico y experimental. Arch Inst Card Mex 1970; 40: 752.

Meinertz T, Lehender M, Honhloser S. Prevalence of ventricular arrhythmias during silent myocardial ischemia. Cardiovasc Rev Rep 1988; 34: 64.

Melgarejo A, Galcera A, Vades M et al. Significación pronóstica del bloqueo AV completo en pacientes con infarto agudo de miocardio inferior. Un estudio en la era trombolítica. Rev Esp Cardiol 1997; 50: 397.

Menown L, McKenzie G, Adgey A. Optimizing the initial 12-lead electrocardiographic diagnosis of acute myocardial infarction. Eur Heart J 2000; 21: 275.

Michaelides A, Psomadakai ZD, Aigyptiadout MN, Richter D, Andrikopoulos G, Dilaveris P. Significance of exercise-induced changes in leads AVR, V5 and V1: discrimination of patients with single or multivessel coronary artery disease. Clin Cardiol 2003; 26(5): 226–30.

Mirvis DM, Goldberger AL. Electrocardiography. In: Braunwald E, Zipes D, Libby P (eds.) Heart Disease. Philadelphia: WB Saunders, 2001.

Mitamura H, Ogawa S, Muurayama A, Fujii I, Handa S, Nakamura Y. Two dimensional echocardiography approach to the localization of myocardial infarction: echocardiographic, electrocardiographic and coronary arteriographic correlations. J Cardiogr 1981; 11(3): 779–90.

Moffa PJ, Del Nero E, Tobias NM, et al. The left anterior septal block in Chagas' disease. Jap Heart J 1982; 23: 163–165.

Mohlenkamp S, Hort W, Ge J, Erbel R. Update on myocardial bridging. Circulation 2002; 106: 2616.

Mont L, Cinca J, Blanch P et al. Predisposing factors and prognostic value of sustained monomorphic ventricular tachycardia in the early phase of acute myocardial infarction. J Am Coll Cardiol 1996; 28: 1670.

Moon JC, De Arenaza DP, Elkington AG, Taneja AK, John AS, Wang D. The pathologic basis of Q-wave and non-Q-wave myocardial infarction: a cardiovascular magnetic resonance study. J Am Coll Cardiol 2004; 44: 554.

Morrow DA, Antman EM, Charlesworth A et al. TIMI risk score for ST-elevation myocardial infarction: a convenient, bedside, clinical score for risk assessment at presentation: an intravenous PA for TIMI II 11 trial substudy. Circulation 2000a; 102: 2031.

Morrow DA, Antman EM, Giugliano RP et al. A simple risk index for rapid initial triage of patients with ST-elevation myocardial infarction: an InTIME II substudy. Lancet 2000b; 358: 1571.

Moss AJ, Zareba W, Hall WJ. Prophylactic implantation of a defibrillator in patients with myocardial infarction and reduced ejection fraction. N Engl J Med 2002; 346: 877.

Myers GB, Howard A, Klein M, Stofer E. Correlation of electrocardiographic and pathologic findings in anteroseptal infarction. Am Heart J 1948a; 36: 535.

Myers GB, Howard A, Klein M, Stofer BE. Correlation of electrocardiographic and pathologic findings in lateral infarction. Am Heart J 1948b; 37: 374.

Myers G, Howard AK, Stofer BE. Correlation of electrocardiographic and pathologic findings in posterior infarction. Am Heart J 1948; 38: 547.

Nesto R, Kowaldruk G. The ischemic cascade: temporal sequence of hemodynamic, electrocardiographic, and symptomatic expressions of ischemia. Am J Cardiol 1987; 57: 23C.

Newby DE, Wright RA, Labinjoh C et al. Endothelial dysfunction, impaired endogenous fibrinolysis, and cigarette smoking: a mechanism for arterial thrombosis and myocardial infarction. Circulation 1999; 99(11): 1411.

Newby KH, Thompson T, Stebbins A et al. Sustained ventricular arrhythmias in patients receiving thrombolytic therapy: incidence and outcomes. The GUSTO Investigators. Circulation 1998; 98: 2567.

Nikus KC, Bayés de Luna A, Clemmensen P et al. Electrocardiographic patterns present at patient admission in acute coronary syndromes: a statement for healthcare professionals from a committee appointed by the International Society for Holter and Non Invasive Electrocardiography. Submitted.

Nikus KC, Eskola MJ, Niemela KO, Sclarovsky S. Modern morphologic electrocardiographic interpretation – a valuable tool for rapid clinical decision making in acute ischemic coronary syndromes. J Electrocardiol 2005; 38: 4.

Nikus KC, Eskola MJ, Niemela KO, Sclarovsky S. How to use ECG for decision support in the catheterization laboratory: cases with ST-segment depression acute coronary syndrome. J Electrocardiol 2004; 37: 247.

Nikus KC, Eskola M, Sclarovsky S. ECG presentation of left main or severe 3 vessel disease in ACS. J Electrocardiol 2006; 39: 568.

Nikus KC, Eskola MJ, Virtanen VK. ST-depression with negative T waves in leads V4–V5 – a marker of severe coronary artery disease in non-ST elevation acute coronary syndrome: a prospective study of angina at rest, with troponin, clinical, electrocardiographic and angiographic correlation. Ann Noninvasive Electrocardiol 2004; 9: 207.

Okamoto N, Simonson E, Ahuja S, Manning G. Significance of the initial R wave in lead A VR of the electrocardiogram in the diagnosis of myocardial infarction. Circulation 1967; 35: 126.

Okin PM. Electrocardiography in women: taking the initiative. Circulation 2006; 31(113): 464.

Oliva PS, Hammill SC, Edwards WD. Cardiac rupture, a clinically predictable complication of acute myocardial infarction: report of 70 cases with clinicopathologic correlations. J Am Coll Cardiol 1993; 22: 720.

O'Rourke RA, Brundage BH, Froelicher VF et al. American College of Cardiology/American Heart Association Expert Consensus Document on electron-beam computed tomography for the diagnosis and prognosis of coronary artery disease. J Am Coll Cardiol 2000; 36(1): 326–40. Review.

Pahlm O, Chaitman B, Rautaharju P, Selvester R, Wagner G. Comparison of the various electrocardiographic scoring codes for estimating anatomically documented sizes of single and multiple infarcts of the left ventricle. Am J Cardiol 1998; 81: 809.

Palmeri ST, Harrison OG, Cobb FR et al. A QRS scoring system for assessing left ventricular function after myocardial infarction. N Engl J Med 1982; 306(1): 4–9.

Pantridge JF, Webb SW, Adgey AA. Arrhythmias in the first hours of acute myocardial infarction. Prog Cardiovasc Dis 1981; 23: 265.

Pastor Torres L, Pavón Jiménez R, Reina Sánchez M, Caparrós Valderrama J, Mora Pardo J. Unidad de dolor torácico: seguimiento a un año. Rev Esp Cardiol 2002; 55: 1021.

Patel OJ, Gomma AH, Knoght CJ et al. Why is recurrent myocardial ischaemia a predictor of adverse outcome in unstable angina? An observational study of myocardial ischaemia and its relation to coronary anatomy. Eur Heart J 2001; 22: 1991.

Peraira JR, Segovia J, Oteo JF, Ortiz P. Síndrome de la discinesia apical transitoria con una complicación inhabitual. Rev Esp Cardiol 2002; 55: 1328.

Perloff J. The recognition of strictly posterior myocardial infarction by conventional scalar electrocardiography. Circulation 1964; 30: 706.

Petrina M, Goodman SG, Eagle KA. The 12-lead electrocardiogram as a predictive tool of mortality after acute myocardial infarction: current status in an era of revascularization and reperfusion. Am Heart J 2006; 152(1): 11.

Phibbs B, Marcus F, Marriott HJ, Moss A, Spodick DH. Q-wave versus non-Q wave myocardial infarction: a meaningless distinction. J Am Coll Cardiol 1999; 33: 576.

Piccolo E, Zuin G, Di Pede F, Gasparini G. L'elettrocardiograma nelle sindromi ischemiche acute. Padua: Editorial Piccin, 2001.

Pinney SP, Rabbani LE. Myocardial infarction in patients with normal coronary arteries: proposed pathogenesis and predisposing risk factors. J Thromb Thrombolysis 2001; 11: 11.

Plas F. Guide du cardiologie du sport. Paris: Baillier, 1976.

Polizos G, Ellestad MH. The value of upsloping ST depression in diagnosing myocardial ischemia. Ann Noninvasive Electrocardiol 2006; 11: 237.

Ponce G, Romero JL, Hernández G et al. El infarto sin onda Q en cirugía cardíaca valvular convencional. Diagnóstico mediante la troponina I cardíaca. Rev Esp Cardiol 2001; 54: 1175.

Pons-Lladó G, Carreras F. Atlas of Practical Applications of Cardiovascular Magnetic Resonance. New York: Springer, 2005.

Pons-Lladó G, Leta-Petracca R (eds.). Atlas of Non-Invasive Coronary Angiography by Multidetector Computed Tomography. New York: Springer, 2007.

Porter A, Sclarovsky S, Ben-Gal T, Herz I, Solodky A, Sagie A. Value of T-wave direction with lead III ST-segment depression in acute anterior wall myocardial infarction: electrocardiographic prediction of a 'wrapped' left anterior descending artery. Clin Cardiol 1998; 21: 562.

Previtali M, Repetto A, Scuteri L. Dobutamine induced severe midventricular obstruction and mitral regurgitation in left ventricular apical ballooning syndrome. Heart 2005; 91(3): 353.

Prieto JA, González C, Hernández MA, De la Torre JM, Llorca J. Predicción electrocardiográfica de la localización de la lesión en la arteria descendente anterior en el infarto agudo de miocardio. Rev Esp Cardiol 2002; 55: 1028.

Prineas RJ, Grandits G, Rautaharju PM et al. Long-term prognostic significance of isolated minor electrocardiographic T-wave abnormalities in middle-aged men free of clinical cardiovascular disease (The Multiple Risk Factor Intervention Trial [MRFIT]). Am J Cardiol 2002; 90: 1391.

Pursuit trial: inhibition of platelet glycoprotein IIb/IIIa with eptifibatide in patients with acute coronary syndromes. The PURSUIT Trial Investigators. Platelet glycoprotein IIb/IIIa in unstable angina: receptor suppression using integrilin therapy. N Engl J Med 1998; 339: 436.

Quyyumi AA, Crake T, Rubens MB, Levy RD, Rickards AF, Fox KM. Importance of 'reciprocal' electrocardiographic changes during occlusion of left anterior descending artery: studies during percutaneous transluminal coronary angioplasty. Lancet 1986; 1: 347.

Rasouli ML, Ellestad MH. Usefulness of ST depression in ventricular premature complexes to predict myocardial ischemia. Am J Cardiol 2001; 87: 891.

Rautaharju PM. ST segment deviation counterpoise – a different perspective. J Electrocardiol 2006a; 39: 160a.

Rautaharju PM, Kooperberg C, Larson JC, LaCroix A. Electrocardiographic abnormalities that predict coronary heart disease events and mortality in postmenopausal women: the Women's Health Initiative. Circulation 2006; 113: 473.

Rautaharju PM, Park L, Rautaharju FS, Crow R. A standardized procedure for locating and documenting ECG chest electrode positions: consideration of the effect of breast tissue on ECG amplitudes in women. J Electrocardiol 1998; 31: 17.

Reddy CV, Cheriparambill K, Saul B et al. Fragmented left sided QRS in absence of bundle branch block: sign of left ventricular aneurysm. Ann Noninvasive Electrocardiol 2006; 11: 132.

Reeder GS, Gersh BJ. Modern management of acute myocardial infarction. Curr Probl Cardiol 2000; 25: 677.

Reiffel J, Bigger T. Pure anterior conduction delay: A variant fascicular block. J of Electrocardiology 1978; 11: 315.

Reimer K, Lowe J, Rasmussen M, Jennings R. The wave front phenomenon of ischemic cell death. Myocardial infarct size vs duration of coronary occlusion in dogs. Circulation 1977; 56: 786.

Reinig MG, Harizi R, Spodick OH. Electrocardiographic T- and u-wave discordance. Ann Noninvasive Electrocardiol 2005; 10: 41.

Rios JC (ed.). Clinical Electrocardiographic Correlations. Philadelphia: FA Davis, 1977.

Roberts WC, Gardin JM. Location of myocardial infarcts: a confusion of terms and definitions. Am J Cardiol 1978; 42: 868.

Rodriguez MI, Anselmi A, Sodi Pallares O. The electrocardiographic diagnosis of septal infarction. Am Heart J 1953; 45: 525.

Roe MT, Parsons LS, Pollack CV, Jr, et al.; National Registry of Myocardial Infarction Investigators. Quality of care by classification of myocardial infarction: treatment patterns for ST-segment elevation vs non-ST-segment elevation myocardial infarction. Arch Intern Med 2005; 165: 1630–6.

Roig S, Gomez S, Fiol M et al. Spontaneous coronary artery dissection causing acute coronary syndrome: an early diagnosis implies a good prognosis. Am J Emerg Med 2003; 29: 549.

Rosenbaum MB, Blanco HH, Elizari MV, Lazzari JO, Davidenko JM. Electrotonic modulation of the T wave and cardiac memory. Am J Cardiol 1982; 50: 213.

Rosenbaum MB, Elizari MV, Lazzari JO. Los Hemibloqueos. Buenos Aires: Editorial Paidos, 1968.

Rosiak M, Bolinska H, Ruta J. P wave dispersion and P wave duration on SAECG in predicting atrial fibrillation in patients with acute myocardial infarction. Ann Noninvasive Electrocardiol 2002; 7: 363.

Roth A, Miller HI, Glick A, Barbash GI, Laniado S. Rapid resolution of new right bundle branch block in acute anterior myocardial infarction patients after thrombolytic therapy. Pacing Clin Electrophysiol 1993; 16: 13.

Roth D, Weiss AT, Chajek-Shaul T, Leibowitz D. ST-deviation patterns in recurrent myocardial infarctions. Am J Cardiol 2006; 98(1): 10.

Rukshin V, Monakier D, Olshtain-Pops K, Balkin J, Tzivoni D. QT interval in patients with unstable angina and non-Q wave myocardial infarction. Noninvasive Electrocardiol 2002; 7: 343.

Ryan TJ, Antman EM, Brooks NH et al. 1999 update: ACC/AHA Guidelines for the Management of Patients with Acute Myocardial Infarction: executive summary and recommendations: a report of the American College of Cardiology/American Heart Association Task Force on Practice Guidelines (Committee on Management of Acute Myocardial Infarction). Circulation 1999; 100: 1016.

Sadanandan S, Hochman S, Kolodzjez A et al. Clinical and electrocardiographic characteristics of patients with combined anterior and inferior ST segment elevation in the initial ECG during acute myocardial infarction. Am Heart J 2003; 146: 653.

Sadony V, Korber M, Albes G et al. Cardiac troponin I plasma levels for diagnosis and quantitation of perioperative myocardial damage in patients undergoing coronary artery bypass surgery. Eur J Cardiothorac Surg 1998; 13: 57.

Sagie A, Sclarovsky S, Strasberg B et al. Acute anterior wall myocardial infarction presenting with positive T waves and without ST segment shift. Electrocardiographic features and angiographic correlation. Chest 1989; 95(6): 1211–15.

Santoro GM, Valenti R, Buonamici P et al. Relation between ST-segment changes and myocardial perfusion evaluated by myocardial contrast echocardiography in patients with acute myocardial infarction treated with direct angioplasty. Am J Cardiol 1998; 82: 932.

Sapin PM, Musselman DR, Dehmer GJ, Cascio WE. Implications of inferior ST segment elevation accompanying anterior wall myocardial infarction for the angiographic morphology of the left anterior descending coronary artery morphology and site of occlusion. Am J Cardiol 1992; 69: 860.

Satran D, Henry CR, Adkinson C, Nicholson CI, Bracha Y, Henry TD. Cardiovascular manifestations of moderate to severe carbon monoxide poisoning. J Am Coll Cardiol 2005; 45: 1513.

Savage R, Wagner G, Ideker R, Podolsky S, Hackel D. Correlation of postmortem anatomic findings with electrocardiographic changes in patients with myocardial infarction. Circulation 1977; 55: 279.

Saw J, Davies C, Fung A, Spinelli JJ, Jue J. Value of ST elevation in lead III greater than lead II in inferior wall acute myocardial infarction for predicting in-hospital mortality and diagnosing right ventricular infarction. Am J Cardiol 2001; 87: 448.

Schamroth L. The Electrocardiology of Coronary Artery Disease. Oxford: Blackwell Scientific, 1975.

Schinkel AF, Bax JJ, Boersma E et al. Assessment of residual myocardial viability in regions with chronic electrocardiographic Q-wave infarction. Am Heart J 2002; 144: 865.

Schmitt C, Günter L, Scmieder S, Karch M, Neuman FJ, Schömig A. Diagnosis of acute myocardial infarction in

angiographically documented occluded infarct vessel: limitations of ST elevation in standard and extended ECG leads. Chest 2001; 120: 1540.

Scholte OP, Reimer W, Simoons ML et al. Cardiovascular disease in Europe. Euro Heart Surv, 2006. Available at: http://www.escardio.org.

Schwartz PJ, Zaza A, Grazi S et al. Effect of ventricular fibrillation complicating acute myocardial infarction on long-term prognosis: importance of the site of infarction. Am J Cardiol 1985; 56: 384.

Sclarovsky S. Electrocardiography of Acute Myocardial Ischemia. London: Martin Dunitz, 1999.

Sclarovsky S, Nikus KC, Birnbaum Y. Manifestation of left main coronary artery stenosis is diffuse ST depression in inferior and precordial leads on ECG. J Am Coll Cardiol 2002; 40: 575.

Sclarovsky S, Rechavia E, Strasberg B et al. Unstable angina: ST segment depression with positive versus negative T wave deflections – clnical course, ECG evolution, and angiographic correlation. Am Heart J 1988; 116: 933–41.

Shandling AH, Kern L, McAtee P, Switzenberg S. The prevalence of cardiac ectopy in elderly patients with echocardiographically normal hearts is not increased by significant coronary artery disease. J Electrocardiol 2006; 39: 232.

Shu J, Zhu T, Yang L, Cui C, Yan GX. ST-segment elevation in the early repolarization syndrome, idiopathic ventricular fibrillation, and the Brugada syndrome: cellular and clinical linkage. J Electrocardiol 2005; 38: 26.

Sejersten M, Birnbaum Y, Ripa RS et al. Electrocadiographic identification of patients with ST-elevation acute myocardium infarction benefiting most from primary angioplasty versus fibrinolysis: results from the DANAMI-2 trial. Circulation 2004; 110: III–409.

Sejersten M, Ripa RS, Maynard C et al. Usefulness of quantitative baseline ST-segment elevation for predicting outcomes after primary coronary angioplasty or fibrinolysis (results from the DANAMI-2 trial). Am J Cardiol 2006; 97: 611.

Selvanayagam J, Kardos A, Nicolson D et al. Anteroseptal or apical myocardial infarction: a controversy addressed using delayed enhancement cardiovascular magnetic resonance imaging. J Cardiovasc Magn Reson 2004; 6: 653.

Selvester RH, Wagner GS, Hindman NB. The Selvester QRS scoring system for estimating myocardial infarction size: the development and application of the system. Arch Intern Med 1985; 145: 1877.

Sevilla O, Wagner N, Anderson W et al. Sensitivity of a set of myocardial infarction screening criteria in patients with anatomically documented single and multiple infarcts. Am J Cardiol 1990; 66: 792–5.

Sgarbossa E, Pinski S, Gates K, Wagner G. Early ECG diagnosis of acute myocardial infarction in the presence of ventricular paced rhythm. Am J Cardiol 1996a; 77: 423.

Sgarbossa EB, Birnbaum Y, Parrilo JF. Electrocardiographic diagnosis of acute myocardial infarction: current concepts for the clinician. Am Heart J 2001; 141: 507.

Sgarbossa EB, Pinski SL, Barbagelata A et al. Electrocardiographic diagnosis of evolving acute myocardial infarction in the presence of left bundle branch block. GUSTO-l (Global Utilization of Streptokinase and Tissue Plasminogen Activator for Occluded Coronary Arteries) Investigators. N Engl J Med 1996b; 334: 481.

Shalev Y, Fogelman R, Oettinger M, Caspi A. Does the electrocardiographic pattern of anteroseptal myocardial infarction correlate with the anatomic location of myocardial injury? Am J Cardiol 1995; 75: 763.

Shen Wei, Tribouilloy C, Lesbre JP. Relationship between electrocardiographic patterns and angiographic features in isolated left circumflex coronary artery disease. Clin Cardiol 1991; 14: 720.

Shen Wei, Xing Hui, Wang Man, Gong Lan. Myocardial infarction due to isolated left circumflex or right coronary artery occlusion. Chin Med J 1991; 104: 369.

Sherif NE. The rsR' pattern in left surface leads in ventricular aneurysm. Br Heart J 1970; 32: 440.

Singer DH, Ten Eick RE. Aberrancy: electrophysiologic aspects. Am J Cardiol 1971; 28(4): 381–401.

Singh M, Reeder GS, Jacobsen SJ, Weston, S, Killian J, Roger VL. Scores for post-myocardial infarction risk stratification in the community. Circulation 2002; 106: 2309–14.

Sodi Pallares D, Bisteni A, Medrano G, Ayola C. Electrocardiography and Vectorcardiography. New York: Grune & Stratton, 1960.

Sodi Pallares D, Calder R. New Bases of Electrocardiography. St Luis: Mosby Company, 1956.

Sodi Pallares D, Rodríguez H. Morphology of the unipolar leads recorded at the septal surface: its application to diagnosis of left bundle branch block complicated by myocardial infarction. Am Heart J 1952; 43: 27.

Sones FM, Jr, Shirey EK. Cine coronary arteriography. Mod Concepts Cardiovasc Dis 1962; 31: 735–8.

Spodick DH. Q-wave infarction versus ST infarction: nonspecificity of electrocardiographic criteria for differentiating transmural and nontransmural lesions. Am J Cardiol 1983; 51: 913.

Starr J, Wagner G, Draffin R, Reed J, Walston A, Behar V. Vectocardiographic criteria for the diagnosis of anterior myocardial infarction. Circulation 1976; 53(2): 229.

Starr J, Wagner G, Draffin R, Reed J, Walston A, Behar V. Vectocardiographic criteria for the diagnosis of inferior myocardial infarction. Circulation 1974; 59: 829.

Stern S (ed.). Silent Myocardial Ischemia. London: Martin Dunitz, 1998.

Stern S, Tzivoni D. Early detection of silent ischaemic heart disease by 24-hour electrocardiographic monitoring of active subjects. Br Heart J 1974; 36: 481.

Steuer J, Horte LG, Lindahl B, Stahle E. Impact of perioperative myocardial injury on early and long-term outcome after coronary artery bypass grafting. Eur Heart J 2002; 23: 1219.

Sugiura T, Iwasaka T, Ogawa A et al. Atrial fibrillation in acute myocardial infarction. Am J Cardiol 1985; 56: 27.

Sullivan VO, Klodever Z, Edwards J. Correlation of ECG and pathological findings in healed myocardial infarction. Am J Cardiol 1978; 42; 724.

Surawicz B (ed.). Chou's Electrocardiography in Clinical Practice, 5th edn. Philadelphia: WB Saunders, 1996.

Surawicz B, Uhlewy H, Borun R et al. Task force I: standardization of terminology and interpretation. Am J Cardiol 1978; 41: 130.

Sutherland SE, Gazes PC, Keil JE, Gilbert GE, Knapp RG. Electrocardiographic abnormalities and 30-year mortality among white and black men of the Charleston Heart Study. Circulation 1993; 88: 2685.

Takatsu F, Osugui J, Nagaya T. Is it possible to rule out extensive anterior myocardial infarction in the absence of abnormal Q wave in lead I and a VL? Effect of inferoapical extension of infarction over apex. Jpn Circ J 1986; 50: 601.

Takatsu F, Osugui J, Ozaki Y, Nagaya T. Relationship between abnormal Q waves in lead aVL and angiographic findings – a study to redefine 'high lateral' infarction. Jpn Circ J 1988, 52: 169.

Takatsu F, Osugui J, Tatsuji F, Watari M, Nagaya T. Vectocardiographic criteria for diagnosis of high lateral infarction. Jpn Circ J 1989; 53: 1072.

Tamura A, Kataoka H, Mikuriya Y. Electrocardiographic findings in a patient with pure septal infarction. Br Heart J 1991; 65: 166.

Tamura A, Kataoka H, Mikuriya Y, Nasu M. Inferior ST segment depression as a useful marker for identifying proximal left anterior descending artery occlusion during acute anterior myocardial infarction. Eur Heart J 1995a; 16: 1795.

Tamura A, Kataoka H, Nagase K, Mikuriya Y, Nasu M. Clinical significance of inferior ST elevation during acute anterior myocardial infarction. Br Heart J 1995b; 74: 611.

Theroux P, Waters DD, Halphen C, Oebaisieux JC, Mizgala HF. Prognostic value of exercise testing soon after myocardial infarction. N Engl J Med 1979; 301: 341.

Thiele H, Kappl MJ, Conradi S, Niebauer J, Hambrecht R, Schuler G. Reproducibility of chronic and acute infarct size measurement by delayed enhancement-magnetic resonance imaging. J Am Coll Cardiol 2006; 47: 1641.

Tranchesi J, Teixera B, Ebaid M, Bocalandrio I, Bocanegra J, Pileggi F. The vectocardiogram in dorsal or posterior myocardial infarction. Am J Cardiol 1961; 7: 505.

Tulloch J. The electrocardiographic features of high posterolateral myocardial infarction. Br Heart J 1952; 14: 379.

Uhley HN, Rivkin L. ECG patterns following interruption of main and peripheral branches of canine left bundle. Am J Card 1964; 13: 41.

Uhley HN. The quadrifascicular nature of the peripheral conduction system in cardiac arrhythmias. In: Dreifus L, Likoff W (eds) Cardiac Arrhythmias. Grune – Stratton. New York 1973.

Uchida A, Moffa P, Pérez–Riera A. Exercise induced left septal fascicular block. Indian pacing and electrophysiology Journal 2006; 6: 135.

Uyarel H, Cam N, Okmen E et al. Level of Selvester QRS score is predictive of ST-segment resolution and 30-day outcomes in patients with acute myocardial infarction undergoing primary coronary intervention. Am Heart J 2006; 151: 1239.e1.

Visner MS, Arentzen CE, Parrish DG et al. Effects of global ischemia on the diastolic properties of the left ventricle in the conscious dog. Circulation 1985; 71: 610–19.

Wackers F, Lie KL, David G, Durrer D, Wellens HJ. Assessment of the value of the ECG signs for myocardial infarction in left bundle branch block by thallium. Am J Cardiol 1978; 41: 428.

Wagner GS, Bahit MC, Criger O et al. Moving toward a new definition of acute myocardial infarction for the 21st century: status of the ESC/ACC consensus conference. European Society of Cardiology and American College of Cardiology. J Electrocardiol 2000; 33(suppl): 57.

Wagner GS, Hinohara T. QRS scoring systems for estimating ventricular function. J Am Coll Cardiol 1984; 3: 1106.

Wagner GS, Pahlm O, Selvester R. Consideration of the 24-lead ECG to provide ST elevation myocardial infarction equivalent criteria for acute occlusion. J Electrocardiol 2006; 30: S62.

Wagner GS. Marriot's Practical Electrocardiography, 10th edn. Philadelphia: Lippincott Williams & Wilkins, 2001.

Wagner GS, Limb T, Gorgels A et al. Consideration of pitfalls in the current ECG standards for diagnosis of myocardial ischemia/infarction in patients who have acute coronary syndrome. Cardiol Clin 2007. In press.

Wagner G, Lim T, Gettes L et al. Consideration of pitfalls in and omissions from the current ECG standards for diagnosis of myocardial ischemia/infarction in patients who have acute coronary syndromes. Cardiol Clin 2006; 24(3): 331–42, vii. Review.

Wang L, Feng ZP, Kondo CS, Sheldon RS, Ouff HJ. Developmental changes in the delayed rectifier K Channels in mouse heart. Circ Res 1996; 79(1): 79–85.

Warner R, Hill N, Sheehe P, Mookherjee S. Improved electrocardiographic criteria for diagnosis of inferior myocardial infarction. Circulation 1982; 66: 422.

Warner R, Hill NR, Mookherjee S, Smulyan H. Diagnostic significance for coronary artery disease of abnormal Q waves in the 'lateral' electrocardiographic leads. Am J Cardiol 1986; 58: 431–5.

Watanabe J, Nakamura S, Sugiura T et al. Early identification of impaired myocardial reperfusion with serial assessment of ST segments after percutaneous transluminal coronary angioplasty during acute myocardial infarction. Am J Cardiol 2001; 88: 956.

Wellens HJ. The value of the right precordial leads of the electrocardiogram. N Engl J Med 1999; 340: 381.

Wellens HJ, Connover HP. The ECG in Emergency Decision-Making. Philadelphia, PA: WB Saunders, 2006.

Wellens HJ, Gorgels A, Doevendans PA. The ECG in Acute Myocardial Infarction and Unstable Angina. Boston: Kluwer Academic, 2003.

Wellens HJJ. Recognizing those ECG that distinguish you as a smart clinician. Cardiosource Rev J 2006; 15: 71.

Wenger W, Kligfield P. Variability of precordial electrode placement during routine electrocardiography. J Electrocardiol 1996; 29: 179.

West of Scotland Coronary Prevention Study. Identification of high-risk groups and comparison with other cardiovascular intervention trials. Lancet 1996; 348: 1339.

Westerhout CM, Fu Y, Lauer MS et al. Short- and long-term risk stratification in acute coronary syndromes: the added value of quantitative ST-segment depression and multiple biomarkers. J Am Coll Cardiol 2006; 48: 939.

Wilde AA, Antzelevitch C, Borggrefe M et al. Proposed diagnostic criteria for the Brugada syndrome: consensus report. Circulation 2002; 106: 2514.

Wilkins ML, Pryor AD, Maynard C et al. An electrocardiographic acuteness score for quantifying the timing of a myocardial infarction to guide decisions regarding reperfusion therapy. Am J Cardiol 1995; 75(8): 617–20.

Willems JL, Abreu-Lima C, Arnaud P et al. The diagnostic performance of computer programs for the interpretation of electrocardiograms. N Engl J Med 1991; 325: 1767.

Wiviott SD, Morrow DA, Frederick PD, Antman EM, Braunwald E; National Registry of Myocardial Infarction. Application of the thrombolysis in myocardial infarction risk index in non-ST-segment elevation myocardial infarction: evaluation of patients in the National Registry of Myocardial Infarction. J Am Coll Cardiol 2006; 47(8): 1553.

Wong CK, French JK, Andrews J et al. Usefulness of the presenting electrocardiogram in predicting myocardial salvage with thrombolytic therapy in patients with a first acute myocardial infarction. Eur Heart J 2002a; 23(5): 399.

Wong CK, French JK, Aylward PE et al.; HERO-2 Trial Investigators. Patients with prolonged ischemic chest pain and presumed-new left bundle branch block have heterogeneous outcomes depending on the presence of ST-segment changes. J Am Coll Cardiol 2005; 46(1): 29.

Wong CK, French JK, Aylward PE, Frey MJ, Adgey AA, White HD. Usefulness of the presenting electrocardiogram in predicting successful reperfusion with streptokinase in acute myocardial infarction. Am J Cardiol 1999; 83(2): 164.

Wong CK, French JK, Krucoff MW, Gao W, Aylward PE, White HD. Slowed ST segment recovery despite early infarct artery patency in patients with Q waves at presentation with a first acute myocardial infarction: implications of initial Q waves on myocyte reperfusion. Eur Heart J 2002b; 23(18): 1449.

Wong CK, Gao W, Raffel OC, French JK, Stewart RA, White HD; HERO-2 Investigators. Initial Q waves accompanying ST-segment elevation at presentation of acute myocardial infarction and 30-day mortality in patients given streptokinase therapy: an analysis from HERO-2. Lancet 2006a; 367(9528): 2061.

Wong CK, Gao W, Stewart RA et al.; Hirulog Early Reperfusion Occlusion (HERO-2) Investigators. Risk stratification of patients with acute anterior myocardial infarction and right bundle-branch block: importance of QRS duration and early ST-segment resolution after fibrinolytic therapy. Circulation 2006b; 114(8): 783.

Wu E, Judd RM, Vargas JD, Klocke FJ, Bonow RO, Kim RJ. Visualization of presence, location, and transmural extent of healed Q-wave and non-Q-wave myocardial infarction. Lancet 2001; 357: 21.

Yamaji H, Iwasaki K, Kusachi S et al. Prediction of acute left main coronary artery obstruction by 12 lead electrocardiography: ST segment elevation in lead VR with less ST segment elevation in lead VI. J Am Coll Cardiol 2001; 48: 1348.

Zafrir B, Zafrir N, Gal T et al. Correlations between ST elevation and Q waves on the predischarge electrocardiogram and the extent location of MIBI perfusion defects in anterior myocardial infarction. Ann Noninvasive Electrocardiol 2004; 9: 101.

Zairis MN, Manousakis SJ, Stefanidis AS et al. C-reactive protein levels on admission are associated with response to thrombolysis and prognosis after ST-segment elevation acute myocardial infarction. Am Heart J 2002; 144: 782.

Zalenski RJ, Rydman RJ, Sloan EP et al. Value of posterior and right ventricular leads in comparison to the standard 12-lead electrocardiogram in evaluation of ST-segment elevation in suspected acute myocardial infarction. Am J Cardiol 1997; 79: 1579.

Zehender M, Utzolino S, Furtwangler A et al. Time course and interrelation of reperfusion-induced ST changes and ventricular arrhythmias in acute myocardial infarction. Am J Cardiol 1991; 68: 1138.

Zimetbaum PJ, Josephson ME. Use of the electrocardiogram in acute myocardial infarction. N Engl J Med 2003; 348: 933.

Zimmerman, HA. The Auricular Electrocardiogram. Springfield: Charles C Thomas, 1968.

Index